Health, Technology and Society

Medicine, health care, and the wider social meaning and management of health are undergoing major changes. In part this reflects developments in science and technology, which enable new forms of diagnosis, treatment and delivery of health care. It also reflects changes in the locus of care and the social management of health. Locating technical developments in wider socio-economic and political processes, each book in the series discusses and critiques recent developments in health technologies in specific areas, drawing on a range of analyses provided by the social sciences. Some have a more theoretical focus, some a more applied focus but all draw on recent research by the authors. The series also looks toward the medium term in anticipating the likely configurations of health in advanced industrial society and does so comparatively, through exploring the globalization and internationalization of health.

More information about this series at
http://www.palgrave.com/gp/series/14875

Anna Lydia Svalastog
Srećko Gajović • Andrew Webster
Editors

Navigating Digital Health Landscapes

A Multidisciplinary Analysis

palgrave
macmillan

Editors
Anna Lydia Svalastog
Faculty of Health and Welfare
Østfold University College
Halden, Norway

Andrew Webster
Department of Sociology
University of York
York, UK

Srećko Gajović
Department of Histology and Embryology
Croatian Institute for Brain Research
University of Zagreb School of Medicine
Zagreb, Croatia

Health, Technology and Society
ISBN 978-981-15-8205-9   ISBN 978-981-15-8206-6 (eBook)
https://doi.org/10.1007/978-981-15-8206-6

This Palgrave Macmillan imprint is published by the registered company Springer Nature Singapore Pte Ltd.
The registered company address is: 152 Beach Road, #21-01/04 Gateway East, Singapore 189721, Singapore

Series Editors' Preface

Medicine, healthcare and the wider social meaning and management of health are undergoing major changes. In part this reflects developments in science and technology, which enable new forms of diagnosis, treatment and the delivery of healthcare. It also reflects changes in the locus of care and burden of responsibility for health. Today, genetics, informatics, imaging and integrative technologies, such as nanotechnology, are redefining our understanding of the body, health and disease; at the same time, health is no longer simply the domain of conventional medicine, nor the clinic. The "birth of the clinic" heralded the process through which health and illness became increasingly subject to the surveillance of medicine. Although such surveillance is more complex, sophisticated and precise as seen in the search for "predictive medicine", it is also more provisional, uncertain and risk-laden.

At the same time, the social management of health itself is losing its anchorage in collective social relations and shared knowledge and practice, whether at the level of the local community or through state-funded socialized medicine. This individualization of health is both culturally driven and state sponsored, as the promotion of "self-care" demonstrates. The very technologies that redefine health are also the means through which this individualization can occur—through "eHealth", diagnostic tests and the commodification of restorative tissue, such as stem cells, cloned embryos and so on.

This series explores these processes within and beyond the conventional domain of "the clinic" and asks whether they amount to a qualitative shift in the social ordering and value of medicine and health. Locating technical developments in wider socio-economic and political processes, each book discusses and critiques recent developments within health technologies in specific areas, drawing on a range of analyses provided by the social sciences.

The series has already published more than 20 volumes that have explored many of these issues, drawing on novel, critical and deeply informed research undertaken by their authors. In doing so, the books have shown how the boundaries between the three core dimensions that underpin the whole series—health, technology and society—are changing in fundamental ways.

Anna Lydia Svalastog, Østfold Gajovic and Andrew Webster, the editors of this new contribution to the series, have brought together an international and multidisciplinary group of scholars to reflect on what the changing digital health landscape means for patients, healthcare professionals, policy makers and designers of the techniques underpinning public and private digital systems. As such, this volume builds on earlier contributions to the series that focus on digital technologies (Wathen et al. 2008; Balka et al. 2009; Oudshoorn 2011). Such technologies have opened up new ways not only to distribute health information, but they also offer possibilities for data and information to be shared and interpreted so that new knowledge can be created. They also change the relationships between those who have been traditionally characterized as simply users of information and those who produce it.

The editors use the metaphor of "landscape" to help readers safely navigate their ways in this rapidly changing environment. In the Introduction, Svalastog, Gajovic and Webster explain how information and knowledge interact to produce this landscape. Information refers to the diverse range of health data, diverse in both form (text, numbers, images) and source (patient experiences, clinical observations, patient records, medical experiments, policy documents, etc.), all of which can be found circulating on the Internet. Knowledge is used to capture the ways in which users interpret, organize and mobilize information as they navigate the digital landscape. Furthermore, knowledge encompasses online/offline entanglements involving a myriad of health-related devices, people and information in specific local contexts that in turn generate diverse health/patient narratives.

This volume provides a valuable contribution for those wishing to understand how digital technologies are affecting the design, implementation and use of digital systems to manage health information in different contexts. The contributors have a wide variety of backgrounds, including STS (science and technology studies), information science, biomedicine, law and ethics, anthropology, social policy and computer science, working in more technical aspects of tracking and visualizing data and information on the Internet. The authors of the chapters position themselves from their own disciplinary perspectives in the knowledge landscape, making it richer and more diverse. They are also linked to the "Navigating Knowledge Landscapes" international network that has been supported by the Norwegian Research Council and Østfold University College.

York, UK — Andrew Webster
Maastricht, The Netherlands — Sally Wyatt

References

Balka, E., Green E., & Henwood, F. (eds.) (2009). *Gender, health and information technology in context*. Basingstoke: Palgrave Press.

Oudshoorn, N. (2011). *Telecare technologies and the transformation of healthcare*. Basingstoke: Palgrave Macmillan.

Wathen, N., Wyatt, S., & Harris, R. (2008). *The go-betweens in a changing socio-technical landscape*. Basingstoke: Palgrave Macmillan.

Contents

Notes on Contributors

Manna Alma is senior researcher at the Department of Applied Health Research of the University Medical Center Groningen, the Netherlands. She is trained as a human movement scientist and an experienced qualitative researcher. She specializes in qualitative research methods for understanding personal health experiences. She is a member of the DIPEx International network, which is engaged in the collection, analysis and application of patients' narratives worldwide, and leads the Dutch DIPEx research group. She also is a trainer in qualitative research methodology.

Hege Kristin Andreassen is head of department at the Centre for Women's and Gender Research at UiT The Arctic University of Norway and associate professor at the Center for Care Research, NTNU. Her research interests are in the intersection of health, gender and technology, where she is an active writer and supervisor. Andreassen is PI in the Norwegian research team affiliated to DIPEX International.

Milena D. Bister holds a PhD in sociology and works at the intersection of science and technology studies, the anthropology of knowledge and urban anthropology. Her research explores socio-material orderings of mental health and illness in public mental healthcare practices and urban living. Milena is a member of the "Laboratory: Anthropology of Environment Human Relations", Institute for European Ethnology,

Humboldt University of Berlin, and lecturer in European ethnology at the University of Vienna.

Siv-Britt Björktomta holds a PhD in social work and is a senior lecturer at CESAR (Centre for Social Work), Department of Sociology, Uppsala University, Sweden. Her research interest is children and young people regarding different aspects of family relations, focusing on the use of parental authority/power and different forms of violence. A new research area is digital transformations and the possibilities created by social media and the effect on children and young people's lives from the perspective of social work. Dr. Björktomta has considerable experience in teaching social work.

Anne Leonora Blaakilde holds a PhD in ethnology and folklore from the University of Copenhagen, Denmark. She is an associate professor at Roskilde University, Centre for Health Promotion Research, also in Denmark. Blaakilde's expertise is within humanities and health studies, in particular cultural gerontology, and she has researched a broad range of subjects from this perspective. As a folklorist, she is a specialist in narrative and performance studies.

Ana Borovečki is associate professor at Andrija Štampar School of Public Health, School of Medicine, University of Zagreb, Croatia. She has backgrounds in medicine, philosophy and comparative literature. She got a European master of bioethics degree from the Catholic University of Leuven, Belgium, and PhD degree from Radboud University in Nijmegen, the Netherlands. Her field of work is medical ethics, bioethics especially issues of patients' rights, ethics in research and ethical issues in healthcare delivery.

Iñigo de Miguel Beriain is Ikerbasque research professor at the University of the Basque Country UPV/EHU and holds a doctorate in law and a doctorate in philosophy. He is the author of six books on bioethics and medical law and more than a hundred articles and book chapters on these issues. He has participated in more than ten EU-funded projects on bioethics since 2004, and he is coordinating the PANELFIT project (https://www.panelfit.eu/).

Antske Fokkens is Associate Professor in Computational Linguistics at the Vrije Universiteit Amsterdam. She obtained her PhD from Saarland University working on methodology for grammar engineering. Since she moved to the Vrije Universiteit in 2012, her main line of research has been methodology for computational linguistics in digital humanities and computational social sciences. She has worked on multiple interdisciplinary projects including BiographyNet, NewsReader and a personal VENI grant project on identifying stereotyping.

Srećko Gajović is professor and head of the Department of Histology and Embryology at the University of Zagreb School of Medicine and Section for Neurogenetics, Medical Genetics, and Regenerative Neuroscience at the Croatian Institute for Brain Research. He is one of the founders of the Navigating Knowledge Landscapes international interdisciplinary network, which deals with how innovative knowledge is communicated in the digital society. He was coordinator of EU-FP7 project "GlowBrain" and established preclinical in vivo imaging platform (GlowLab) for brain research.

Aleksandra Głos holds doctor of law (2017) and master of philosophy (2012) degrees, from Jagiellonian University. Part of her studies she accomplished at Ruprechts-Karls-Universität Heidelberg and Humboldt Universität zu Berlin. Recently, she is a fellow at the *Institute* for *Human Sciences* (IWM) in Vienna and a visiting scholar at the Hastings Centre Bioethics Research Institute. She specializes in bioethics, social and legal philosophy. She works at the Collegium Medicum of Jagiellonian University and at the Tischner Institute, Kraków, Poland.

Heidi Aarum Hansen holds a PhD in social work and is a senior lecturer at the Department of Health and Welfare Sciences, Østfold University College, Norway. Dr. Aarum Hansen has experiences from practical social work with children and families. Her research area is children and Norwegian child welfare, focusing on social workers' work in supporting parents. A new research area is social welfare services in digital society and the challenges children's navigation on social media entails for practical social work. Dr. Aarum Hansen has considerable experience in teaching social work.

Hrvoje Jurić works as a full professor at the Department of Philosophy, Faculty of Humanities and Social Sciences, University of Zagreb, teaching ethics and bioethics. He is chief secretary of the Croatian Centre of Excellence for Integrative Bioethics and president of the Croatian Bioethics Society, as well as an active member of different scientific, cultural and social projects and initiatives. Besides numerous scientific articles and essays in Croatian and international journals and books, he has written three monographs and was a co-editor of three books.

Kishan Kariippanon is a medical doctor, a public health practitioner and an early career researcher in the intersection of health innovation and digital and mobile technology. He approaches technology and design with ethnographic methods drawing from his doctoral study in anthropology on the use of mobile technology and social media in a remote Aboriginal community in Northern Australia. He is active in the start-up space, as research partner and innovation lead.

Denis Kos works as a teaching and research assistant at the Centre for Integrative Bioethics and the Department of Information and Communication Sciences, Faculty of Humanities and Social Sciences, University of Zagreb. At the same university, he attends the PhD programme in information sciences. His articles have been published in domestic and international scientific and professional journals primarily on the topics of information literacy and knowledge organization.

Marko Kos works as a teaching and research assistant at the Centre for Integrative Bioethics and the Department of Philosophy, Faculty of Humanities and Social Sciences, University of Zagreb. He is a PhD candidate at the same faculty teaching on the topics of philosophy of technology and bioethics. He writes articles, reviews and commentaries in the fields of ethics, bioethics and philosophy of technology in Croatian, German and English languages.

Lucie Klůzová Kráčmarová (PhD) is at Palacky University Olomouc, Olomouc University Social Health Institute, Czechia, and is a qualitative researcher with a doctorate in clinical psychology. She is dedicated to qualitative studies of lived experiences of illness (e.g. cancer, IBD, ADHD, epilepsy, nightmares) conducted within the international DIPEx project. She participated in qualitative research on experiences of children and parents with primary healthcare systems within an international collaborative project "Models of Child Health Appraised".

Tomas Krilavičius is chief scientist at the Baltic Institute of Advanced Technology and head of the Applied Informatics Department at Vytauto Didžiojo University, Lithuania. His main research interests are application of artificial intelligence in defence and security applications, fintech and other areas, language technologies and scientific infrastructure. He is a member of NATO STO IST panel and several NATO STO workgroups, as well as Lithuania's representative at CapTech Information, EDA.

Joyce Lamerichs is assistant professor and senior researcher at the Department of Language, Literature and Communication at Vrije Universiteit in Amsterdam. She is trained as a researcher in science and technology studies and moved to discursive psychology and conversation analysis to study health interactions. Her research interests centre around the ways in which people describe concerns to do with health and illness in different mediated forms, with a special interest in identity work and mental health. She studies family consultations in intensive care units in several university medical centres in the Netherlands.

Martin Maiden has over 30 years of experience in the UK NHS and academia translating basic science into public health benefits, especially in vaccines, vaccination and food safety. This has included leading and participating in national and international studies, investigating the impact of vaccines and developing widely adopted approaches and bioinformatics platforms for exploiting genomic approaches. He has more than 20 years' experience in training for health professionals and capacity building, especially in Europe and Africa

Predrag Pale has an educational background and 35 years of experience in electrical engineering and computing research and industry. He has a rich understanding of Internet technology and cybersecurity and has expertise in envisioning future technological development. He combines this with his passion for teaching and learning and his profound interest in psychology to research human interaction with technology and the benefits and undesired side effects and consequences. One of his research interests relates to learning through web browsing.

Øystein Ringstad is an associate professor at Østfold University College, Norway, Faculty of Health and Welfare. He has worked as a physician in neurology and clinical rehabilitation. For about 20 years he has been teaching medical and science subjects and ethics for health and welfare students. His research includes a dissertation on patient autonomy in clinical rehabilitation and papers on patient autonomy in chronic disease.

Melike Şahinol is a senior research fellow at the Orient-Institut Istanbul affiliated with the Max Weber Foundation and head of the research area "Human, Medicine and Society". Şahinol studied sociology, political science and psychology at the University of Duisburg-Essen and received her doctorate in 2015 in sociology at the Eberhard Karls Universität Tübingen. Şahinol received several grants and fellowships, including one at the programme on "Science, Technology and Society" (STS) at the Kennedy School of Government, Harvard University. Her research interests lie in the field of sociology of technology and the body, medical sociology and crip technoscience. In her project "Additive Manufacturing: Enabling Technologies in the Childhood", she analyses the development of 3D printed prosthesis for children and disability beyond the technological fix narrative from a crip technoscience perspective.

Kate Senior is a medical anthropologist with extensive (20 years+) experience working with people in remote Aboriginal communities. Her work focuses on how people live and understand health and well-being and the barriers they face when accessing health services. Recently Kate's research has focused on the health and well-being of Indigenous adolescents, and in 2012 Kate was awarded an Australian Research Council Future Fellowship to explore young people's lived experiences of the social determinants of health.

Jana Šimenc is a medical anthropologist exploring eHealth/digital health; the relationship between (new) technology, health, innovations and people; and the social dimensions of organ donation. As a researcher, she made substantive contributions to more than ten scientific and applied international projects. She has conducted fieldwork in

Southeastern Europe and Turkey. Šimenc holds a PhD in anthropology from the University of Ljubljana. From 2016 to 2018 she was a postdoctoral research fellow at the Scientific Research Centre of Slovenian Academy of Sciences and Arts.

Dina Simunic is at the Department of Wireless Communications at the University of Zagreb, Faculty of Electrical Engineering. She served as editor-in-chief of the *Journal of Green Engineering* and is editorial board member of the international scientific journal *JOSE*. She served as a chair and vice-chair of pre-competitive research framework of the European Union's COST programme for more than ten years. She served as a vice-chair and technical secretary of COST 244bis: Biomedical Effects of Electromagnetic Fields. She served as a vice-chair of the Croatian Telecommunication Council and is chair of the National Standardization Committee for Telecommunications and of the Board of National Standardization. Dr. Simunic has more than 100 publications in journals and conferences.

Anna Lydia Svalastog is Professor of Psychosocial Work at Østfold University College, Norway. Svalastog received her PhD from Uppsala University in 1998 and became an associated professor at the Faculty of Humanities at Umeå University in 2005. Her research concerns cultural analysis of everyday behaviour and public perception combining empirical analysis with conceptual and theoretical elaboration and research history. Svalastog has initiated and coordinated several national and international research networks and co-edited five previous anthologies.

Margaret Varga is a visual analytics specialist at the University of Oxford Zoology Department. She has over 140 publications. Her extensive research interests include visual analytics, visualization, uncertainty analysis and big data analysis. Some of her research includes transforming inherently non-visual complex data into intuitive visual presentation for interactive exploration and analysis. She is chairman of the NATO Exploratory Visual Analytics Research Task Group, and in 2019 she received the NATO Scientific Achievement Award.

Piek Vossen is a full-time professor at the Vrije Universiteit Amsterdam. He is leading a group of researchers that develop software which automatically reads texts and models its content for machine reasoning. He coordinated several European projects, among which the NewsReader project that created reading machines in four languages to extract from millions of news articles what happened, who is involved, where and when. Through NewsReader, many different lenses, called perspectives, are created on the same events from the different sources. In 2013, Vossen received the Spinoza Prize (the most prestigious scientific prize in the Netherlands). He used this prize to set up a research framework for understanding-language-by-machines. This framework aims to model human communication and understanding in robot models.

Helena Webb is an interdisciplinary researcher working at the University of Oxford. She is interested in how individuals interact with each other and with technologies in different kinds of settings. She has conducted work on healthcare interactions in eye care, obesity care and the conduct of surgical procedures. She has also studied various features of online interactions and is part of a project exploring the use of social robots for purposes including health and social care.

Andrew Webster is emeritus professor in the Sociology of Science and Technology at the University of York, UK. He was founder and director of SATSU for 30 years. He has also directed various national research programmes on novel biomedical technologies and regenerative medicine. His main interest is in understanding how emergent technologies are, or are not, adopted in clinical settings, and through this work developed, with his colleague John Gardner, the model of "institutional readiness" which is now adopted by NHS trusts introducing advanced therapies in the cell and gene therapy area. He is also executive secretary of the Association for Studies in Innovation Science and Technology (AsSIST-UK). With Sally Wyatt he has been co-editor of the Palgrave *Health, Technology and Society* series.

List of Figures

1

Introduction: A Multidisciplinary Approach to the Digital Landscape

Anna Lydia Svalastog, Srećko Gajović, and Andrew Webster

This book explores the ways in which people in the digital society search, find, select and build health-related knowledge. In the area of health communication, health literacy has been a key public health strategy. Literacy implies that information is understood, so that what is being read is transformed from information to knowledge. The general trust in this strategy is mirrored in the mass of online distribution of medical advice websites, healthy living sites, research reports, alternative medicine

A. L. Svalastog (✉)
Faculty of Health and Welfare, Østfold University College, Halden, Norway
e-mail: anna.l.svalastog@hiof.no

S. Gajović
Department of Histology and Embryology, Croatian Institute for Brain Research, University of Zagreb School of Medicine, Zagreb, Croatia
e-mail: srecko.gajovic@hiim.hr

A. Webster
Department of Sociology, University of York, York, UK
e-mail: andrew.webster@york.ac.uk

A. L. Svalastog et al. (eds.), *Navigating Digital Health Landscapes*, Health, Technology and Society, https://doi.org/10.1007/978-981-15-8206-6_1

communities, advocacy groups, personalised health apps, and so on. In short, information needs to be integrated in a knowledge landscape to be understood. Thus an analytical distinction between information and knowledge seems important. The dissemination of information—facts, conclusions, guidelines, examples and so on—intends to inform and help, to affect peoples' behaviour towards what the sender perceives as good health, or a good choice. Without literacy, such information is piecemeal and disaggregated, and the basis on which to choose what to follow is unclear.

To make sense of information is never a straightforward process. Digital systems enable an individual to access vast amounts of online information in relation to health—medical advice websites, healthy living sites, research reports, alternative medicine communities, advocacy groups, personalised health apps and so on. At the same time however, beyond being simply a consumer of information, individuals or groups create and curate health information (Zeibland 2012; Harris and Wyatt 2015; Harris et al. 2016; Nettleton et al. 2011) related to specific disease areas, patient experiences (such as the international DiPEX network), or research outside of formal science processes (Rabeharisoa et al. 2013). The interactive and joint process of understanding can help transform information into knowledge, and has become a more and more important strategy for public health. One can assume that the interactive processing of online health information is of key importance for the understanding of non-interactive online health information, helping the individual to transform information into knowledge that can be discussed, agreed upon and also criticised. As the population ages and chronic conditions become more common, there is also an increasing use of online health management tools to self-monitor personal health as well as the use of telemedicine to monitor and indeed treat people remotely (Oudshoorn 2011). The need for the patient to understand, as treatment is moved to the home, is increasingly important. Digital systems also generate and marshall personal health data, as in electronic medical records, gene and tissue banks, and related health and care databases. They also mobilise multiple data sources, seen as a democratising of forms of expertise and information yet also critiqued as reproducing existing or creating new forms of social hierarchy and exclusion (Lupton 2014).

The online dissemination, construction, production and distribution of health-related knowledge does not only present information, it shapes information, by implicitly or explicitly defined categories and the meaning of health/health risks, and the borders too between the normal and abnormal. Being involved in online health-related interactions, the border between the 'clinical' and the experiential, between the person as passive and active, as patient and non-patient is deconstructed. It makes it important to understand how these processes work and how they are performative and productive. To understand the bases of these processes also requires an understanding of the digital 'landscape' itself, how it is constructed (the basic components and principles organising the elements into systems), and its dynamics—how people make sense of it and navigate its socio-technical contours. What are the opportunities, risks and concerns seen and experienced by those travelling in this landscape? How can we develop a rich sense of its topography and the routes people take in traversing it? Are there ways in which this can be done which reduce risks, which offer greater accountability? Together, we can understand these processes as reflecting the play of different forms of 'health agency', within institutional, cultural and personal contexts.

In exploring these issues, the book complements the three texts already published in the Health, Technology and Society Series which, in turn, describe how telecare technologies transform the home and public places into spaces of care (Oudshoorn 2011), the gendered socio-technical relations of ICTs (Information and Communication Technologies), in healthcare (Balka et al. 2009) and the role of intermediaries in health (Wathen et al. 2008). This book provides detailed analysis of the health information landscape, its geography, journeying through it, and how to 'travel safely'. The book offers a critical yet constructive perspective on the ways in which health information can be understood and managed.

The defining feature of the book is its *multidisciplinary* approach to these issues. We have brought together those working in STS (science and technology studies), information science, biomedicine, law and ethics, anthropology, social policy and those working in more technical aspects of tracking and visualising data and information on the internet. This ensures the book can help to build a broad framework which has both analytical depth and diverse implications for policy and practice.

The authors of each of the chapters were asked to approach their particular chapter through a shared metaphorical lens—that of the knowledge landscape—to ensure that this concept serves as an integrative framework for the book as a whole. Each chapter offers its own commentary on the 'landscape' within which to situate its particular disciplinary contribution towards the integrative metaphor of 'landscape' itself.

In the book we argue that the digital health landscape reflects and is contextually *produced* through the interplay between information and knowledge. There is an important distinction between the two: we treat information as the diverse range of health data (textual, statistical, observational, policy-related, etc.) that can be found circulating on the internet, and knowledge as the ways in which users interpret, organise, curate and deploy this information as they navigate the digital landscape. Moreover, knowledge encompasses highly contextual online/offline entanglements, engagements and practices that in turn produce diverse health/patient narratives that shape and help explain a person's life experiences. In this sense, as argued in Chap. 6, online/offline entanglements generate different *affordances* for individuals and so possibilities for action.

The importance and integrated presence of digital communication and services has rearranged and transformed public health services (Burke-Garcia and Scally 2014) and private life and the meaning of patienthood (Erikainen et al. 2019). Early on, telehealth initiatives were launched for long-distance consultation or monitoring of health practices (for example consulting for diagnostic purposes, or to secure clinical expertise to monitor advanced surgery). In addition, telephone hotlines soon became an integrated part of these practices, not least for mental health issues, child abuse and violence against women. The online dissemination of information and communication has established a new situation where new search engines such as Google and YouTube make information and knowledge available. The online flood of information is in turn subject to algorithms organising search results, often driven by commercial interests that reproduce digital capitalism (Sharon 2018). Some filters are easier to grasp, like parental control filters, or spam filters for e-mail accounts. For key search engines the filters/algorithms organising our online search are business secrets. As social media depend on their users, a company can be pushed to adjust their algorithm, or if they resist, public debate can draw attention to unwanted consequences, as we have seen in the public discussions about what and who is permitted to disseminate what content on Twitter, Facebook and Instagram. There is a wide range of uses of online information, from public health officials, patient groups, enterprises selling health products, nutrition advisors, alternative medicine, religious groups and those peddling highly dubious information. In this context, knowledge and the ability to navigate and critically read the flood of information available online, is a key challenge for public health strategies, individual well-being and safety. The chapters in this book explore the ways in which different users search and make sense of the digital information they access.

Background to the Book: Navigating Knowledge Landscapes

The Navigating Knowledge Landscapes (NKL) network was launched in 2015, initiated as a follow-on activity to the COST Action 1001 *Bio-objects and their governance*, which was supported by the European Commission between 2010 and 2014 (Vermeulen et al. 2012): the concept of the 'bio-object' is now widely explored in academic papers drawing on STS and other perspectives (see, e.g. Holmberg and Ideland 2016; Tamminen and Vermeulen 2019; Williams and Brown 2015). Within the Action debate over how people engage with the digital was one of the core themes, especially in regard to issues surrounding governance and regulation. This led to the establishing of the NKL network after the completion of the Action with a continued key focus on how to navigate health-related knowledge in the present situation of online information, communication and services. Researchers from all corners of academic training—social science, the humanities, natural science, law, religious studies, engineering, and researchers with a background in practices including medicine, nursing, social services and social work—were brought together, and depending on which topic that was understood as most pressing, small multidisciplinary collaborations were established and together we started to build a multidisciplinary collaboration on health navigation and knowledge in the digital society.

Navigation and *Knowledge Landscapes* (KL) became the two key terms that kept the variety of what became integrated NKL-work together. Through a series of investigations and analyses, the complexity of communication, health-related knowledge and practices in the present globalised and digitalised society has been discussed and investigated (see Svalastog et al. 2015). The broad ongoing aim of the network is to establish a multidisciplinary academic and research-based conversation, and to develop trans-disciplinary work into the multifaceted field of health and health-related work. Reflecting the variety of topics, and the practical, theoretical and philosophical perspectives needed to address this complexity, the key terms have been elaborated in diverse and constructive ways.

In this book, depending on the topic being discussed, the KL has been explored in considerable empirical detail, as areas of health-related knowledge in offline and/or online environments. In other chapters, KL is itself an object of analysis in respect to the questions it raises for legal, ethical and broader governance domains. Knowledge landscapes are multiple and not fixed in either digital time or space, and different encounters with the Internet will create novel and complex landscapes for users. Hence, we need, as one of the chapters in the book argues, to understand the socio-technical 'geography' of the KL. We now outline the structure of the book and summarise the contribution of the different chapters.

Structure of the Book

The book is structured into three main parts after this introductory chapter, and each section has a short overview that captures the main lessons that can be drawn across the section chapters, and in what ways these point to shared issues cutting across the discrete disciplinary contributions.

The first part, *Mapping the Digital Health Landscape*, comprises four chapters that discuss the broad aspects that make up the digital health landscape and how this might be understood from a variety of perspectives. The first chapter by Svalastog et al. on 'Narrative Genre and Health in the Digital Society', draws on folklore, social anthropology, socio-linguistics and narrative ethics approaches to explore the presentation and function of what are seen to be 'personal health narratives' in different contexts. The chapter discusses those found within clinical settings in doctor–patient interaction, personal blogs and news media. These can be understood as discrete 'genres', though all of them intended to be performed. The narratives that populate the web are created by different social actors and are reproduced through the various social media and related channels found there. These can create considerable traction as they become more widely shared over time and are reproduced through different information networks in the knowledge landscape, and so move beyond the original context within which they were created (such as a personal blog or clinical encounter). These narratives circulate in the digital landscape and are shown to draw on wider cultural identities and practice and become touchstones for other users of the web to help explain their own health experiences.

In their chapter on the law, Beriain and his co-authors examine how a legal perspective can be used to explore and help address how very different types of narrative can be found on the knowledge landscape—those deliberately acting as dis-information and others that can be characterised as mis-information, pointing out that the boundaries between these two can be blurred. How might the law help to distinguish, police and handle these two, and what steps have already been taken at the European and national levels to do this? They show how the issues that are raised have direct effects on patient–clinician relations and how steps can be taken to help assuage and deal with both of these problems in the digital health landscape.

The fourth chapter by Kos et al. continues the broad theme of mapping by discussing the development over recent years of new approaches in bioethics and how these can be used to interrogate the forms of both information and knowledge found in the digital landscape. They argue for a form of bioethics that seeks to integrate different forms of knowledge and through this help build what is called an 'orientational' approach to knowledge, and thereby health. They discuss the ways in which such a perspective goes beyond and is critical of the often-seen reductionism of science and technologies, and what counts as 'information'. Navigating knowledge landscapes then involves the development of a bioethical literacy among citizens based on open, reflexive forms of knowledge.

The final chapter in Part I is a more reflective essay from the perspective of a biomedical scientist, Gajović, that endeavours to unpack the concept of a 'geography' of the knowledge landscape: what does this mean in terms of the temporal and spatial aspects of information and its flow across different terrains? How does it assume the mantle of knowledge and authority? It begins by discussing the shift from medical paternalism to patient-centred medicine then moves to a more detailed discussion of a linear to a non-linear, interactive basis for knowledge and information exchange, the complexities this throws up on the web in terms of temporal and spatial dynamics, and how in turn this is reflected in changes in the expectations people have in regard to digital health.

Part II of the book, *Journeys in the Knowledge Landscapes*, provides an opportunity to drill down into more detailed empirical work on how people engage with the digital health infrastructure. The six chapters explore various themes in this broad area, with a number examining diverse digital-user communities. Chapter 6, the first chapter in this section, by Lamerichs et al. draws on very detailed empirical work on patient experiences, extending and bringing to life the role and function of narratives seen in Chap. 2. Drawing on social anthropology and communication studies, the chapter asks how does person-centred access to health-related knowledge engender quite specific journeys (for example in regard to different conditions) across the landscape, and how do these redefine the meaning of health and well-being. It does so by discussing the community of users associated with the DiPEX website which hosts and makes available many thousands of patient experiences. A similar account of the ways in which online communication can be empowering can be found in Chap. 9.

Chapter 7 by Senior and her colleague, offers an appreciation of Aboriginal ways of navigating knowledge landscapes, and represents an analysis from within medical anthropology of an indigenous community in Australia and how they engage with and travel across the online health landscape. The chapter discusses the tension to the co-existence and potential dialogue between the Western bio-medical model and traditional health and well-being practices. The authors offer a critique of the design and delivery of online 'mHealth' and the need to rethink the current approach to move towards more genuine two-way exchange between remote Indigenous communities and medical advisors/practitioners.

Chapter 8, by Bister, tackles the question of the use of digital systems for mental healthcare in Germany. Adopting an approach that combines STS with material-semiotic theory, Bister examines the ways in which policy and care are (or are not) co-ordinated in daily service provision in the city of Berlin. She shows how health documentation affects health practices, as episodes in a community care are transformed into entries in a digital documentation system, and 'how the entries travel and in which kind of actions they again translate'. The chapter reveals the ways in which production of information within institutional settings both document and hide actual care practices and can be seen as a material-semiotic practice embedded in a localised digital system.

Chapter 9 by Šimenc deploys an anthropological ethnography to examine in detail one of the major social media platforms, Facebook, to ask how people navigate the site when seeking the way out of (biomedically unexplained) pain and poor treatment of rare disease. Rare diseases pose particular problems for patients (and medics alike) given the uncertainties around diagnosis, prognosis and the (biological and social) boundaries of the disease itself. Sufferers of rare disease are often 'invisible' to medicine so seek alternative sources of advice through the web. Drawing on her empirical work in Slovenia, Šimenc provides a critically constructive analysis of the value of social media for those in need of information and whether and if so how this can become a form of personal knowledge, her account based on the story of 'Eva'.

The last two chapters in this section offer analyses of formal eHealth interventions directed towards different demographics. Chapter 10 by Şahinol focuses on Turkish authorities' policy to deploy eHealth to manage patient records. Combining expertise in STS and medical informatics, Şahinol compares these formal eHealth interventions—which she understands as 'socio-(bio-)-technical systems'—with patients' own attempts to build their own frameworks for a personal intervention or management of their condition. The final chapter in this section by

Björktomta and Hansen examine eHealth through the lens of social policy and welfare studies, asking how professional interventions from within social welfare practice can assist in regard to children's health information needs. In particular the authors ask how might existing and new forms of knowledge be organised and operationalised in present and future social work through an engagement with social media, and in what ways does this affect responsibilities and governance within professional practice?

Part III, *Travelling Safely*, offers three chapters that provide more applied, practical insight into the ways in which technical analyses of the health knowledge landscape can help users navigate more safely and so better address users' needs, and how that process might be mapped. Chapter 12 deploys expertise from the discipline of information science and digital humanities and the tool of natural language processing techniques to track and map patterns of communication on the web. It does so to follow debates over online vaccination. Chapter 13 by Simunic and Pale brings together two authors with expertise in the areas of bio-electromechanics and wireless communication and computing. They discuss the 'internet of (medical) things' and the dangers, risks and threats likely to be confronted while navigating this particular domain found within the health knowledge landscape. The final chapter by Varga and Webb from within the field of Visual Analytics provides an introduction to the area and how it can be used to interrogate movement in the digital landscape providing visual re-descriptions of data flows in the health knowledge landscape. By drawing on recent work in regard to specific ehealth applications, visual analytics and social care practices, each of the chapters points to ways in which we can help build a more responsible and accountable digital health infrastructure.

References

Balka, E., Green, E., & Henwood, F. (Eds.). (2009). *Gender, health and information technology in context*. Basingstoke: Palgrave Press.

Burke-Garcia, A., & Scally, G. (2014). Trending now: Future directions in digital media for the public health sector. *Journal of Public Health, 36*(4), 527–534.

Erikainen, S., Pickersgill, M., Cunningham-Burley, S., & Chan, S. (2019). Patienthood and participation in the digital era. *Digital Health, 5*(1), 15–25.

Harris, A., Kelly, S., & Wyatt, S. (2015). Autobiologies: Making sense of engagements with healthcare technologies. *Journal of Medical Humanities & Social Studies of Science and Technology, 7*(2), 71–86.

Harris, A., Kelly, S., & Wyatt, S. (2016). *CyberGenetics: Health genetics and new media*. London: Routledge.

Holmberg, T., & Ideland, M. (2016). Imagination laboratory: Making sense of bio-objects in contemporary genetic art. *The Sociological Review, 64*(3), 447–467.

Lupton, D. (2014). *Digital sociology*. New York: Routledge.

Nettleton, S., Burrows, R., O'Malley, L., & Watt, I. (2011). Health e-types? *Information, Communication and Society, 7*(4), 531–553.

Oudshoorn, N. (2011). *Telecare technologies and the transformation of healthcare*. Basingstoke: Palgrave Macmillan.

Rabeharisoa, V., Moreira, T., & Akrich, M. (2013). *Evidence-based activism: Patients' organisations, users' and activist's groups in knowledge society*. Accessible online at https://hal-mines-paristech.archives-ouvertes.fr/hal-00822864/document

Sharon, T. (2018). When digital health meets digital capitalism, how many common goods are at stake? *Big Data & Society, 5*, 2.

Svalastog, A. L., Allgaier, J., & Gajović, S. (2015). Navigating knowledge landscapes: On health, science, communication, media, and society. *Croatian Medical Journal, 56*(4), 321–323.

Tamminen, S., & Vermeulen, N. (2019). Bio-objects: New conjugations of the living. *Sociologias, 21*(50), 156–179.

Vermeulen, N, Tamminen S, and A, Webster. (2012). Bio-Objects - Life in the 21st Century, London: Ashgate.

Wathen, N., Wyatt, S., & Harris, R. (2008). *The go-betweens in a changing socio-technical landscape*. Basingsoke: Palgrave Macmillan.

Williams, R., & Brown, N. (2015). Cord blood banking: Bio-objects on the borderlands between community and immunity. *Life Sciences, Society and Policy, 11*(1), 1–18.

Zeibland, S. (2012). Health and illness in a connected world. *Milbank Quarterly, 90*, 219–249.

Part I

Mapping the Digital Health Landscape

In the first part of this book, we approach some broad themes of the digital society that directly concern health and how they can, and indeed in regard to ethics and the law, shape knowledge landscapes: these are health narratives, law, ethics and temporal/spatial dimensions. Each chapter discusses its topic from a specific disciplinary perspective, and here, we draw out some cross-cutting themes. Multidisciplinarity searches for a diversity of analytical angles and the contributions they can make to a shared problematic or meta-theme—here understanding knowledge landscapes. We can see how the authors have focussed on very specific issues, but these can be given additional value through exploring common themes, values and analytical framings.

A common meta-theme found across all four chapters is the recent shift from paternalistic to person-centred medicine and care, and the complex relationship between person-centred care and the digital society. The first chapter concerns the personal health narratives that individuals voice in the knowledge landscape. If Michel Foucault pointed out how sex was a key topic of 'talk', and an overall discourse of the Victorian era in the nineteenth century, one might say that personal health narratives are a topic of 'talk' that reflects health as an overall discourse at the present time. By focusing on personal narratives, the attempt to document and make sense of health is done through narratives that are told that presuppose some kind of dialogue between social actors. The second chapter approaches legal challenges in the intersection of personal medicine and the digital overload of information and the challenges identifying and policing misinformation and disinformation, both more extensive in the context of personalised medicine. The third chapter calls for a new, integrative bioethics that addresses challenges such as those made particularly acute and more complex where singular sources of authority and trust no longer hold. The last chapter portrays the geography of knowledge landscapes as multi-layered, where communication is multi-directed, constantly shifting and filtered by algorithms shaping information about personal medicine.

We can also see multidisciplinary elements in how the chapters draw on collaborations between the authors of a chapter and/or by an author being actively involved in research outside their main area of competence. To acknowledge the relevance of disciplines outside one's own main line of work reflects a preparedness to listen, listening to the variety of expressions a cultural expression might take (Chap. 2), listening to knowledge from social sciences to inform legal work, (Chap. 3), listening to insights from a wide range of disciplines when approaching ethics (Chap. 4) and listening to non-medical research to facilitate dialogue in medical doctor–patient situations (Chap. 5).

2

Narrative Genre and Health in the Digital Society

Anna Lydia Svalastog, Anne Leonora Blaakilde, Øystein Ringstad, and Joyce Lamerichs

Introduction: Personal Health Narrative as Genre

In this chapter we argue that personal health narratives (PHN) work as a narrative genre of key importance in present day society. As society has become digital and global, personal stories have entered the public sphere

A. L. Svalastog (✉) • Ø. Ringstad
Faculty of Health and Welfare, Østfold University College, Halden, Norway
e-mail: anna.l.svalastog@hiof.no; oystein.ringstad@hiof.no

A. L. Blaakilde
Centre for Health Promotion Research, Roskilde University, Roskilde, Denmark
e-mail: ablaa@ruc.dk

J. Lamerichs
Language, Literature and Communication, Vrije Universiteit Amsterdam, Amsterdam, The Netherlands
e-mail: j.m.w.j.lamerichs@vu.nl

A. L. Svalastog et al. (eds.), *Navigating Digital Health Landscapes*, Health, Technology and Society, https://doi.org/10.1007/978-981-15-8206-6_2

through homepages and social media. In addition, societal institutions (the media as well as a variety of public and private institutions) use PHN when communicating content. As the PHN is used for different purposes in different contexts we have found it important to argue for discrete PHN sub-genres. Our argument is that the context in which the PHN is told is formative, and that the PHN carries with it aims that differ and carries different meanings of importance. In addition, the authorship of a PHN is affected by the context in which it is presented. The examples we have chosen are drawn from the clinical situation, blogs and edited news media. In the clinic, the PHN is told from the point of view of the practitioner. Within the blog, the PHN is told from the point of view of the individual or group running the blog. In the news media, the PHN is selected by the newspaper though told by the individual. To reflect the variety of PHN contexts and the effect they have on the aim, content and function of PHN, the concept of PHN-subgenre opens up elaboration of specific audiences, editors and co-authors.

Construction and interpretation of meaning is multifaceted. In order to be informative, any piece of information needs context. When we misunderstand words, information or context, the meaning is lost or distorted. In this chapter, we lean on a hermeneutical tradition where meaning is understood as a result of interpretative processes, and where interpretative contexts (for example medical knowledge or knowledge about the history of a person) are understood as essential for the interpretative outcome. It is from this angle we approach the presence of PHN in present society, and the question of how these stories have become important and gained significant functions in the digital society. The chapter draws on folklore, social anthropology and socio-linguistics/discourse analysis to explore these processes, and does so to contribute to the book's overall understanding of the digital landscape and voices heard therein.

Personal Health Narratives

According to the American folklorist, Sandra Dolby Stahl, a personal narrative is a prose narrative relating a personal experience, usually told in first person (Stahl 1989: 12). This means that the narrative embeds a perception of a specific author (Bakhtin 1986), providing a certain truth-value to the story. Our focus is on personal health narratives (PHN) as they are increasingly used to inform conversations and understandings of health in digital health discourses, distributed in both offline and online contexts. As a field of narratives we recognise PHNs, and respond to them in ways that show expectations of both format and content. In this chapter we underline that the function and politics of PHN is context dependent, and thus the PHNs need to be categorised into discrete sub-genres. The main argument in this chapter is that the profound presence of PHN in present society is significant, and that the concept of genre and sub-genre is helpful when and if we want to recognise and understand them.

Drawing on folklore, where genre has been used to categorise oral folk traditions that have culturally specific format and content, we emphasise the importance of a known format, and the performing of the narrative (Koski et al. 2016: 18–30). When folk genre is performed, people already know the format, maybe even the content. The performance is an act that involves the listener or audience, as it is also a communal act. Whether the person is asked to perform, or him/herself initiates the performance, it is still a communal act, which can also be said about the different examples of PHN we present in this chapter. For example, increasingly PHNs appear in online blogs, such as in 'Illness blogs', as 'online accounts of the course of a disease is an example: they are unsolicited first person narratives, which are publicly accessible and allow for author-reader interactivity' (Tshuma 2012: A68). As in other examples below, the content of PHN appears as a narrative that tells something authentic about a person that is put forward to be confirmed or criticised by its audience. In addition to sub-genre reflecting particular narrative contexts, and because the distribution of online PHNs is global, the person encountering the PHNs is always interwoven in social, cultural, historical and economic-political contexts when interpreting the PHNs (Leslie et al. 2008; Allgaier and Svalastog 2015). This is of particular importance to those who use PHN to distribute public health or other information. Thus, the sharing of PHNs also needs to be understood in terms of the contexts of relevance to the person encountering the PHN. This is an approach that includes culture as fundamental, in contrast to, for example, a more traditional health literacy approach.[1] In this chapter we approach the profound presence of PHN in society through discussing these narratives and their contexts, to understand their meaning and impact, their contextually defined function as well as common features. We argue that the PHN is a vital genre in the broader area of personal narratives, and that the presence and importance of this genre both reflects and challenges structuring organisational principles and values in present society. Our analysis focuses on empirical examples that document the use of PHN in order to contribute towards work in this text and elsewhere that explores diverse forms of health knowledge in the present and digital society. In this chapter we ask: Do PHNs help people navigate towards better or more knowledge? If so, knowledge for whom or towards what purpose? An initial question is therefore: How, where and why are these stories told?

Background: Digital Health and Personal Health Narratives

Today, the health concerns of individuals are structured by a variety of practices and different types of traditions and discourses. In the online realm, old and new understandings are presented simultaneously, and this creates a synchronic landscape of new and old understandings of health (Svalastog et al. 2017). One form of discourse is based on current research, including new diagnoses and treatments. A second discourse, sometimes overlapping with Western medical discourse, is traditional medicine, or so-called alternative medicine including acupuncture, chiropractic, meditation, homeopathy and so on (Brosman et al. 2018). In addition, there are local cultural systems (Kleinman 1978), new religious movements, and the knowledge among individuals about their own health and family history. In this picture of health discourses, we have activists and lobbyists concerned with single issues (e.g. concerns with

[1] Culture is here not approached as a totality, but used as a concept that makes it possible to appreciate the importance of 'thick descriptions' (C. Geertz) when approaching health and health narratives. See earlier reference Allgaier and Svalastog 2015 on cultural complications in communicating information on the Ebola outbreak 2015.

pharmaceuticals—vaccines, new drugs, or potential benefits or risks generated from new technology or products). Lobbyists and activists are explicitly challenging a specific subject, for example proposing particular (biomedical) explanations and treatment, or work to change established health knowledge and public health recommendations. Both the patient and the health professional are embedded in the variety of discourses mentioned above. In the online domain, the private and professional person searching for information can experience an overload of information derived from different and often conflicting sources. During their lifetime, individuals will occupy different positions, as a receiver of health care and health services, a private or professional health carer, or administrating health services for family or friends or for the public. This is also the context in which the PHN is told/published and given importance.

The sharing and searching for information and knowledge are reflecting each individual's responsibility and options in present society.[2] The multi-directedness of how information and stories travel, reflects a deconstruction of the hierarchical organisation of knowledge, and the former distinction between professional health workers and the individual health agent.

Genre

PHN can be claimed to be a certain kind of genre, and in the humanities, genre is a concept that points towards fine art and popular culture. The meaning of, and boundaries between genres, for example what constitute journalism and news, and what is propaganda, or what constitutes a novel, and what is autobiographical, is an ongoing public debate as well as an academic exercise that mirrors the relation between genre and knowledge, norms and values, and the social and cultural importance of genre. The 'tellability' of a personal narrative is in part tied to categories attributed to experience (Shuman 2005: 16–17).

[2] Present society has also seen that there are people that do not want information (Palant 2019). And §17 in the GDPR *Right to erasure ('right to be forgotten')*. This law is meant to facilitate privacy options in the further context of forced interrelatedness brought on citizens by the digital society (https://gdpr-info.eu/art-17-gdpr/).

Genre refers to formal criteria as well as to content. Research in sociolinguistics has examined generic conventions in different types of discourse and shown how genres are constructed so as to serve particular communicative purposes (Bauman 1984). The rise in digital formats, however, has also shown a rise in hybrid genres, and it is no longer a simple task to relate genres to singular communicative purposes (Bhatia 2004; Frow 2014). We still use generic conventions to make sense of what we read: 'Genre guides interpretation because it is a constraint on semiosis, the production of meaning; it specifies which types of meaning are relevant and appropriate in a particular context, and so makes certain senses of an utterance more probable, in the circumstances, than others' (Frow 2014: 101). Examples of how particular genres have a formal structure and expected content are numerous, though we seldom discuss or reflect upon the phenomenon itself, on how much our lives and society, communication and interpretations rely on genre, on genre expectations, on the function of particular genres in present society, and on the impact of genre in our daily lives, which might illustrate that 'all understanding of verbal meaning is necessarily genre-bound' (Hirsh 1976: 76).

Definition: Personal Health Narratives

In a health context, we define a PHN as a story linking personal health knowledge to a wider story of the person's life, experiences and contexts. The situating and/or integrating of health information and knowledge in a person's life creates this narrative, one that is situated in a specific time and space, which makes the narrative a carrier of information concerning more than the narrator herself (Ricoeur 1991). Life stories are complex and constantly revised. In the constellation of each person's life, worldview and conditions, there is a need to situate and/or integrate new information gains from professionals as well as from other sources, offline as well as online. Integration of new information and its embedding in forms of knowledge is a complex process. In a longitudinal study of women who had received an abnormal cervical smear and who were referred for further investigation and treatment, it was shown that information needs, as well as the sources of information that were preferred (both offline and online), varied during the different stages of treatment

(Dubbeldam 2016). We are interested in ways in which PHNs function as a carrier of *organised* information, that is, as knowledge in contexts where health is communicated, with a specific narrative form and content (genre). As we shall see, it seems as if the complexity of the PHN as a type of the personal narrative genre enables transportation of crucial information to and between professionals, the public and individual health agents.

Empirical Examples: PHN Sub-genre

In the section below, we discuss and examine PHN as they have been produced in different settings. When studying PHN, our focus will be on the content and function of the stories in the sub-genres of: clinical situations, in the format of blogs, and as stories published in traditional news.

In Clinical Situations

Patients' PHNs are essential in the communication between patients and health care practitioners in the clinical setting. Because this kind of communication is protected by strict rules of confidentiality, it is possible for the patient to talk about private matters such as bodily dysfunctions or troubling thoughts and emotions that in other settings would have been inappropriate, evoking feelings of shame and humiliation. Worries about health and disease may be discussed openly, even if they may seem strange and irrational in other contexts and genres.

In such conversations, the clinical practitioner may have different approaches to the patient's PHN. The immediate approach is to listen to the patient's questions and then analyse the patient's health problem in terms of professional knowledge. The practitioner 'translates' and re-tells the patient's PHN in the categories and language of professional knowledge. Accordingly, there will be two different narratives about the patient's health problem: the patient's PHN and the professional account based on relevant theory and professional practice. This duality may influence the ongoing communication in different ways, as Hunter (1991) describes in her study of doctors' stories. If the doctor answers the patient's questions by telling the medical narrative about her health problem, it will be the patient's task to integrate this story into her own narrative. Many patients will find this difficult if the two narratives seem incommensurable. They may think that the doctor ignores or misunderstands essential parts of the story. They will not be convinced and may feel even more isolated and suffering than before the consultation (Hunter 1991: 142–143). The cooperation between patient and doctor will fail.

Empirical studies have shown that patients often have their own opinions and concerns regarding the explanation of the symptoms. They may fear serious and potentially life-threatening diseases with devastating consequences for themselves and their families (Lang et al. 2000). Patients also may have specific expectations regarding information, support, diagnoses and treatment (Geurts et al. 2017). If the practitioner does not recognise or underestimate the importance of such perceptions, patients' expectations and needs may remain unmet (Nettleton 2005).

It is also quite common that patients do not disclose medically relevant information to clinicians. Such information may mean that they disagree with clinicians' recommendations or do not understand their instructions, that they have unhealthy habits, or use irregular medication. Some common reasons for not telling this are that patients do not want to be embarrassed, to be judged or paternalised, or to be perceived as difficult patients. They may also fear that clinicians should find them 'stupid' (Levy et al. 2018).

On the other hand, when patients and clinicians manage to communicate well in spite of different perspectives and narratives, the two stories may supplement and enrich each other. The importance of focusing directly on patients' PHNs is discussed in the literature about narrative in medicine and health care (Brody 2002; Charon 2006; Hurwitz et al. 2004; Frank 2013). Firstly, focusing directly on this narrative can improve the immediate outcome of the clinical work. Secondly, the patient's health narrative may also be an expression of her efforts to cope with chronic disease.

The immediate outcome of the clinical consultation is not only a question of correct diagnosis and treatment. The patient also needs answers to her questions, and to have her fears and concerns addressed. Patients' satisfaction with clinical consultations is linked to the fulfilment of their prior expectations (Bowling et al. 2013; Jaworski et al. 2017). In order to recognise and address or fulfil such expectations, practitioners will have to listen carefully to what the patient tells them. Often the clinical evaluation results in recommendations about treatment and changes in the patient's daily habits, for instance, to stop smoking, lose weight or exercise more systematically. Letting the patient first tell about her everyday routines and preferences and then discuss possible changes, may be both an effective and respectful way of helping the patient to make changes in her daily life. The patient will be the one who chooses and takes responsibility for the changes she wants to make.

Often patients find that their lives are permanently changed by chronic disease. Sometimes these changes are dramatic and invasive, with major losses of physical or mental abilities and perhaps risk of an early death. Sometimes such losses are only frightening possibilities that patients try to prepare for or avoid thinking about. Reactions of grief and depression are common. However, how serious this is to the individual person, is not only a question of objective measures of quality and length of life. The personal significance of the disease is expressed in the person's story about her health and illness.

When we feel well and healthy, we can tell stories about our lives that fulfil our own and others' demands and expectations. We may align our stories to social and cultural perceptions of what counts as a happy and successful life. By telling coherent and rational stories about ourselves, we show that we are in control and can cope. However, particularly in serious and chronic disease, these stories are threatened. Brody (1994) discusses this in an article called 'My story's broken – can you help me fix it? Medical ethics and the joint construction of narrative'. Patients need help, also to heal their broken stories. Health care practitioners can contribute to this by listening carefully in a supportive manner. Professional knowledge about causes, treatment possibilities and prognosis can be useful for the patient who struggles to restore basic feelings of hope, belonging and self-respect.

Agich (2003) sees self-biographical narratives as something that we may revise and re-construct when life is changed. We tell different stories about ourselves under different circumstances and at different phases of life in order to make sense of the present situation. This is not only an individual process, but also a social action and negotiation of meaning. Other people may contribute to this process with their own interpretations and help the patient restore meaning in a life that is changed by chronic disease.

In the clinic, the PHN has a multitude of functions, and it is part of a co-production of knowledge. It ensures communication between the doctor and the patient, makes vital health information available, together with concerns, circumstances and values of importance to the patient and for successful treatment. Discrepancies between, for example, the doctor's need for information from the patient, societal norms and the patient's life situation may cause the patient editing out vital information. This may reflect patients' worries of losing the ownership of their own life by telling a fuller story. On the other hand, the clinic and the medical doctor may also be the one facilitating a safe space where aspects of the narrative, related to shame, disappointment or worry, can be allowed, told and even explored and reconstructed in new ways, as an integral part of the person's health narrative and life story. The sub-genre of PHN in the clinic comes with a twist. Though it is the patent's narrative, when digitalised in the format of the patient's health record (discussed more fully in Chap. 10), the PHN is told by and from the point of view of the medical doctor. As the clinical situation is the context of this sub-genre, it will be an implied context of importance for PHN from the clinic when these stories are transported into other arenas, like blogs or other forms of social media.

In the following section we explore how the patient's PHN is configured when it leaves the clinic and engages with the digital domain.

Presenting a Positive Subjectivity[3]: The Case of Ostomy Blogs

The advantages of the Internet as a space for people to talk about issues concerning their health and illness and to receive support, to be able to cross boundaries of time and place, and to have access to multiple perspectives have been well documented. So are the disadvantages, such as

[3] The notion of 'positive subjectivity' was coined by Broom and Whittaker (2004) in their study of how people with diabetes use moral language to talk about the ways in which they manage their illness. It is a useful notion to understand some of our empirical work on ostomy blogs.

the short-time membership of participants in many online discussions and ongoing debates about anonymity and the credibility of the information shared online (Wright et al. 2011).

Empirical studies have mostly focused on mapping online interactions in terms of the social support they offer, often by comparing the online environment to face-to-face interaction (Wright et al. 2011). A more elaborate view of what actually happens in online support groups or in other platforms where people share the story of their illness is however, still needed (Paulus et al. 2016). We need a systematic attempt to explore the range of online illness narratives, their formats and how they are being told in different online environments. In addition, as the nature of the empirical work on online environment is sometimes described as theoretically under-developed, we also need a linkage to broader theoretical frameworks (Wright and Bell 2003; see also Wright et al. 2011 for an overview).

In this section a case-study is presented to show what the field of discourse analysis (DA) may offer to the study of online PHNs (Koteyko and Hunt 2016). A DA approach starts from the idea that language is not merely a referential system for describing the world, but such an approach would argue that when we use language 'we are saying and doing and being' (Gee 2014). When we use language we say things that enact our identities; we may say scholarly things and enact our identity as a scholar; we may say 'carer' things (as in caring for a parent who is ill) and enact our identity as a carer. Discourse analysis looks at how people put things together in sentences and how these different combinations say different things. For example, the sentence 'I feel responsible for my husband's health' does something else, and enacts different identities when compared with a sentence that consists of roughly the same words, but has a different syntax: 'my husband makes me feel responsible for his health'. These examples show that with the language or discourse we use we actively construct particular versions of who we are in text and talk. With this focus, the DA approach is representative of a constructivist approach on language that treats language as performative (Gee 2014).

PHNs offer a rich terrain for exploring such performative identity work (Antaki and Widdicombe 1992), and authors of illness blogs might also use these online conversation spaces in ways they are not able to find anywhere else (Wright et al. 2011). Examples of how people create or enact identities online are, for example, posts to an online support group that establish legitimate membership of the community of people with eating disorders (Stommel and Lamerichs 2014), or highlighting one's long-standing experience with diabetes, which creates 'authority' and truth-value when offering advice on how to manage the condition (Koteyko and Hunt 2016; also Bakhtin 1986).

The focus in this section lies on exploring the language used in blogs, which are often compared to online diaries. Blogs consist of frequently updated entries, latest contributions displayed on top, in which people relate their illness story (Jaworska 2018). The study used as key example here consists of 25 blogs that were collected from different platforms, and from male and female authors who had various conditions that ultimately led to ostomy surgery. The United Ostomy Associations of America (UOAA) describes ostomy surgery as a 'procedure that allows bodily waste to pass through a surgically created stoma on the abdomen into a prosthetic known as a 'pouch' or 'ostomy bag' on the outside of the body or an internal surgically created pouch for continent diversion surgeries. An ostomy may be necessary due to birth defects, cancer, inflammatory bowel disease, diverticulitis, incontinence and many other medical conditions' (UOAA, June 1, 2019).

Bloggers might begin their personal health narrative by describing their illness history and their struggles with, for example, inflammatory bowel disorder, Crohn's disease or cancer, which have all led to the point where ostomy surgery has become unavoidable. In the analysis, the study explored the language used by bloggers when they write about their condition leading up to their ostomy surgery and also beyond the surgery. The study found that bloggers pervasively use a 'transformative narrative' (cf., Horton-Salway 2018). This type of narrative is constructed in a way that shows how the ostomy, after a long period of struggle, and an initial period of getting used to a new situation (with what are presented as minor adaptation problems), has now resulted in a 'new normal'. In this new situation, the bloggers highlight the positive qualities of the ostomy, stressing the renewed, sometimes extraordinary possibilities it has brought them in their lives (Lamerichs and Van Hooijdonk forthcoming).

An interesting feature in these blogs has to do with the blurring of contexts (Davis and Jurgenson 2014; Litt 2012), which is a characteristic of many public online environments. As is the case with social media in general, publicly available illness blogs blur the lines between the public and private, the professional and personal, and thus the many different selves and situations in which individuals may find themselves (Davis and Jurgenson 2014). This blurring of contexts is also visible in the ways in which bloggers orient to their 'imagined audience', or the people with whom the blogger envisages to communicate with the blog (see Litt 2012 for an overview). This study found that the audience was often activated by a call from the blogger to lift the stigma on ostomies or to explicitly counter the view that life with an ostomy bag was fraught with difficulties. It might be that this position of 'advocacy' stimulates the bloggers in our data to tell 'transformative stories' about having reached a state of the new normal, or to tell how they have come to terms with illness and ostomy surgery and have succeeded in doing so (cf., Mattingly 2010).

If we consider the nature of these ostomy blogs from a more critical perspective, it might be that these stories mostly reflect positive personal stories of coping. What they do not offer is a narrative that offers a perspective other than the mainstream views of coping, or less positive accounts of problems one might encounter. In the dataset, the accounts of choosing invasive surgery are predominantly told from the perspective of how they have been a solution to live a normal life again, and this enables them geared mostly to lifting the taboo on ostomies and ostomy surgery. Moreover, the study shows that some of the bloggers consider themselves 'advocates' for the decision to undergo ostomy surgery. The dominant online voices regarding representations in ostomy blogs thus seem to be the voices of those who have successfully coped with their condition and their surgery. Bloggers also address issues related to ostomy surgery and how to 'manage the bag', but to a lesser extent; this however might be a topical area where the blogging offers a conversation space to address stigma and shame surrounding ostomies.

The fact that bloggers address their audience in a way that fits the position of advocate to overcome stigma related to ostomies, also shows that it is important to know the goals or communicative purpose of the authors of a blog, which makes it recognisable as a genre (see Bhatia

2004). This allows readers, analysts, health professionals and possibly also other parties to arrive at a better understanding of what these personal health narratives represent, and to be able to contextualise them in the larger landscape of available illness narratives.

Personal Health Narratives in Public Media

Between the ongoing debate about fake news and agents who have a public information task (journalists, governmental bodies, public agencies, public institutions, public services, etc.), the PHN has found its place, and one of its functions is to position itself as a carrier of truthful information with societal importance.[4] This 'truthful' information may be for or against generally accepted medical opinion, depending upon the PHN and the editorial policy of the media source. The PHN describes the history and contexts of a particular health-related issue. In the public media, the intention is explicitly to illuminate the chosen health issue, and aspects of societal or political importance. The narrative is told, because the narrator finds it important, and the news media or public media distributing the narrative is confirming the societal impact of the narrative by printing it. This is a newer genre, in that such PHN would not commonly be published 30 or more years ago. In order to show how a personal health narrative may aim at the general, we will present an example of a personal health narrative told by a national daily news media distributed on the news media's online platform.

Example: Ida Maria Børli Sivertsen 'I do not need to be drunk to be creative'

December 2015 *Aftenposten*, one of the main national online and offline newspapers in Norway, published an article written by the Norwegian

[4] In this chapter we focus on the presence and potency of PHNs. We do not focus on illness narratives that have risen as a new phenomenon of societal concern, as for example eating disorder groups on Instagram. See, for example, the BBC series of articles on this topic, https://www.bbc.com/news/uk-47637377.

rock star Ida Maria Børli Sivertsen.[5] This was not an interview where a journalist had found a story to illuminate a case. The text was written on the author's own initiative, and the story was told in her own words (Sivertsen 2015). Aftenposten was the Norwegian counterpart in the Panama papers' network of newsrooms, and it is a key contributor to the agenda of political and societal news and debates in Norway. Ida Maria Børli Sivertsen is a globally known rock music artist, known by her first names Ida Maria.

Ida Maria starts her texts by stating 'Two weeks ago, one of my American rock colleagues, Scott Weiland, died, as so many before him, of an overdose … now, his family has approached the Rolling Stone Magazine, begging people to stop glorifying his addiction'. Ida Maria continues by declaring 'My history is in many ways parallel to that of Scott Weiland, but with a twist. I am still alive – to the joy and indignation of many'. She goes on by describing her tour life in 2007–2009 in the UK, Norway and USA, and how Colombia Records had paid for her, and other artists' use of sex, drugs and rock 'n roll. She writes that the Company had special credit cards to pay for the partying, and that a PR-lady followed the musicians around to get hold on scandals to print. She tells how journalists got her drunk to make her talk negatively about other artists. Then Eva Maria continues telling about details describing what the tour life did to her body. 'At 24 my digestion system was ruined. My body did not want to absorb food, but I thought, "…well, it is a lot of nutrition in liquid …" I did not have an alcohol problem, but a career problem. My career disturbed my drinking.' She then describes a negative spiral leading to severe obesity and alcoholism, and how she moved to Los Angeles, because they had liquor stores that were open all night. In the USA, after years in northern Norway, London, Stockholm and Oslo, she finally met sober colleagues, and she says that the Grammy organisation MusiCares, with their tailored programme for rehabilitation of musicians with an alcohol problem, saved her. She then describes alcoholism as a disease, and she ensures that help is available. She says, 'Now

[5] Ida Maria Børli Sivertsen, Jeg trenger ikke være full for å være kreativ. Available at https://www.aftenposten.no/meninger/kronikk/i/4BEE/kronikk-jeg-trenger-ikke-vaere-full-for-aa-vaere-kreativ-ida-maria

it is time to build a similar organisation in Norway. I am ready'. She underlines that her personal experience is that one does not need to be drunk to be creative, confirming Weiland's parents' statement in the Rolling Stones Magazine, as she lists the music she is involved with and has produced after she became sober. In the final part of this personal health narrative of Ida Maria, there is a longer passage of stories with different outcomes, and some references to her friend Iggy Popp, and other rock colleagues, including Amy Winehouse and a bar-dancing moment back in 2007, as she says, four years proceeding Amy's death. The text ends with 'Rest in peace Amy. Rest in peace Scott'.

When we claim that PHNs are important in the digital society, our understanding of what PHN contains is important. This includes how facts are made important, and how certain narrative features seem to characterise PHNs and provide them with importance for individuals and society at the same time.

Ida Maria's story was quickly distributed across different platforms, in social media as well as in traditional TV media, including the most prominent Scandinavian talk show Skavland, with key cuts from the show now stored on YouTube (Ida Maria 2016; Skavland Feb 26th 2016). Though Ida Maria wrote her story herself, and it was published in a newspaper, which includes the newspaper's online version, the text is closer to traditional *oral genres* than written text genre, regarding the form of words used, that is, *everyday language* more than formal language. A genre, in an oral tradition, consists of *variants* of narratives, and an oral narrative is always *performed* anew, in accordance to the specific context and time of each performance. As with narratives belonging to an oral genre, Ida Maria's story slightly varied, as she retold it in different contexts. The variations reflected where and when the story was told, how it was interconnected to previous presentations of the story, and to the different approaches that for example Skavland, as a host of a TV show, had when she told the story to him. The key elements of the story stayed the same.

Ida Maria's story about her own alcoholism was obviously a *personal* and *individual* narrative, reflecting her experiences of choices she and others had made for her, experiences of a lack of help to get sober, and experiences of help and options that later became available for her. She links her personal narrative to a wider set of already known stories about addictions and deaths of other rock musicians. In several regards Ida Maria's narrative embeds a knowledge claim and authority (see earlier discussions on the relation between 'author' and 'authority' above). Her narrative represents many layers, such as a personal story, an illness and recovery narrative about addiction as a phenomenon, and particular aspects of present culture (for instance the romanticisation of addiction, rock music and creativity), and her narrative furthermore touches upon a societal aspect revealing lack of organised help for musicians with addiction. She has an *agenda*, and in addition to the awareness and general changes she will achieve, she suggests a specific initiative to establish a new organisation in Norway after a US model, the organisation where she herself became sober.

There are *two levels intertwined* in Ida Maria's story: the individual and particular levels, and the societal and general levels. The complexity and authenticity of the individual experience is what gives bearing as key arguments for societal and general arguments. The narrative aims at disseminating knowledge, and it aims at suggesting societal changes based on the authentic knowledge presented.

To Tell What One Is, and Societal Relevance

Ida Maria's story is one example of a PHN told on her own initiative in a main newspaper with editorial practices and an editor-in-chief. The narrative is personal, told within the frame of her individual life story, filled with details pointing towards a specific theme (addiction). At the same time, it strives to achieve awareness, and to contribute to further societal, cultural and institutional changes. Ida Maria's story is not unique, but it is an example of a narrative type, PHN, of the genre personal narrative, that has become an integral part of, and thus a typical and expected story in, traditional news media. The distribution of Ida Maria's story was quick and reached far outside the national newspaper where she first told her story.

The impact of a PHN is something more complex and difficult to estimate, but like all stories entering the public domain, a PHN becomes a potential resource in the public discourse, in addition to work as a resource for those searching for examples and experience concerning addiction. An example of the potency of PHN is the story of Nini Stoltenberg. In Norway, and regarding drug addiction, the story of Nini Stoltenberg, the little sister of former prime minister of Norway, and then chief of NATO, Jens Stoltenberg, is well known, and Nini Stoltenberg's telling of her story of addiction is recognised as the key reason for the present politics towards medical assisted use of heroin in the Social Democratic Party of Norway (Arbeiderpartiet https://www.arbeiderpartiet.no/politikken/heroinassistert-helsehjelp-og-lar/).

As for Ida Maria, it was Nini Stoltenberg herself who initiated the telling of her narrative. In the present society such stories are invited and appreciated, a phenomenon which confirms that PHNs are important and represent more than personal destinies.

The criteria for getting access to telling one's PHN in traditional news media are not fame and age. This is shown in another personal health story from Aftenposten which is about suicide (Vignes 2014). This story is also very detailed and personal at the same time as it claims knowledge regarding the phenomenon of suicide, and general conclusions are drawn about the institutionalised hindrances for insights (i.e. patient-doctor confidentiality). This narrative underlines the societal and cultural importance of openness, and why it is important, even necessary to repeal, or even go beyond it and deconstruct the shame that the narrator in this case has described as an obstacle causing silence for all parties involved. Aftenposten also provided a special page for debate articles from people under the age of 21, and the stories published include young peoples' personal health narratives (https://www.aftenposten.no/meninger/sid/).

Suicide and mental health have become a key theme for PHNs published in traditional news media. It also includes stories where those left behind are the ones telling the person's and family's story. In these stories, the PHN is contextualised by the complexity of health and life in culture and society, and its aim is to inform and educate, presupposing an understanding (from the narrator and publisher) that the story is informative and educating. PHNs, in these settings, are something other than traditional politics, though they aim at discussions including implications of societal services and institutions.

The traditional nationwide newspapers, now both in online and offline formats, focus on reporting politics, societal and academic news, in ways that document the news, investigate their truthfulness and tie them to present and past power agents and structures. News media are organised in editorial groups with a main editor-in-chief, thus claiming knowledge and truthfulness as key tools in their function as the fourth independent leg of modern democracy.[6] It is thus interesting to notice how news media have become an arena for PHNs written by the concerned individual himself/herself, often in the format of a debate article/a commentary, usually signed with a full name.

Health Literacy and Citizenship

The present organisation of health services and information in today's European society is strongly linked to citizenship. In the EU citizen's rights and obligations, a person is a key agent herself/himself, expected to make informed choices, including choices regarding health and medical treatment when signing contracts of informed consent. The 2014 Special EU Barometer 460 *European citizen's digital health literacy* report confirms the importance of the Internet when people search for information and seek answers to their health requests. (The Special EU barometer 460 Attitudes towards the impact of digitisation and automation on daily life.)

We know the potency of individual stories in a genre context, in particular the importance of novels, whether fictional novels like *Uncle Tom's Cabin*, or autobiographic, like Anne Frank's diary. As a genre, the personal narrative is conveying meaning that transgresses the individual person himself/herself. Women's magazines represent a long tradition for the printing of personal lay stories, including personal health narratives, and as a societal phenomenon, personal health narratives are nothing new. However, the use of them in public news media is quite novel, not the

[6] The public discussion about social media and fake news is a topic in itself, and the counter strategies are many, including an EU-financed citizen project (Media for Citizens—Citizens for Media; http://www.cimusee.org/).

least with its online visibility, ability to share between online platforms, and thus easy access in social media.

The variety of social-media platforms, and the possibility to share between online platforms, reflects recent and rapid technological developments in the digital society, starting out from Web 1.0 situation, where the world wide web (www) made it possible to build and reach homepages through web addresses, to the introduction of search engines (like Google), and new software introducing Web 2.0 with social media platforms that made interactive communication and co-production of online content possible. The ongoing development of hardware and software has made transportation of information between devices and the sharing between platforms easy and an everyday activity for online users. This is mirrored in the ways PHNs travel, and in the way these narratives are presented. Former distinctions between public and private, between news media and popular culture, are intertwined and blurred (see the reference to collapsed context above, Zappavigna 2012). For example, the suicide of a young girl is presented in the Swedish women's magazine *Amelia*, and the PHN told contains the narrative of Johanna's own suicide note, plus her brother Johan's original message from Facebook, presenting Johanna's suicide story and text. The PHN of Johanna contains the personal and contextual details discussed above, and it is linked to her brother's present work on mental health, because he is now explicitly taking on a role to ensure openness and knowledge about suicide, and to contribute to changes in society (Näs 2016).

Regarding the complexity of actual interaction and (co-)production of health content in the digital society, understanding PHNs is at the heart of the challenges that concerns health literacy and citizenship.

Concluding Remarks

The PHN, as we define it in this chapter, is a complex and compact story told in a variety of contexts. We could have easily added more examples, for example healthtalk.uk, or other research-based homepages presenting PHNs to inform about public health issues. However, our intention is not to document the overall presence of a broad variety of personal health narratives, but to create awareness about PHN and their function Ziebland and Wyke (2012). Taken together, all of the different sub-genres of PHN presented in this chapter are at work in society, though the sub-genres' primary aim differ. The PHN in the clinical setting aims at the patient's well-being and health, and how to achieve necessary change, located in specific circumstances and relations, and tied to personal preferences and choices. The PHN on blogs and homepages are aiming at public health issues that concern groups, societal knowledge, awareness and policymaking. The PHN in news media are aiming at political dimensions, underpinnings and consequences regarding health and well-being. As they are all PHNs, to approach them as sub-genres helps clarify the impact, potency and aims.

Based on our examples in this chapter we can draw some general conclusions about the PHN genre. PHN is intended to be heard by a person or an audience, it includes elements of the teller's life, is presented as authentic and truthful, and as a container of information that makes the individuality and complexity of health visible, implicating a kind of authority as well as a human interrelatedness between the narrator and the listener or reader. PHNs are of importance to both online and offline contexts. A PHN functions as a vehicle for private and clinical counselling and public health information, and it provides a way to explain practices, premises, and organisational models for public health, and their effect on the individual. When distinguishing between PHN sub-genres, the close relation between sub-genre and contexts can be understood more thoroughly. This is important because there is also a need to be cautious and aware of the context's impact, and the sub-genre as a carrier of aims. In addition to being carriers of specific content related to a person's life and circumstances, PHNs reflect a societal emphasis on citizenship, patient participation principles, and the co-production of health knowledge.

In the Navigating Knowledge Landscapes' (NKL) vocabulary, PHNs have become an important vehicle for dissemination of knowledge about health and health-related issues in the digital society. The spread and impact of the PHN reflects societal demands and rights that include health and well-being, citizenship, personalised medicine, narrative medicine and ethics. PHNs have plural functions. One function is that PHNs enable people to navigate towards knowledge about health and well-being, whether it concerns personal health or societal aspects of it. And the different sub-genres of PHN elaborate different aspects of the PHN. The PHN in present society reflects how communication and relations work in the digital society. The PHN has an intention, and its discursive direction seems to aim at helping, or enlightening, guiding, and ensuring that people navigate health and health-related issues in a particular way. We suggest that when the societal importance and potency of the PHN today is acknowledged, a next step could be to discuss risk and misuse, for example linked to further discussions on fake news versus news, or PHN versus illness-stories, or research on how collective narratives also become drivers that form personal narratives (Shuman 2005). The presence of PHNs reflects how health and the relation between the individual and society is at the centre of ongoing societal attention and discussion, and how it is an integral part of people's life, including consultation and medical treatment. The PHN is a key strategy for societal agents, professionals and individuals alike, but the telling and interpreting of personal health narratives work differently in different contexts. In the clinical setting, the PHN is part of a co-production of personal health narratives, and it is tied to a personal-professional relation. The clinic can be a place for further elaboration and extension of a PHN, as well as a place for reduction, revision or hiding, and in both cases, the success or failure to co-produce a PHN has impact on the life and well-being of the patient. The PHN in the clinic is digitalised by the practitioner, because when entering the patient's health record, the PHN is told from the point of view of the medical doctor. In the blogs discussed in this chapter, the PHN is told by people sharing similar health conditions and procedures. In this context the blogs seem to strengthen coping, at the same time as the blogs have a normative mission, as agents that work for the procedure they themselves have chosen. The PHN as an identity project is personal and political, thus resisting stories that might argue for other procedures based on other experiences than the ones that are put forward and discussed on the blog. The presence of PHN in edited news media underlines the societal, cultural and/or political importance of PHN in today's society, and the truth-value they are given. But most of all, the PHN in news media mirrors how health and individual life is a societal matter that negotiates knowledge, power, policies, norms and values: democratic rights, understandings of health and well-being and society's responsibility in all of this.

Stories have a long tradition as an acknowledged way of expressing knowledge in academic disciplines such as theology, history, law and medicine (i.e. parables, cases, biographies). Modern epistemology also sees narratives as a basic structure of knowledge. However, in matters concerning health and disease, the public versions of such stories have been dominated by the stories told by professionals and health authorities, often devaluing or simplifying individual or deviant experiences. Personal health narratives have typically been restricted to the protected space of confidentiality between patient and clinician. Still, persons are expected to be in charge of their own lives, both as a right to autonomy and a responsibility to cope. In this situation, modern digital communication makes it possible for individuals to publish their personal health narratives, to get to know others' experiences, and for clinicians to see more of the whole picture of what their patients' lives are like.

Genre can be defined along lines of culture, and so can the different sub-genres. To present a PHN, one needs to recognise the fundamental importance of language and meaning, and how it is contextually situated. Both the clinic and the blogs and media stories discussed in this chapter are providing context on within which PHNs might be framed and mobilised. The PHN genre is concerned with knowledge; it strives to organise information in informed and systematic ways, by telling a story that others can follow and also discuss. The PHN genre pays attention to details, relations and processes, and it is told to affect and/or change the reader's or listener's perception and actions, societal organisation, and the part of present culture that the narrative problematises. The PHN is a potent part of present public discourse. As such, we find it important to understand the meaning in and of these particular stories, as well as to recognise and reflect upon the new status and potency of PHN, its pathways in society, the attention and audiences it has, its impact and influence, and its contribution to the production of meaning and culture, in the lives of people, groups and for society at large. The presence of PHN reflects health as a key societal issue. The content of PHNs that we present, reflect important aspects of present society, not the least how health information and choices about health have become an individualised responsibility. The content of PHNs and the online and offline arenas where PHNs operate also reflect a society where services and knowledge production and communication are driven forward by the continuing development of new technology and software, regarding both services and communication. PHN is performed and received as a story that reflects or brings information that is of general value, as it is implied that health is a bodily-mental-spiritual state of what it is to be a human being. If our argument that PHN is narrative that is recognisable as a genre in present society is accepted, we can draw on knowledge about oral narratives as it has been dealt with in regard to folk tradition, how narratives work, travel and change, how identification of repertoire can be of importance to cultural and societal analysis and how contexts and performance (audience and interaction) are defining for the narrative's meaning and function.

References

Agich, G. J. (2003). *Dependence and autonomy in old age: An ethical framework for long-term care*. Cambridge: Cambridge University Press.

Allgaier, J., & Svalastog, A. L. (2015). The communication aspects of the Ebola virus disease outbreak in Western Africa – Do we need to counter one, two, or many epidemics? *Croatian Medical Journal, 56*(5), 496–499.

Antaki, C., & Widdicombe, S. (1992). *Identities in talk*. London: Sage Publications.

Arbeiderpartiet: Heroinassistert helse og LAR. https://www.arbeiderpartiet.no/politikken/heroinassistert-helsehjelp-og-lar/, July 2th 2019.

Attitudes towards the impact of digitisation and automation on daily life, The Special EU barometer 460. https://ec.europa.eu/digital-single-market/en/news/attitudes-towards-impact-digitisation-and-automation-daily-life, July 2th 2019.

Bakhtin, M. M. (1986). *Speech genres and other late essays* (trans: McGee, V. W., and ed: Emerson, C., & Holquist, M.). Austin: University of Texas Press.

Bauman, R. (Ed.). (1984). *Verbal art as performance*. Prospect Heights: Illinois Waveland Press, Inc.

Bhatia, V. K. (2004). *Worlds of written discourse: A genre-based view*. London: Continuum.

Bowling, A., Rowe, G., & McKee, M. (2013). Patients' experiences of their healthcare in relation to their expectations and satisfaction: A population survey. *Journal of the Royal Society of Medicine, 106*(4), 143–149. https://doi.org/10.1258/jrsm.2012.120147.

Brody, H. (1994). "My story is broken; Can you help me fix it?": Medical ethics and the joint construction of narrative. *Literature and Medicine, 13*(1), 79–92.

Brody, H. (2002). *Stories of sickness*. New York: Oxford University Press.

Broom, D., & Whittaker, A. (2004). Controlling diabetes, controlling diabetics: Moral language in the management of diabetes type 2. *Social Science & Medicine, 58*(11), 2371–2382. https://doi.org/10.1016/j.socscimed.2003.09.002.

Brosman, C., Vuolanto, P., & Brodin Danell, J.-A. (Eds.). (2018). *Complementary and alternative medicine: Knowledge production and social transformation*. Basingstoke: Palgrave Macmillan.

Charon, R. (2006). *Narrative medicine: Honoring the stories of illness*. Cary: Oxford University Press.

Davis, J. L., & Jurgenson, N. (2014). Context collapse: Theorizing context collusions and collisions. *Information, Communication & Society, 17*(4), 476–485. https://doi.org/10.1080/1369118X.2014.888458.

Dubbeldam, I. (2016). De dokter vertelt mij wel wat er loos is. In *Een kwalitatief Onderzoek naar patronen in het informatiegedrag van zorggebruikers Proefschrift*. Amsterdam: Vrije Universiteit Amsterdam.

Frank, A. W. (2013). *The wounded storyteller: Body, illness, and ethics* (2nd ed.). Chicago: University of Chicago Press.

Frow, J. (2014). *Genre*. London: Routledge.

Gee, P. (2014). *An introduction to discourse analysis: Theory and method*. London: Routledge.

Geurts, J. W., Willems, P. C., Lockwood, C., van Kleef, M., Kleijnen, J., & Dirksen, C. (2017). Patient expectations for management of chronic non-cancer pain: A systematic review. *Health Expectations: An International Journal of Public Participation in Health Care and Health Policy, 20*(6), 1201–1217. Retrieved from https://www.ncbi.nlm.nih.gov/pubmed/28009082. https://www.ncbi.nlm.nih.gov/pmc/PMC5689237/. https://doi.org/10.1111/hex.12527.

Hirsh, J. D., Jr. (1976). *Validity in interpretation*. New Haven: Yale University Press.

Horton-Salway, M. (2018). Voices of experience: Narrative lives and selves. In M. Horton-Salway & A. Davies (Eds.), *The discourse of ADHD, the language of mental health*. London: Palgrave Macmillan.

Hunter, K. M. (1991). *Doctors' stories: The narrative structure of medical knowledge*. Princeton: Princeton University Press.

Hurwitz, B., Greenhalgh, T., & Skultans, V. (2004). *Narrative research in health and illness*. Malden: BMJ Books.

Ida Maria. (2016). Ida Maria:—Karrieren kom i veien for drikkinga mi. At YouTube https://www.youtube.com/watch?v=_eW9iHj1xa0

Jaworska, S. (2018). Bad mums tell the 'untellable': Narrative practice and agency in stories about postnatal depression on Mumsnet. *Discourse, Context & Media, 25*, 25–33.

Jaworski, M., Rzadkiewicz, M., Adamus, M., Chylinska, J., Lazarewicz, M., Haugan, G., Lillefjell, M., Espenes, G. A., & Wlodarczyk, D. (2017). Primary care patients' expectations regarding medical appointments and their experiences during a visit: Does age matter? *Patient Preference and Adherence, 11*, 1221–1233. https://doi.org/10.2147/ppa.S133390.

Kleinman, A. (1978). Concepts and a model for the comparison of medical systems as cultural systems. *Social Science & Medicine*, in ParB: Medical Anthropology, *12*: 85–93.

Koski, K., Frog, M., & Savolainene, U. (2016). Genre – Text – Interpretation. Multidisciplinary Perspectives on Folklore and Beyond. *Studie Fennica Flkloristica, 22*, Turenki: Hansaprint Oy. https://doi.org/10.21435/sff.22.

Koteyko, N., & Hunt, D. (2016). Performing health identities on social media: An online observation of Facebook profiles. *Discourse, Context & Media, 12*, 59–67.

Lamerichs, J., & Van Hooijdonk, C. (forthcoming). "Mijn stoma is een #superstoma": een analyse van narratieve blogs over stoma's. [My Ostomy is a #superostomy": An analysis of narrative ostomy blogs], in Tijdschrift voor Taalbeheersing.

Lang, F., Floyd, M. R., & Beine, K. L. (2000). Clues to patients' explanations and concerns about their illnesses: A call for active listening. *Archives of Family Medicine, 9*(3), 222.

Leslie, B., Harris, R., Chavez, D., Fear, J., & Gill, P. (2008). 'Everybody is talking at me': Situating the client in the info(r)mediary work of health professionals. In N. Wathen, S. Wyatt, & R. Harris (Eds.), *Mediating health information. The go-between in a changing socio-technical landscape*. London: Palgrave Macmillan.

Levy, A. G., Scherer, A. M., Zikmund-Fisher, B. J., Larkin, K., Barnes, G. D., & Fagerlin, A. (2018). Prevalence of and factors associated with patient nondisclosure of medically relevant information to clinicians. *JAMA Network Open, 1*(7), e185293–e185293. https://doi.org/10.1001/jamanetworkopen.2018.5293.

Litt, E. (2012). *Knock,Knock*. Who's there? The imagined audience. *Journal of Broadcasting & Electronic Media, 56*(3), 330–345. https://doi.org/10.1080/08838151.2012.705195.

Mattingly, C. (2010). *The paradox of Hope: Journeys through a clinical borderland*. Berkeley: UCP.

Näs, L. (2016). Johanna tog sitt liv – nu vill lillebror att du läser avskedsbrevet. In Amelia Sept 19th 2016. https://www.amelia.se/artiklar/johanna-tog-sitt-liv-nu-vill-lillebror-att-du-laser-avskedsbrevet/, July 2th 2019.

Nettleton, S. (2005). 'I just want permission to be ill': Towards a sociology of medically unexplained symptoms. *Social Science and Medicine, 62*(2006), 1167–1178.

Palant, A. (2019). Are there also negative effects of social support? A qualitative study of patients with inflammatory bowel disease. *BMJ Open, 9*(1).

Paulus, T., Warren, A., & Lester, J. N. (2016). Applying conversation analysis methods to online talk: A literature review. *Context, Context & Media, 12*, 1–10.

Ricoeur, P. (1991). Narrative identity. *Philosophy Today, 35*(1), 73–81.

Shuman, A. (2005). Collective memory and public forgetting. In *Other people's stories. Entitlement claims and the critique of empathy*. Champaign: University of Illinois Press.

Sivertsen, I. M. B. (Dec 12th 2015, updated Dec 17 2015). Jeg trenger ikke være full for å være kreativ. In Aftenposten Dec 12 2015. https://www.aftenposten.no/meninger/kronikk/i/4BEE/Kronikk-Jeg-trenger-ikke-vare-full-for-a-vare-kreativ%2D%2DIda-Maria, July 2th 2019.

Skavland, F. (2016). Interview: Ida Maria. In NRK (Norwegian Broadcasting). https://tv.nrk.no/serie/skavlan/2016/KMTE50000816, July 2th 2019.

Stahl, S. D. (1989). *Literary folkloristics and the personal narrative*. Bloomington: Indiana University Press.

Stommel, W., & Lamerichs, J. (2014). Interaction in online support groups. Advice and beyond. In H. E. Hamilton & W. S. Chou (Eds.), *The Routledge handbook of language and health communication* (pp. 198–211). London: Routledge.

Svalastog, A. L., Donev, D., Kristoffersen, N. J., & Gajović, S. (2017). Concepts and definitions of health and health related values in the knowledge landscapes of the digital society. *Croatian Medical Journal, 58*(6).

Tshuma, N., Aboulela, S., Chowdhury, F., Macken, L., Kamperidis, N., Goodhand, J., & Lindsay, J. (2012). Content analysis of illness blogs posted online by patients with IBD. *Gut, 61*(suppl 2), A68–A69. https://doi.org/10.1136/gutjnl-2012-302514a.159.

United Ostomy Associations of America (UOAA). Accessed via www.ostomy.org on June 1, 2019.

Vignes, O. (2014). Det er ingen som trur at toastmasteren skal gjere sjølvmord. In Aftensposten April 22th 2014, updated April 25th. https://www.aftenposten.no/meninger/kronikk/i/BdPv/Det-er-ingen-som-trur-at-toastmasteren-skal-gjere-sjolvmord, July 2th 2019.

Wright, K. B., & Bell, S. B. (2003). Health-related support groups on the Internet: Linking empirical findings to social support and computer-mediated theory. *Journal of Health Psychology, 8*, 37–52.

Wright, K. B., Johnson, A. J., Bernard, D. R., & Averbec, J. (2011). Computer-mediated social support. Promises and pitfalls for individuals coping with health concerns. In T. L. Thompson, R. Parrott, & J. F. Nussbaum (Eds.), *The Routledge handbook of health communication* (pp. 349–362). London: Routledge.

Zappavigna, M. (2012). Enacting identity in microblogging through ambient affiliation. *Discourse & Communication, 8*(2), 209–228.

Ziebland, S., & Wyke, S. (2012). Health and Illness in a connected world: How might sharing experiences on the Internet affect people's health. *Millbank Quarterly. A Multidisciplinary Journal of Population Health and Health Policy, 90*(2), 219–249. https://doi.org/10.1111/j.1468-0009.2012.00662.x.

3

Legal Aspects of Knowledge Landscapes in Healthcare

Iñigo de Miguel Beriain, Ana Borovečki, and Aleksandra Głos

Introduction

The practice of medicine is one of the human activities that have undergone significant changes in the last 50 years. During this period, we have witnessed the transition from a basically paternalistic model, in which the patient was no more than the object of the application of medical science, to a new framework based on the idea of informed consent. In this new

I. de Miguel Beriain (✉)
GI Derecho y Genoma Humano RG Law and the Human Genome, UPV/EHU, Leioa, Spain

Ikerbasque, Basque Foundation for Science, Bilbao, Spain
e-mail: INIGO.DEMIGUELB@ehu.eus

A. Borovečki
Andrija Štampar School of Public Health, School of Medicine, University of Zagreb, Zagreb, Croatia

A. Głos
Jagiellonian University, Kraków, Poland

A. L. Svalastog et al. (eds.), *Navigating Digital Health Landscapes*, Health, Technology and Society, https://doi.org/10.1007/978-981-15-8206-6_3

paradigm, the patient—now empowered—is configured as the centre of medical care; it is the patient who makes the final decision on whether to receive a treatment on the basis of adequate information. Traditionally, this fundamental requirement—the acquisition of adequate information—was covered mainly through the construction of a doctor–patient relationship in which the latter relied on the information provided by the former and then decided on the option that best suited his or her preferences among those proposed by the doctor. This established a relationship between the doctor and patient based on trust and mutual cooperation that, typically, was based on the recognition of the health professional's better knowledge of medical science.

This framing of the relationship was subject to some criticism however. Indeed, authors such as Kreindler (2015) have pointed out that "The seemingly benign concept of patient-centred care can easily become a weapon on an intergroup battlefield. Understanding this dimension may help organizations resolve the intergroup tensions that prevent collective achievement of a patient-centred system" (p. 44). In the last few years, however, the patient-centred care model has changed dramatically due to the emergence of technologies that have substantially altered issues such as access to information, the volume of available data or the relevance of sources. This not only provides some advantages to both patients and healthcare professionals but also creates strong dysfunctions (Meghachandra and Devi 2014).

For patients, access to information that in previous times was not available can adequately complement the knowledge transmitted by healthcare professionals who, all too often, do not have enough time to explore in depth the pathologies of each patient. It must be emphasised that patients have, in theory, all the time at their disposal to focus on a single pathology, while practitioners have to contemplate a range that encompasses thousands of diseases. This makes it sometimes true that a patient knows more than a doctor about a particular pathology. This circumstance rather defies one of the main hypotheses of medical practice and is not always well accepted by the professional who has to provide healthcare.

This is not, however, the most pressing problem that has arisen in recent times. For every patient who manages to have a good understanding of his or her pathology, there are many more who end up being guided by imprecise—if not clearly mistaken or misleading—information (Bynum 2008). Indeed, one of the problems we are currently facing is no longer a lack of information, but rather an excess of it. Furthermore, the difficulty of contrasting the available sources creates great anxiety in patients who often end up demanding treatments from a doctor that have no scientific validity whatsoever, proposing unrealistic diagnoses or assuming a risk perspective that is very far removed from reality (Nuffield Council on Bioethics 2014).

This situation often creates a scenario far removed from medical best practice. As Fiske et al. (2018) have written, "new types of mistrust within doctor–patient relationships have been documented and partly blamed on more—yet often unreliable—health information from sources outside of traditional clinical realms" (p. 39). The consequences of this end up being patients' frequent recourse to self-medication, conflicts and even physical aggression to healthcare professionals, as well as a substantial increase in the stress to which health professionals are subjected (Bernburg et al. 2016). These circumstances create such a difficult scenario that sometimes a physician may end up agreeing to request unnecessary tests to avoid coming into conflict with the patient, which is conduct that not only borders on malpractice but also brings unnecessary economic cost to the public health system. This constitutes what has been called "wish-fulfilling medicine" (Buyx 2008)—that is to say, medicine adapted to what the patient demands, although its real usefulness is not clear. It is also quite clear that medicine *à la carte* does not really resolve these situations. We are currently witnessing a boom in direct-to-consumer tests, online diagnostics and telemedicine that often increase healthcare costs when the disconcerted patient forces their doctor to confirm or deny results via unnecessary new tests (Annes et al. 2010).

The primary aim of this chapter is to address a key question in this scenario: how might information availability be better managed so that the patient can relieve his or her anxiety and cooperate efficiently with healthcare professionals while avoiding all of the problems generated by an excess of information and health supply in the virtual space? While other chapters in this book also explore this issue using a variety of disciplinary approaches, here we deploy a socio-legal perspective and ask how the law might engage with this area. We therefore analyse the existing legal framework at the EU level and explore policy options proposed to enhance the current situation, including considerations of the role to be played by content providers, healthcare givers and providers, patient associations or newly created roles such as that of health information counsellors (HICs).

A Preliminary Distinction: Disinformation and Misinformation

One must begin the analysis of the role to be played by law in improving patients' access to reliable information by recognising an undeniable premise: law cannot be the unique response to this main challenge. Freedom of expression is a fundamental human right, as we will show in depth in the following discussion. Therefore, legal restrictions to this right must be proportional, legitimate and proven necessary as the least restrictive means to pursue what they are aimed at. Under these conditions, the main question arises of when could we consider that such restrictions to freedom of expression would be both legitimate and necessary.

It is difficult to identify this precisely. Tracing a clear distinction between two different concepts—disinformation and misinformation—may help here. Disinformation includes "all forms of false, inaccurate, or misleading information designed, presented and promoted to intentionally cause public harm or for profit" (High Level Group on Fake News and Online Disinformation 2018). Misinformation, meanwhile, refers to "unintentionally false or inaccurate information" (Wardle and Derakhstan 2017). Misinformation is usually covered by the right to freedom of expression, and the law may find it difficult to deal with the issues this might create. Disinformation, however, is often considered an attack on the public interest that must be confronted by the law, even criminal law. In other words, we usually assume that it is legitimate for the law to prohibit disinformation, because it violates fundamental legal rights, a situation that set limits to freedom of expression. We can therefore arrive at a preliminary conclusion: legal tools can be efficient in prosecuting disinformation, while misinformation creates a challenge that is hard to address through the law.

There are circumstances that may make things more difficult. Unfortunately, in practice, it is not easy to distinguish whether something should be considered disinformation or misinformation. For instance, if a terrorist group plans to cause harm by creating fake news about a false pandemic, if someone disseminates inaccurate medical information to earn huge sums of money or if a clinic offers stem cell therapies that do not work at all, we might clearly consider these to be examples of disinformation. Obviously, these cases might be driven by different criminal purposes, but they would all share a common element: the intention to cause public harm or earn money by purposefully providing false, inaccurate or misleading information. There are, however, some other cases in which this distinction is not so clear. Homoeopathy and the information that some providers could bring about its real utility may be one example of this—and perhaps makes it easier to imagine how difficult it could be to distinguish disinformation and misinformation. We must therefore clarify in advance that, although we are dividing our analysis into two parts corresponding to the legal response to both types of conduct, in practice it might be very difficult to determine these boundaries.

Fighting Disinformation with Legal Tools

As mentioned, although misinformation constitutes a clearly censurable practice, it is difficult to fight from a legal point of view, because it stands very close to (if not directly in) the territory of freedom of speech. Indeed, the European legal framework is marked by the fundamental moral tension between freedom and responsibility. Article 11.1 of the Charter of the Fundamental Rights of the European Union, which, with the entry into force of the Lisbon Treaty in 2009, gained the same binding legal status as the European Union treaties, emphasises the importance of freedom of expression as follows: "Everyone has the right to freedom of expression. This right shall include freedom to hold opinions and to receive and impart information and ideas without interference by public authority and regardless of frontiers" (Charter of the Fundamental Rights of the European Union 2019). Similar is the sense of Article 10 of the European Convention on Human Rights (ECHR), which underpins the activity of the Council of Europe and binds its Member States. The first paragraph acknowledges the salience of freedom of expression, while the second points to the duties and responsibilities attached to its exercise.

It is of course true that responsibility may impose restrictions or penalties prescribed by law and necessary in a democratic society, which can be justified inter alia by the interest of public safety and the protection of health (Charter of the Fundamental Rights of the European Union 2019). However, the jurisprudence of the European Court of Justice (ECJ) has specified that these eventual limits of the freedom of speech must be interpreted "restrictively" and "reserved for the purposes of a "pressing social need" and with a "relevant and sufficient" justification" (Connolly/Commission (C 274/99) §41). Moreover, as the ECJ states, "the restrictions must be prescribed by legislative provisions which are worded with sufficient precision to enable interested parties to regulate their conduct, taking, if needed be, appropriate advice" (Connolly/Commission (C 274/99) §42). This legal framework clearly shows the underlying philosophical tension between freedom of expression and the right to be properly (and responsibly) informed, as well as showing how sensible and "soft" the legal instruments applied to such cases should be. Nevertheless, this evidence does not mean that laws can do nothing to reconcile freedom of speech with the defence of basic public goods, such as the right to adequate, evidence-based healthcare.

Indeed, in the EU and its Member States, there are a number of legal tools that have been approved in the last two years to fight disinformation, such as the Communication on Tackling Illegal Content Online, the Recommendation on Measures to Effectively Tackle Illegal Online Content or the Communication on a European Approach to Tackling Online Dissemination. To this must be added the proposed Regulation on the Prevention of the Dissemination of Terrorist Content Online.

At the national level, it might be worth highlighting some legal actions introduced in countries such as Germany. In October 2017 the Network Enforcement Act (NetzDG, *Gesetz zur Verbesserung der Rechtsdurchsetzung in sozialen Netzwerken*, also known as the "Facebook Act") entered into force; this act facilitates the imposition of a fine of 50 million euros on social media platforms that fail to remove content that is manifestly unlawful within 24 hours of receiving the complaint. For content that is offensive but in a less manifest manner, a seven-day assessment period is allowed, and failure to comply with this may also lead to a company being fined.

In France, a bill on disinformation was passed in 2018 that reinforced the principle of transparency by obliging social media platforms to disclose who sponsored particular content and for what amount of money. The companies failing to fulfil this obligation could face a fine of €75,000. However, only a week after the Parliament approved it, senators from the French Republican Party (LR) and the Centrist Union group appealed to the Constitutional court over the law, and the bill is still pending.

The Czech Republic created a special Centre Against Terrorism and Hybrid Threats at the Ministry of the Interior. The aim of the Centre is to monitor threats directly related to internal security, which also include disinformation campaigns also related to internal security. Based on its monitoring work, the Centre evaluates detected challenges, comes up with proposals for substantive and legislative solutions and implements them where possible (Centre Against Terrorism and Hybrid Threats 2019). It also disseminates what it regards as accurate information and counters the false statements by, for example, publicising available facts and debunking fake stories. As the Ministry emphasises, the Centre will not force the "truth" on anyone, or censor media content; neither will it remove content from the Internet or other (printed) media.

It appears, therefore, that there are several legal tools, both at the EU and the Member State level, aimed at fighting disinformation. Most of them, however, tackle particularly worrying types of disinformation, such as terrorist attacks or disinformation (or influence) operations—that is, commercially or politically motivated manipulation strategies, a variant of intentional disinformation at a much greater scale (Policy Department for Economic, Scientific and Quality of Life Policies 2018, p. 5).

However, not all varieties of disinformation should lead to a block on the spread of information via hard law initiatives, because this would dramatically impoverish our democracy and society. Indeed, the regulator would then be promoting practices that violate freedom of expression and other fundamental rights, leading to censorship, online surveillance "and other misguided responses that can backfire substantially, and that can be used by purveyors of disinformation in an 'us vs. them' narrative that can de-legitimize responses against disinformation and be counter-productive in the short and long run" (High Level Group on Fake News and Online Disinformation 2018).

On the other hand, it is necessary to keep in mind that offences related to disinformation often include in their wording a reference to actions directed "to intentionally cause public harm or for profit". Intention therefore plays a key role in determining whether the diffusion of false information about health can be considered disinformation. The problem is that, too often, the intention to provide inaccurate information to harm or to profit is not clear. Providers are usually well aware of the legal framework and often avoid conveying an obvious falsehood. Rather, they opt for a certain ambiguity that induces error but does not inevitably cause it. For instance, laboratories sometimes promote their genetic tests by providing patients with information that is only partially accurate but could hardly be defined as deceitful. In such cases, it is quite difficult to prove that disinformation as such exists, so sanctions would not be applicable. As a result, penal or administrative law based on fines or penalties might be an inadequate tool to fight disinformation of this type.

Alternative tools might work equally well without affecting freedom of speech. In this respect, the Policy Department for Economic, Scientific and Quality of Life Policies of the European Parliament distinguished three main policy types advisable for this intricate task: (1) the promotion of responsible behaviours in disseminating the information among providers of information, (2) the enactment of a proactive media policy aimed at promoting pluralism and exposure of diverse content among its recipients and (3) as the Department formulates it, improving media literacy and supporting user behaviours that "can take the form of 'hyper-nudges', i.e. ways to focus the attention of end users on a diverse set of contents, and to discourage them from sharing non-verified content" (Policy Department for Economic, Scientific and Quality of Life Policies 2018, p. 21).

The most decisive legal action undertaken by the European Commission that can be subsumed under the first of the above categories—"promotion of responsible behaviour among information providers"—was issuing the EU Code of Practice on Disinformation. This unprecedented document was signed by the most relevant private stakeholders in the field including Facebook, Google, Twitter and Mozilla, as well as professional associations representing both Internet platforms and the advertising industry. The Code applies to cases of disinformation—as opposed to misinformation—defined as a "veritably false or misleading information". To be counted as disinformation, a piece of information must *cumulatively* fulfil the conditions of (1) being "created, presented and disseminated for economic gain or to intentionally deceive the public" and (2) being a possible cause of "public harm, intended as threats to democratic political and policymaking processes as well as public goods such as the protection of EU citizens' health, the environment or security" (EU Code of Practice on Disinformation 2018).

The sting in the Code is therefore aimed at political and issue-based advertising on social media. Obviously, the second category applies to healthcare issues in a more direct way, but this does not mean that the category of political advertisement remains unrelated. There are many potential (or real) situations when ostensibly false or misleading information could be used for political aims, such as to spread political and social anxiety (Broniatowski et al. 2018). An example of such a case would be the social media rumours circulating during the outbreak of Ebola in 2014, which, as Chou et al. (2018) have argued, triggered hostility towards healthcare workers and hindered control of the epidemic. The most repressive of the provisions of the Code is the commitment of its relevant signatories not to accept remuneration from, or otherwise promote, accounts and websites that consistently misrepresent information about themselves (EU Code of Practice on Disinformation 2018, Commitment II A.).

There are also many other, softer, means designed to counter the spread of disinformation. Most important, in the context of healthcare, are those directed at empowering consumers and the research community. The signatories have committed to invest in products, technologies and programmes that may both prioritise relevant, authentic and authoritative information and help individuals make more informed decisions about the trustworthiness of the provided information (EU Code of Practice on

Disinformation 2018, Commitment II D.). They have also agreed to cooperate with academics and civil society organisations (including an independent network of fact-checkers) in their good faith efforts to track disinformation and understand its impact (EU Code of Practice on Disinformation 2018, Commitment II E.). The discussed commitments are, undoubtedly, a very soft and low-interference form of legal intervention into the practice of diffusion of information on social media; however, as the Code envisages various means designed to monitor and enhance the effectiveness of its implementation—such as signatories' annual self-assessment duties and regular follow-up meetings—they may bring positive results. It may thus be hoped, that, in the long term, the actions and commitments undertaken in the Code may also increase the transparency of information provided in the area of healthcare and improve people's media-related health literacy.

Another important legal tool for facing the challenges posed by the tension between the right to free expression and responsibility, underlying the EU legal framework, is the latest opinion of the European Committee of the Regions on tackling online disinformation, which strongly emphasises the salience of the latter—obligatory—aspect of freedom. As the Committee rightly points out (Opinion of the European Committee of Regions 2019), the hallmark of social media is an inherent lack of responsibility caused by the fact that, unlike "traditional" media—which are governed by professionals (journalists, editors and administrators) who must regularly account for the content they create—information disseminated on social media is created by non-professionals and often highly anonymised (with its authors being not only unknown but difficult to identify).

To counterbalance this inherent lack of accountability on social media platforms, the Committee formulates four governmental strategies to fight disinformation, including the following: (1) increasing transparency, (2) promoting the diversity of information sources, (3) developing a system for assessing the reliability of information sources and (4) introducing civic education programmes. The latter dimension to improve users' media-related literacy is regarded by the Committee as the best long-term solution and investment by regional and local government is strongly advised.

This is also potentially the most productive strategy in the domain of healthcare, where both providers and patients could profit from improved media-related skills. This claim may be strengthened by the annual Edelman Trust Report, which in 2018 for the first time investigated the (declining) levels of trust in healthcare and formulated the following conclusion (among many others): to maintain patients' trust in today's post-truth era, healthcare should be "their own publishers" (Edelman 2018). As the report states, information provided by health companies is usually viewed as credible, whereas, on the global level, only 53% of people trust health news reported by the media. Therefore, health companies should "leverage their own channels to share their stories" rather than leave this task to the media. Leveraging such channels should mean not only creating attractive and commercially productive Internet profiles but also providing the public with reliable, evidence-based medical information. The potential improvement in social media usage from healthcare professionals must go together with the general effort to increase health literacy among individual patients whose unskilled consultation with "Doctor Google" (Bryan 2019) may bring many detrimental effects to their personal, as well as to the public, health. However, there is one caveat to his approach. The whole Eurobarometer survey series reflect how peoples' opinions are not based on knowledge alone, but rely on values and preferences of different types. There is more than dis- or misinformation that will guide the reading of health-related information, and thus literacy will be an answer for some, but may be not as crucial as one might think (Eurobarometer: Survey Series—GESIS).

Misinformation: An Extremely Challenging Scenario for the Law

The above-described legal means are aimed at fighting disinformation. Misinformation, as a much more subtle and nuanced phenomenon, is, in the light of the fundamental place of freedom of expression in European democracies, much more difficult to tackle from a legal perspective. As misinformation is spread without any intention to deceive the public, the application of repressive legal means would be misplaced in most of cases. However, the above-discussed documents already provide a wide and interesting repertoire of proactive legal strategies that could be successfully applied in the domain of healthcare. These are (1) increasing transparency, (2) proactive media policy on the side of healthcare providers and (3) introducing civic education programmes. To these might be added some alternative but potentially useful tools in the context of healthcare, such as the creation of a new type of professionals: the so-called health information counsellors.

Increasing Transparency

The first of these policies is one of the most popular strategies (European Commission 2016) being introduced to re-establish declining trust (Edelman 2017) in many European democracies. It is important and potentially effective in the political realm, which is characterised by an inherent conflict of interest often leading to many mis-statements and malpractices that, as such, should be kept under public scrutiny. In an apparently golden era of democracy (when the Cold War has already been "won", and Eastern Europe liberated for the democratic model, as Francis Fukuyama declared in his "end of history" thesis (Fukuyama 1992)), Piotr Sztompka (2000) has formulated a famous, and often quoted (Warren 2018), paradox of democracy: trust in democracy is based on the mechanisms of institutionalised mistrust, such as judicial review, civil disobedience and checks and balances, provided that—and this is the second paradox—they are not used too eagerly.

The politics of transparency is one of the mechanisms of "institutionalised mistrust" that is most open to the public and particularly apt for our contemporary "post-truth" (Flood 2016) times, where the overflow of information has diminished its credibility and transparency. It must be remembered, however, that Sztompka's paradox has a second side: these mechanisms cannot be used over-zealously and too often, because they can yield an adverse effect. This adverse effect consists of "crowding out" (Bohnet et al. 2001) genuine, interpersonal or institutional, trust by overprotective or overly coercive legal mechanisms.

The necessary limits of the culture of transparency are wisely indicated by Ivan Krastev (2013) in the context of contemporary democracy, as well as in the already classic work by Onora O'Neill on autonomy and trust in bioethics. As O'Neill insightfully stated: "Members of the public can access information about the remit, membership, current work and reports of public bodies. Major companies, universities and charities provide increasing amounts of information on their websites (…). Yet despite all these changes, and all these measures of improving trustworthiness, public trust still falters" (O'Neill 2002).

It is beyond doubt that in an era of increasing malformation, some transparency measures should also be taken in healthcare. This could take the form of a network of medical fact-checkers designed to counter specific medical kinds of misinformation, such as debunking and correcting paramedical "revelations" on alternative, miracle therapies, unproven wellness supplements advertised by celebrities or ubiquitous irrational and anti-vaccination arguments that are so widely spread on social media. Because healthcare is one of the most significant institutions of public trust, it is important to implement policies of transparency with due, healthcare-specific caution. Rather than multiplying the mechanisms of institutionalised distrust, more effort should be invested in the proactive and educative media policies described below.

Enacting Responsible and Proactive Policy on Social Media

The second recommended strategy would be to enact a responsible and proactive policy on social media. In the case of healthcare, this could mean creating partnerships among healthcare entities, trusted social media influencers, marketing firms and technology companies. The aim of such a partnership would be to establish diverse online channels disseminating accurate, evidence-based medical information in an accessible and Internet-friendly way.

Another form of this strategy would be to partner with advertisement agencies to create an interactive Internet page (or social platform profile) for a given healthcare entity (as the Edelman report advises: be your own publisher) that would disseminate evidence-based medical data in an interactive way, such as by answering questions posed online by patients, preventing their reliance on their own unprofessional and often distorted interpretation of information they find for themselves on the Internet.

A third implementation of this proactive social media strategy would be contacting social media influencers and asking them to share trustworthy medical content with their followers, which, as Collier (2018) has argued, has already proven to be effective. It is worth mentioning that this type of proactive media policy was explicitly recommended by the Council of the European Union to strengthen cooperation against vaccine-preventable diseases (recommendation 6), which obliged Member States to "increase communication activities and awareness-raising on the benefits of vaccination by: (a) presenting scientific evidence in a form understandable to laypersons, using different context-based strategies, to counter the spread of misinformation, including, for example, through digital tools and partnerships with civil society and other relevant stakeholders; (b) engaging with and offering training for relevant actors, such as healthcare workers, education stakeholders, social partners and the media as multipliers, to fight complacency and increase trust in immunisation"(Council of European Union recommendation of 7 December 2018).

The Education of the Civil Society

The third strategy, strongly emphasised by the opinion of the Committee of Regions described above, is civil education, which, indeed, is the best way to counter both disinformation and misinformation in the long term. A critical and selective approach towards information found on social media is the key to responsible interpretation. Possible educational programmes should not only be directed at patients but also at healthcare workers. Doctors, nurses and medical assistants should be trained to cope with patients' Internet-based convictions in an open, professional and respectful manner (Bella et al. 2008.)

This, however, would require governmental initiatives such as introducing technology-oriented courses within medical studies and special training for current active medical professionals. Some interesting tools have already been developed for this purpose; in Canada, for instance, the CanMEDS framework identifies and describes the abilities physicians require to effectively meet the healthcare needs of the people they serve. These abilities are grouped thematically under seven roles, and a competent physician seamlessly integrates competencies from all six of these: communicator, collaborator, leader, health advocate, scholar and professional. If the physician has mastered these abilities, he or she becomes a medical expert who can provide high-quality, safe, patient-centred care, drawing upon an evolving body of knowledge, clinical skills and professional values (Royal College of Physicians and Surgeons of Canada). Of these, perhaps the most helpful in allowing physicians to deal with information technology are those of physician as communicator, physician as health advocate and physician as a scholar. As communicators, physicians form relationships with patients and their families that facilitate the gathering and sharing of essential information for effective healthcare informed by evidence and guidelines. Physicians explore the patient's perspective, including fears, ideas about the illness, feelings about the impact of the illness and expectations for healthcare and healthcare professionals. The physician integrates this knowledge with an understanding of the patient's context, including socio-economic status, medical history, family history, stage of life, living situation, work or school setting and other relevant psychological and social issues.

As health advocates, physicians contribute their expertise and influence as they work with communities or patient populations to improve health. In this role, physicians support patients in navigating the healthcare system and advocating for patient access to appropriate resources in a timely manner, as well as gathering information about issues and working with patients and their families to develop an understanding of the needs and potential mechanisms to address these needs. As scholars, physicians are expected to demonstrate a lifelong commitment to excellence in practice through continuous learning and by teaching others, evaluating evidence and contributing to scholarship, and they are able to identify pertinent evidence, evaluate it using specific criteria and apply it in their practice and scholarly activities.

Similar considerations should be applicable to nurses, who also play an essential role in healthcare delivery. Core nursing competencies can be described as the ability to understand people and situations. This means that nurses must have the ability to apply knowledge, understand patients' needs and, based on this, develop an adequate clinical judgement. Moreover, they need to have the ability to build supportive interpersonal relationships through communication. Nursing competencies consist of the integration of knowledge, including professional judgement, skills, values and attitudes, which represent an intelligent practical skill set that integrates or combines different factors and issues in complex ways, specific to each circumstance encountered in clinical practice. To acquire nursing competency, nurses must possess the skills and personal traits necessary to perform their duties effectively while integrating multiple elements including the knowledge, techniques, attitude, thinking ability and values that are required in specific contexts (Fukada 2018).

It must therefore be concluded that, by looking at physician and nursing competencies, one finds significant input that could help in communicating and understanding the complexities of big data and health information technologies in today's healthcare delivery system. Should we change healthcare curricula so healthcare providers can also have competencies in health information provision? By looking at the CanMEDS framework and nursing competencies, this would seem to be a reasonable solution.

An alternative tool to improve the education and support of civil society is the inclusion of patients in the processes. Patient associations are efficient agents for improving the performance of the system. They have traditionally provided a supporting role for patients, and their activities are constantly developing and evolving. Historically, the sharing of patients' experiences of their own disease was the key reason for establishing patient associations. Many patient associations still provide face-to-face opportunities to meet and discuss pathologies. However, much interaction now takes place online, through blogs, Internet forums and websites. Patient associations help people to understand their condition(s), and many still provide comprehensive and clear information on paper, but this is being supplemented with websites, videos and social media.

More recently, patient groups have become involved in scientific and therapeutic activism. The concept of the "expert patient" or the "expert of experience" has developed (as is discussed in Chap. 6). The expert patient provides input into research and healthcare using his or her unique expertise as someone with first-hand experience of a disease. Many patient associations have designed processes and methodologies to ensure that their members are fully prepared to get involved in areas such as research and clinical trials and ensure that patients are available to participate wherever needed (European Lung White Book 2019). It therefore seems that patient associations have been able to keep up with the new technological developments and contribute effectively in improving the education and training of patients and civil society in general (Werder 2015).

Alternative Tools

Finally, it is worth mentioning that some authors consider that physicians and nurses are not adequately educated to navigate the complexities that have emerged because of the increasing range and quantity of digital information available for healthcare purposes. This can put significant strain on the healthcare giver–patient relationship. There have been numerous discussions and calls for better training of healthcare providers in big data, assessing treatment options using online resources and comparing information from different online sources. A new profession that would help both healthcare providers and patients has been proposed: the health information counsellor (HIC) (Fiske et al. 2018). The basis of this suggestion is clear: with the advent of big data, the healthcare provider–patient relationship is undergoing a change that appears to be detrimental to the main issue at hand when it comes to this relationship—trust.

This is a familiar scenario. At the end of the twentieth century, with the revolution in genetic and genomic sciences and the introduction of genetic testing, a new strain was placed on the physician–patient relationship. Physicians needed to be able to navigate the complexities of explaining genetic test results to their patients. Additional training was introduced and a new profession founded: genetic counsellors (Skirton et al. 2015).

Now, with the advent of big data, online healthcare services and electronic healthcare records, there is again a need to somehow "help" physicians and (especially) patients better understand and navigate the complexities of modern healthcare delivery through the invention of the health information counsellor (HIC).

What would be the role of the HIC? According to the literature, their role should be broader than that of genetic counsellors. HICs should be prepared to help patients evaluate the reliability of commercially available tests (including genetic tests), assess treatment options and compare information from online sources with physician recommendations. Does this mean that the genetic counsellors should cease to exist as a profession and reinvent themselves as HICs? This remains to be seen (Fiske et al. 2018). There are certainly many ethical issues arising from the new approaches to healthcare delivery that may have an impact on the everyday physician–patient relationship. Can HICs also be a sort of ethical consultant? This is still not clear from the discussions in the literature, although ethical competencies applied in big data settings are necessary for HICs.

When discussing the skills and competencies that HICs should possess, as well as how their training should look, it has been suggested that HIC training should take place in interdisciplinary programmes affiliated with medical schools. The fields of epidemiology, biomedical statistics, genetics/genomics, computer science, science education, social medicine, ethics and health policy should be covered. These programmes should be part of postgraduate training. Persons with degrees in health or natural sciences—including physicians—would be eligible to apply.

It seems that the notion of trust and mutual partnership in the physician–patient relationship may be called into question by the role of HICS, whose purpose is to help both parties muddle through the complexities of digital data in healthcare delivery. Is there really a need for HICs or should we change medical school curricula so that healthcare providers (i.e. physicians and nurses) can also serve the role of HIC? The answer to this question remains to be seen.

Conclusion

Social media and new technologies—including discussion boards, social network sites, blogs and videos—may be excellent tools to guarantee adequate patient-focused healthcare or contribute to improving the healthcare system by providing alternative sources of training and surveillance. However, their use also raises concern about misinformation and disinformation that might cause serious harm to the patient–doctor communication and relationship. Such use might also induce the patient to make wrong decisions on the basis of non-scientific knowledge or even provoke a threat to public health if a patient suffering from a contagious disease refuses treatment due to misguided advice, as happened in some contexts in regard to the COVID-19 virus in 2020. It is therefore perfectly understandable that all collectives involved are increasingly concerned about the need to regulate these activities in a way to serve the interests of all involved.

This chapter contributes towards the book's overall multidisciplinary exploration of the digital health landscape, inasmuch as here this landscape is in part being shaped by the examples of the various new legal interventions in the management of information discussed above. These should help patients, carers and others to navigate this landscape in a more reassured way. In order to fulfil this task, we analysed these issues from the perspective of EU law and policy recommendations on management of information. We provided an updated commentary on the EU legal framework applicable to online activities in the digital environment including the Internet and social networks, in the healthcare context. This comprises topics such as the regulation and policy tools developed by the EU concerning social networking communities and data-sharing platforms that include the sharing of sensitive information, such as health data, as well as the role played by patient organisations in improving available information. In doing so, we have highlighted the main issues and gaps that currently exist and analysed the measures proposed by EU institutions to improve the situation. We discussed a very soft and low-interference form of legal intervention into the practice of diffusion of information on social media, as well as various means designed to monitor and enhance the effectiveness of its implementation. Hopefully, this will serve to guarantee an optimal development of these new technologies, while preserving healthcare workers' interests, patients' health and basic public goods.

Acknowledgements Iñigo de Miguel Beriain's work was supported by the Government of the Basque Country, Grant IT-1066-16, and the EU Commission, H2020 SWAFS Programme, PANELFIT Project, research grant number 788039.

References

Annes, J. P., Giovanni, M. A., & Murray, M. F. (2010). Risks of presymptomatic direct-to-consumer genetic testing. *The New England Journal of Medicine, 363*, 1100–1101.

Bella, L., Harris, R., Chavez, D., Fear, J., & Gill, P. (2008). 'Everybody's talking at me': Situating the client in the info(r)mediary work of the health professions. In N. Wathen, S. Wyatt, & R. Harris (Eds.), *Mediating health information: The go-betweens in a changing socio-technical landscape* (pp. 18–37). London/New York/Melbourne: Palgrave Macmillan UK.

Bernburg, M., Vitzthum, K., Groneberg, D. A., & Mache, S. (2016). Physicians' occupational stress, depressive symptoms and work ability in relation to their working environment: A cross-sectional study of differences among medical residents with various specialties working in German hospitals. *BMJ Open, 6*, e011369.

Bohnet, I., Frey, B. S., & Huck, S. (2001). More order with less law: On contract enforcement, trust and crowding. *American Political Science Review, 95*, 131–144.

Broniatowski, D. A., Jamison, A. M., Qi, S., et al. (2018). Weaponized health communication: Twitter bots and Russian trolls amplify the vaccine debate. *American Journal of Public Health, 108*, 1378–1384. https://doi.org/10.2105/AJPH.2018.304567.

Bryan, J. M. (2019). Trust me, I'm a doctor: Public trust in the Information Age. *Canadian Medical Association Journal* website, http://www.cmaj.ca/content/trust-me-i%E2%80%99m-doctor-public-trust-information-age. Accessed 28 May 2019.

Buyx, A. (2008). Be careful what you wish for? Theoretical and normative aspects of wish-fulfilling medicine. *Medicine, Health Care, and Philosophy, 11*, 133–114.

Bynum, W. (2008). *The history of medicine a very short introduction* (p. 123). Oxford: Oxford University Press.

Centre Against Terrorism and Hybrid Threats. https://www.mvcr.cz/cthh/clanek/centre-against-terrorism-and-hybrid-threats.aspx. Accessed 24 May 2019.

Charter of the Fundamental Rights of the European Union. https://www.europarl.europa.eu/charter/pdf/text_en.pdf. Accessed 24 May 2019.

Chou, W. S., Oh, A., & Klein, W. M. P. (2018). Addressing health-related misinformation on social media. *Journal of the American Medical Association, 320*, 2417–2418. https://doi.org/10.1001/jama.2018.16865.

Collier, R. (2018). Containing health myths in the age of viral misinformation. *Canadian Medical Association Journal, 190*(19), E578. https://doi.org/10.1503/cmaj.180543.

Commission and High Level Expert Group. https://ec.europa.eu/digital-single-market/en/news/final-report-high-level-expert-group-fake-news-and-online-disinformation. Accessed 24 May 2019.

Connolly / Commission (C 274/99). Judgment of the Court of 6 March 2001. Bernard Connolly v Commission of the European Communities.

EC Communication on Tackling Online Disinformation: A European Approach (COM(2018) 236 final). https://eur-lex.europa.eu/legal-content/EN/TXT/?uri=CELEX:52018DC0236. Accessed 24 May 2019.

EC Communication on Tackling Illegal Content Online: Towards an Enhanced Responsibility of Online Platforms (COM(2017) 555 final). https://ec.europa.eu/digital-single-market/en/news/communication-tackling-illegal-contentonline-towards-enhanced-responsibility-online-platforms. Accessed 24 May 2019.

EC Recommendation on Measures to Effectively Tackle Illegal Online Content (C(2018) 1177 final). https://ec.europa.eu/digital-single-market/en/news/commission-recommendation-measures-effectively-tackleillegal-content-online. Accessed 24 May 2019.

Edelman (2017) corresponds to: (2017) Edelman TRUST BAROMETER™- Global Report, at: https://www.slideshare.net/EdelmanInsights/2017-edelmantrust-barometer-global-results-71035413.

EU Code of Practice on Disinformation, 2018. https://ec.europa.eu/digital-single-market/en/news/code-practice-disinformation. Accessed 24 May 2019.

Eurobarometer: Survey Series—GESIS. https://www.gesis.org/eurobarometer-data-service/survey-series/. Accessed 24 Sept 2019.

European Commission. (2016). *Trust. European research. Co-creating Resilient Societies*. Brussels: RTD Publications. OECD. (2017). *Trust and public policy how better governance can help rebuild public trust*. Paris: OECD Publishing. http://www.oecd.org/governance/trust-and-public-policy-9789264268920-en.htm, Published 27 March 2017. Accessed 24 May 2019.

European Lung White Book. (2019). https://www.erswhitebook.org/chapters/patient-organisations-and-the-european-lung-foundation/the-role-of-patient-organisations/. Accessed 24 May 2019.

Fiske, A., Buyx, A., & Prainsack, B. (2018). Health information counselors: A new profession for the age of big data. *Academic Medicine, 94*, 37–41. https://doi.org/10.1097/ACM.0000000000002395.

Flood, A. (2016). 'Post-truth' named word of the year by Oxford Dictionaries. *The Guardian*. https://www.theguardian.com/books/2016/nov/15/post-truth-named-word-of-the-year-by-oxford-dictionaries. Accessed 25 May 2019.

Fukada, M. (2018 Mar). Nursing competency: Definition, structure and development. *Yonago Acta Medica, 61*, 1–7.

Fukuyama, F. (1992). *The end of history and the last man*. New York: Free Press.

High Level Group on Fake news and Online Disinformation. A multi-dimensional approach to disinformation report of the independent high level group on fake news and online disinformation. Luxembourg: Publications Office of the European Union, 2018.

Krastev, I. (2013). *In Mistrust we trust*. New York: TED Conferences. https://www.iwm.at/publications/books/in-mistrust-we-trust/. Accessed 25 May 2019.

Kreindler, S. A. (2015). The politics of patient-centred care. *Health Expectations, 18*, 1139–1150.

Legislation put forward in France to tackle fake news and disinformation, 2018., at https://www.europeansources.info/record/legislation-france-tackle-fake-news-disinformation/. Accessed 25 May 2019.

Meghachandra Singh, M., & Devi, R. (2014). Information overload and patient's reactions. *BMJ, 349*, 5153.

NetzDG (Gesetz zur Verbesserung der Rechtsdurchsetzung in sozialen Netzwerken, Network Enforcement Act), at https://germanlawarchive.iuscomp.org/?p=1245. Accessed 24 May 2019.

Nuffield Council on Bioethics. (2010). *Medical profiling and online medicine: The ethics of "personalised healthcare" in a consumer age*. http://nuffieldbioethics.org/wp-content/uploads/2014/07/Medical-profiling-and-online-medicine-the-ethics-of-personalised-healthcare-in-a-consumer-age-Web-version-reduced.pdf. Accessed 24 Apr 2019.

O'Neill, O. (2002). *Autonomy and trust in bioethics* (p. 137). Cambridge: Cambridge University Press.

Opinion of the European Committee of Regions—Tackling online disinformation: A European Approach (COM(2018) 236 final) https://cor.europa.eu/en/our-work/Pages/OpinionTimeline.aspx?opId=CDR-3908-2018 Commitment II A. https://ec.europa.eu/digital-single-market/en/news/code-practice-disinformation, Accessed 24 May 2019.

Policy Department for Economic, Scientific and Quality of Life Policies. (2018). *The legal framework to address "fake news": Possible policy actions at the EU level.* http://www.europarl.europa.eu/RegData/etudes/IDAN/2018/619013/IPOL_IDA(2018)619013_EN.pdf. Accessed 21 May 2019.

Proposed EU Regulation on Prevention of Dissemination of Terrorist Content Online (COM (2018) 640 final—2018/0331 (COD)), https://ec.europa.eu/commission/sites/beta-political/files/soteu2018-preventing-terrorist-content-onlineregulation-640_en.pdf. Accessed 24 May 2019.

Skirton, H., Cordier, C., Ingvoldstad, C., et al. (2015). The role of the genetic counsellor: A systematic review of research evidence. *European Journal of Human Genetics, 23*, 452–458.

Sztompka, P. (2000). *Trust. A sociological theory*. Cambridge: Cambridge University Press.

The Council of European Union recommendation of 7 December 2018 on strengthened cooperation against vaccine-preventable diseases which recommends to the member states (2018/C 466/01). https://eur-lex.europa.eu/legal-content/EN/TXT/PDF/?uri=CELEX:32018H1228(01)&from=GA. Accessed 24 May 2019.

Wardle, C., & Derakhstan, H. (2017). *Information disorder: Toward an interdisciplinary framework for research and policy making*. Cambridge, MA: Shorenstein Center on Media, Politics and Public Policy at Harvard Kennedy School for the Council of Europe. https://shorensteincenter.org/information-disorder-framework-for-research-and-policymaking. Accessed 24 May 2019.

Warren, M. (2018). Trust and democracy. In E. M. Uslaner (Ed.), *The Oxford handbook of social and political trust* (pp. 75–94). Oxford: Oxford University Press.

Werder, M. (2015). Health information technology: A key ingredient of patient experience. *Patient Experience Journal, 1*, 143–147.

4

Integrative Bioethics and Knowledge Landscapes

Denis Kos, Marko Kos, and Hrvoje Jurić

Over the past 15 years, bioethical discussions in Europe have seen accelerated development. Southeastern European authors, in particular, are attempting to reconfigure bioethics as an innovative concept and project in the field, through gathering various scientific approaches (multidisciplinarity, interdisciplinarity and transdisciplinarity) in an integrated way. The concept of an integrative bioethics starts from the integration of all aspects of life into bioethical debates, both in regard to its content (human and non-human, in biomedical and ecological perspectives) and through an interdisciplinary and "pluriperspectival" integration at the methodological level. Integrative bioethics has considerable comparative

D. Kos (✉)
Faculty of Humanities and Social Sciences, Department of Information and Communication Sciences, University of Zagreb, Zagreb, Croatia
e-mail: dkos@ffzg.hr

M. Kos • H. Jurić
Faculty of Humanities and Social Sciences, Department of Philosophy, University of Zagreb, Zagreb, Croatia

A. L. Svalastog et al. (eds.), *Navigating Digital Health Landscapes*, Health, Technology and Society, https://doi.org/10.1007/978-981-15-8206-6_4

advantages over traditional approaches, and its conclusions could have impacts on different spheres of science and higher education and also, most importantly here, health. Integrative bioethics opposes any scientific and cultural reductionism and criticizes the regimes of total power over knowledge and life (represented by ruling models of techno-science, the economy, politics and media), which is the point where integrative bioethics meets "biopolitical theory", on one hand, and the concept of "knowledge landscapes", on the other hand.

The idea of integrative bioethics synthesizes the ideals found in the current development of bioethics, while expanding the historical perspective of bioethics to avoid ahistorical approaches. In other words, integrative bioethics establishes different theoretical and practical interactions (interdisciplinary, international, intercultural, interreligious and others). The integrative bioethics programme draws in particular on Van Rensselaer Potter's (1971) notion of "the totality of the human survival perspective" allied to Mittelstraß's (1982) concept of "orientational knowledge" to meet the demands of what Čović (2017) and others call a new "historical epoch". It is an essential methodological feature of integrative bioethics that the concrete problems of life and their reproduction are understood via a single framework, which means that the category of life is taken in its entirety—encouraging the inclusion of all sciences and scientific disciplines and scientific and non-scientific approaches but also worldviews and socially proactive practices that can contribute to the debates over the meaning of life and its manipulation made possible through contemporary science and technology (Čović 2017).

One of the main drivers behind bioethics reflects the loss of authority by and trust in contemporary science and its understanding of what being human means. So far, bioethics has provided a response to this "new medical situation" by means of direct moral reflections (called principlism) and then has expanded by the means of ethical reflection within an interdisciplinary frame (Čović 2017: 111).

This chapter will discuss integrative bioethics and its methodological framework, as a principle of bioethical literacy within the complex and shifting landscapes of knowledge within which information and data circulate and are mobilized. To achieve this, we first define integrative bioethics in the context of the global discussion on bioethics and then posit its principles as means to achieve an effective orientation within today's society. In the second part of the chapter, the contemporary biopolitical situation is portrayed through the concept of knowledge landscapes while referring to practices dealing with the problem of navigation and orientation within them.

The Development of Bioethics

The history of bioethics can be organized in three developmental stages, in which there are noticeable shifts in the methodological constitution of bioethics and the determination of the subject area in which it is involved. These developmental changes have been described in the definitions of bioethics found in the first and second editions of the *Encyclopedia of Bioethics* (2003).

These stages of bioethical development start from the initial period signified by the introduction of "new medical ethics" (Beauchamp and Childress 1979) and its interactions with diverse social movements, subsequently expanded into the stage defined by Van Rensselaer Potter's "global bioethics" (Potter 1988) and concluded, as Čović proposes, at the stage of integrative bioethics (Čović 2005).

Bioethicists are still working towards the broadening of the field not only at the methodological level but also on the level of cultural and intercultural reflections that aim at establishing connections between different bioethical approaches. Authors in integrative bioethics provide disciplinary and transdisciplinary outlooks on bioethics while understanding "transdisciplinarity" as scientific endeavours in which "researchers in specific disciplines jointly ask questions related to the subject, form the course of research together, transfer methods from one discipline to another, but also add the implementation of political initiatives, cultural elements and diverse social moments" (Potthast 2008: 261). The societal elements in these debates transform their considerations into biopolitical and cultural questions concerning health, life sciences and medical practice. These might include the following: Is genetic research and gathering of genetic material justifiable without public knowledge and public debate? (cf. Knoppers and Chadwick 2005) Can we and/or should we abandon religious freedoms in the context of self-determination and patient care? Are we ready to dismiss unjustified "vaccination paranoia" as a mere movement in the face of "alternative facts" and other suspicious media and information practices? Integrative bioethics and its discursive and disciplinary practices are an ever-expanding platform for these debates but also a necessary "space" for elaboration of public concerns and scientist-to-public interaction before they become too complex to be dealt with effectively. From the integrative bioethics stance, bioethicists should not forget that even though bioethics might be seen to be a scientific discipline, it sprang to life from the necessities of the present era made visible by the social action of engaged individuals, groups and minorities. Its definition takes into account distinct cultures and culturally based perspectives and introduces to the field a methodology with a higher problem-solving capacity.

In this sense the so-called *quest for health* (cf. Sass 2004) has to be rethought with regard to inter- and transdisciplinary approaches bearing in mind that individual and group agency carries significant meaning when trying to understand the complexity of ethical challenges in the digital era. This means that such expanded approaches to problem resolution in regard to bioethical issues in healthcare also have to be considered in the context of new technological developments.

Pluriperspectivism and Orientational Knowledge

Ante Čović defines integrative bioethics as "an integrative orientative science", that is, as "a pluriperspectival field, in which footholds and measures for orientation in the questions concerning life or the conditions and circumstances of the preservation of life are being created through the interaction of diverse perspectives" (Čović 2005: 150–151).

> Pluriperspectivism means interaction or integration and interpretation of as many different perspectives as possible of what is being viewed, transcribed, discerned, disclosed, and so on, respectively what is being comprehended and explained (Čović 2006; Pavić 2014). Therefore, here we have

> not only the awareness of a multitude of different perspectives on a particular subject, but also awareness of the necessity of integration, and thus a manifestation of many different perspectives in the process of acquiring knowledge, understanding and its evaluation. Only integration of different perspectives allows us to view things 'with many eyes and conscience' (Nietzsche 2002: 150 in Borš 2016) which observers contemplate, and also the emergence of a more complete perspective, a new truth, as the product of the mentioned interrelation of different perspectives ('truths'). But it is important to indicate that multiperspectivism does not start from the fact that all the perspectives are equally valuable, which often is the case in a postmodern perspective, nor does Čović intend to 'reconcile' them, but simply starts from the position that all authentic perspectives are equally deserving of integration through comprehension or explication. So, in contrast to the view that considers all perspectives equally valuable or equally worthless, which ends in relativism or radical scepticism (which ultimately represent nothing but reductionism) – here we are speaking about an approach that 'implies an interactive, or integrative pluralism of perspectives' (Čović 2006: 9), which allows 'a new perspective of more truthful truths'(Borš 2016).[1]

This integrationist approach finds roots for such an orientation in the critique of techno-scientific axis of societal development. Jürgen Mittelstraß (1982) notes that the original idea of science has been forgotten and that science and universities should not only be institutions that reproduce knowledge but also that provide a wider understanding for social life. Moreover, in modern industrial societies, which Mittelstraß calls "technical cultures" (*technische Kulturen*), this wider form of knowledge has almost completely disappeared. Mittelstraß establishes the conceptual distinction between (partial) "knowledge about mastering nature and society" and (universal) "knowledge of orientation in nature and society", which is very clearly summarized in the categorical differentiation between *Verfügungswissen* (usable, instrumental or

[1] In this context Vanja Borš' reference has to be understood as an explication on the interactions of diverse perspectives. When different perspectives meet, more than often they carry a presupposition on truthfulness of their claims (definitions, theories and so on), but it is not possible for all of them to be true. Therefore, pluriperspectivism is a methodological process, a dialectic, that analyses all of the perspectives linked to problem resolution and produces a truth that is not restricted by a monoperspective point of view.

technical knowledge) and *Orientierungswissen* (orientational knowledge) (Mittelstraß 1982: 12). Contemporary, or rather modern, industrial society relying on a technical culture produces only partially usable knowledge of nature and society, ignoring the aforementioned orientational knowledge. A technology-oriented society behaves as a system of relationships merely between technologies, ignoring that society is the people and their interdependencies. In the digital health arena, humans are not perceived as health-seekers, but rather as customers, potential buyers of services and sources of data for biometric data collection.

What the best orientation is, of course, has to be defined. Being a contrast to knowledge about mastering nature and society, orientational knowledge is always based on subjective understanding, prior to any form of what might be regarded as objective knowledge. Hence, the epistemological result of orientation is a perceived truthfulness, which means that anything in the context of orientation which is considered to be true is considered so for subjective reasons. Also then, thinking is to be perceived as a conceptual and orientational act, as a theoretical and practical reasoning (Schildknecht 2008: 140). We should use these notions when our questions relate to orientation, or when it comes to understanding and discerning, instead of reasoning based on a techno-scientific rationality.

Knowledge Landscapes

The focus on knowledge and the precision in understanding the complex contemporary notions of health and life in general on one hand and the focus on orientation as a socially situated practice on the other can be better understood if we seek the strength of some kind of metaphorical discursive moment which would provide an interdisciplinary dialogic framework. One of such moments lies in the innovative concept of knowledge landscapes which considers these issues as spatial relations. This chapter's title points to the need and possibility to connect the concepts of integrative bioethics and the metaphor of *knowledge landscapes*.

The use of metaphors in science has been widely debated, especially as a moment of scientific communication. Taylor and Dewsbury (2018) even go as far as to claim that "metaphors are crucial in the production of knowledge in that they allow us to make concrete connections between abstract concepts and everyday experiences [...] that metaphors shape the mind, structure our experiences, and influence behaviour" (Taylor and Dewsbury 2018: 1; cf. Fox Keller 2003). Their observations were motivated by researching the etymology of the word. "The term metaphor can be traced to the Greek word metaphora, which is derived from meta (meaning 'over') and pherein (meaning 'to carry')" (ibid.). Therefore, by definition, "metaphor is a comparison between two seemingly dissimilar concepts that involves the 'carrying over of a word from its normal use to a new use'" (Richards 1930 in: Taylor and Dewsbury 2018: 1).

The relevance of metaphors in science has many illustrative examples: "Robert Hooke was the first to denote the cell using the term 'cell' when an image of a piece of cork under his microscope reminded him of the small rooms, or cells[...]. Huygens used water waves to theorise that light is wavelike. Arrhenius described the greenhouse effect by referring to his experience with hot pots" (Niebert, Gropengießer 2015: 2 in: Taylor and Dewsbury 2018: 2). These examples point at the unbreakable link between metaphors, scientific language and our cognition. "Lakoff and Johnson's theory of conceptual metaphor posits that the nature of human cognition is metaphorical, and that all knowledge emerges as a result of embodied physical and social experiences. Under this view, metaphors are not mere linguistic embellishments. Rather, they are foundations for thought processes and conceptual understandings that function to map meaning from one knowledge and/or perceptual domain to another" (Lakoff and Johnson 1980 in: Taylor and Dewsbury 2018: 1). Nonetheless, we have to be careful of these linguistic blessings in disguise, "while we may not be able to conceptualize, or communicate, abstract scientific phenomena without employing such metaphors, we must also recognize their limitations [...]. In many ways, the metaphors we rely upon may uphold and reinforce outdated scientific paradigms, contributing to public misunderstandings about complex scientific issues" (Taylor and Dewsbury 2018: 2).

Svalastog and collaborators (2014) argued that the knowledge landscapes metaphor conceptualizes the broader communicative situation in contemporary science. It is concerned with the communication, understanding and distribution of scientific and other forms of knowledge considered in the moment when actual sites of everyday life that contain knowledge from beyond the disciplines become ever more influential and relevant in personal and group decision-making. The concept is also founded upon a democratic agenda to facilitate navigation through the vast universe of information and subsequently produced knowledge at a personal or wider level.

The same authors argue that "today the Knowledge Landscapes appear as confusing sites for gaining information and knowledge, reflecting current changes in the communication infrastructure, research, and political system and industry, and that we need physical and virtual communicative spaces where dialogue seeks to understand and critically discuss the content distributed in the Knowledge Landscapes. We also need to acknowledge that knowledge communication is vital for not only democratic advances and processes, but it is also infused in the everyday life, delivering the democratic principles to all spheres of society, in particular to the field of medicine and health care, not the least due to the new paradigm referred to as personalized medicine. The presence and complexity of the scientific issues in the Knowledge Landscapes are in need of clarification and processing in an open-ended dialogue to gain a qualified perception of the Knowledge Landscape itself, and we need permanent sites for public reflection" (Svalastog et al. 2014: 54). They go on to argue that:

> The need for dialogue and communication regarding innovative science, new technology, and bio-objects goes hand in hand with an urgent need to establish an open ended dialogue to gain a qualified perception of the knowledge. To achieve this we need to identify arenas where these issues can be discussed, not once or as a unique happening but as permanent sites for public reflection. The debate is needed not for policy reasons, but because of the presence and complexity of the scientific issues in a need of clarification and processing. We therefore argue for the creation of communicative spaces where the consequences of innovative knowledge could be discussed without the distortions mentioned before. In such a Knowledge Landscape actors and stakeholders from various arenas (science, the public, industry, politics etc.) should be able to meet and discuss freely and equally.

> In this context, societal dialogue will imply epistemological clarifications, that is, clarification of how scientific knowledge (not only scientific results) is constructed. This will produce a transparent communication that will avoid misunderstanding and confusion, and make a dialogue a joint interpretative project. Hermeneutical ideals from both Habermas and Gadamer underline the fundamental importance of communication and the necessity of reciprocal understanding for conversation, dialogue, and interpretation to be real/true (in contrast to untrue, i.e., represent misunderstandings and confusion). (Svalastog et al. 2014: 56)

So defined, knowledge landscapes evoke both the need for a pluriperspectivist treatment of ethical challenges in the digital society and conceptualize further the idea of "orientation". The orientational act is being metaphorically "embodied" and "physicalized" as *navigation in knowledge landscapes*.

Other fields have used metaphorical thought in the same context. In order to expand the initial focus of library and information sciences on recorded knowledge to the examination of the communicative aspects of information production, authors like Annemaree Lloyd (2010) have used the notion of the information landscape which she defines as "intersubjectively created spaces that have resulted from human interaction, in which information is created and shared and eventually sediments as knowledge" (Lloyd 2010: 9–10). The characterization of information landscapes comes mainly from descriptive research which wants to reveal the state of real human practices. What may be the most relevant thing to consider is that, according to Lloyd's research, information landscapes are not only constituted through print media and information and communication technologies, but they are also constituted through social relations and experiences of practice. This means that there are other kinds of information sources out there—ones that are not so easy to read or easily accessed—the unwritten knowledge embodied in practices and social knowledge of individuals and groups.

Information landscapes act as communicative spaces created by shared experiences of people in mutual interaction with the signs and symbols of their setting (Lloyd 2010). According to Lloyd, when it comes to the ability to navigate an information landscape, we cannot just talk about specific characteristics of individuals and then define them as skills. Rather, we have to look at the complete information practices of individuals or groups in a particular context. She also recognizes that this interpretation has not been congruent with the more traditional library and information sciences understandings. The introduction of "information practices" allows us to pin-point a particular phenomenon which we then approach in research without presuppositions on the nature of that practice or without prescribing what those practices of individuals or groups should be like. The idea is to describe them as they came to be in a particular context. When we talk about what the information practices should look like, Lloyd offers that they refer to knowing "what there is in a landscape and to draw[ing] meaning from this through engagement and experience with information. [...] This ability arises from complex contextual practice, processes, and interactions that enable access to social, physical and textual sites of knowledge" (Lloyd 2006: 2).

An even better characterization of these ideas may be given if we consider her research of health information practices of different people. In an article by Lloyd, Bonner and Dawson-Rose (2014), the authors studied the health information practices of people living with chronic health conditions. The authors argued that health literacy is a socially derived health information practice and that a more complex outlook is needed than the currently dominant one in the field of health literacy—an outlook which would enact the whole person into an information landscape, a holistic outlook. To achieve this, they maintain, health literacy cannot be regarded as a set of skills and has to be recast as a socio-cultural practice. The study had two goals: first, to describe the practices and skills used by people with chronic health diseases to know how these inform their judgements about their health and treatment, and second, to understand what sources they use. The study showed that each of the diseases formed their own information landscape even though there were many similarities. Both groups' initial experience of their landscape was a corporeal experience. They reported that their bodies acted as a reference point for their illness and this stimulated them to seek information that would help them resolve their uncertainties with regard to the information gaps they had and thereby produce what they regard as a robust and stable form of *knowledge* about their condition. On the level of using authoritative sources, participants of both groups stuck to the information given to them by their doctors and viewed the doctor as the health authority. On the level of social information, the most important were the communities of "experts by experience" and their information was the most valued at the social level. When talking about specific information practices of participants, the authors recognized three main areas of activities: orienting, information sharing and creating. Orientation was needed for the participants to become situated in the reality of their illness. It consisted of recognizing what was relevant and finding different kinds of sources available. Orienting also involved "orienting others". The illness affected not only the participants but also their family and friends who had to be informed about certain aspects of the condition. The sharing of information was either professional or peer-to-peer and was used for orientation, for developing relationships with people who have the same illness, for information evaluation, etc. On the level of professional sharing, nurses were seen as important mediators who could explain advice given by doctors in a simpler way. Sharing among peers was used for sharing experiences, expressing solidarity and care for others and a way of sharing different textual resources. The activity of creating was used for keeping track with all the information that was found, but also it was suggested that there is a need to collate all the information and make it available to everyone. The example was the HIV community collecting articles and newspaper clippings on new treatments and side effects; notices of death were collected and passed out among the community which wanted to be informed about these. In both research studies, it is possible to notice that a health literate is not someone who has satisfied a set of decontextualized educational criteria. The descriptions of the information landscapes and practices are deeply connected to the context of participants.

Both discourses expressed through the notions of knowledge and information landscapes treat orientation as their final purpose and understand it as necessarily situated in current communicative and social contexts. Contemporary digital society is facing issues such as ownership, access, privacy, security as well as those related to "the relationship between information and the good of society, the relationship between information providers and the consumers of information" (Moran et al.

2007: 351). The growing trends of algorithmization and big data exploitation change the way citizens access public and private services and the way in which they treat the data they themselves have created and disseminated across the online public domain. This domain of "online life" being largely corporately owned raises questions about exploitative relationships between companies and the public who are compelled to relinquish their personal data and their privacy in exchange for services but also for the very inclusion into this domain whose economic, political and societal import becomes unquestionable. The problems are further exacerbated by the influence of different media and political actors who provide the public with ideologically saturated lies and falsehoods often based on confirmation bias. For the ethicists, these new trends open a wide array of possible problems and traps that make it harder to navigate through already problematic debates such as air pollution and climate change, care for children in fragile and vulnerable settings, vaccination and many other bioethical and biopolitical issues. It is extremely important to analyse how the above-mentioned social situation determines the nature of navigating in health knowledge landscapes affected by both impeding and enabling, culturally, politically and socially shaped knowledge processes.

Biopolitics, Integrative Bioethics and Knowledge Landscapes

Integrative bioethics, as presented in the first part of this chapter, requires answers oriented towards *theoretical*, that is, scientific goals (knowledge of particular sciences and knowledge as an entirety of all the sciences, viewed as a foundation of any human action); *practical*, that is, ethical, political, legal and economic goals (background of the actions); and *technical*, that is, medical, biotechnological and information-technological goals (performing the actions). To put it another way, integrative bioethics is equally interested in questions: What do we know and what can we know at all? What should we do? How should this be done?

Looking at the issues of current manipulation of life both on a small and a large scale,[2] we could say that the logical hierarchy of the above-mentioned questions and answers is turned upside-down. The primacy of the rather narrow and limited technical approach over the reflexive practical approach[3]—which, ideally, should be not only connected to but also situated in the realm of knowledge—causes different problems and is the problem in itself.

One of the consequences of this process is the reduction of knowledge down to information and the reduction of information down to data. Myriads of accidentally collected data do not create the information on a subject matter, just like the possession of single information or information clusters does not mean that we have knowledge on a subject matter, which will offer a foundation for our actions related to this subject matter. The above-mentioned reduction is all but surprising, because it is an expression of the general reductionist model of contemporary science, that is, techno-science as a complex network of natural sciences, mathematics, biomedicine, biotechnologies and information-communication technologies, also called STEM. In other words, the problem is the monopoly of the reductionist and monoperspectivist techno-science. It is the ostensible unity of modern natural sciences and technologies which provides the basis on which it claims to be the only valid form of understanding and directing human and non-human life on the planet (Jurić 2012). It would be only a theoretical issue if such knowledge or, more precisely, such an idea of knowledge would not be a basis or a framework for concrete manipulations of human health and life, as well as the non-human life and the nature in general. It would be only a theoretical issue if techno-science would not operate in alliance with the ruling models of economy and politics, which is currently the case. They are equally reductive in relation to diversity of human views and needs but also equally

[2] For example, biomedical and ecological issues, ranging from cloning Human Genome Project and CRISPR/Cas9 technology, through GM technology in agriculture and "biopiracy" (Shiva 1997), to climate issues and nuclear technology.

[3] A perfect summary of this problem and its implications can be found in Günther Anders who said "The basic dilemma of our age is that 'we are smaller than ourselves', incapable of mentally realizing the realities which we ourselves have produced. Therefore, we might call ourselves 'inverted Utopians': while ordinary Utopians are unable to actually produce what they are able to visualize, we are unable to visualize what we are actually producing" (Anders 1962: 496).

powerful in the terms of their hegemony over human views and needs. Such a kind of monopoly can be compared with what Ivan Illich calls "radical monopoly"—"when one industrial production process exercises an exclusive control over the satisfaction of a pressing need, and excludes nonindustrial activities from competition" (Illich 1975: 66).

However, we can neither analyse nor modify the current economic-political system if we do not understand and modify the underlying systems of knowledge. One of the most impressive examples of such analysis is the biopolitical theory by Michel Foucault who not only developed a critique of dominant models of knowledge and science (Foucault 2002a, b) but has also demonstrated, in the series of his books, how these models function in particular fields of the life-world, especially regarding human life, body, health and sexuality (Foucault 1973, 1979, 1988, 1990, 1992, 2008).

If bioethics should not be reduced to a casuistic approach aimed at palliative measures, then it should broaden its perspective. In connecting the biopolitically based issues of knowledge and sciences with the bioethically considered issues of the manipulation of life and health, help could be found not only in Foucault's analyses but also in Giorgio Agamben's analysis of the "politicization of bare life" (Agamben 1998) and Michael Hardt's and Antonio Negri's analysis of "biopower" as "a form of power that regulates social life from its interior, following it, interpreting it, absorbing it, so that every individual embraces and reactivates this power to his or her own accord", whose "primary task is to administer life", so that it "refers to a situation in which what is directly at stake in power is the production and reproduction of life itself" (Hardt and Negri 2000: 23–24). In such a way we could discover the deeper layers of bioethical problems which are extremely important, but they are usually discussed merely on the level of what can be done technically and what should be done under the unreflected and technically applied moral and legal norms.

On one hand, bioethical issues cannot be perceived only as practical issues (and even less as technical issues), because mechanisms "of control over" and "manipulation of" life and health are basically the mechanisms "of control over" and "manipulation of" knowledge. On the other hand, in biopolitical analysis and critique, we rarely find the answers to the questions "what to do" and "how to act", both generally and in particular situations, according to such insights. It is where biopolitical theory meets the anti-reductionist approach of integrative bioethics. Integrative bioethics opposes not only the questionable and dangerous manipulations of life but also the reductionist approaches to knowledge which enables or even causes such manipulations. What is knowledge at all? How it emerges or how it is created? What systems of knowledge exist or in what systems the knowledge exists? Who rules the knowledge? How and for what purposes the knowledge is used?—these questions on the sources, character and implications of the knowledge should be points of departure not only for the biopolitical theory but also for bioethical reflection, discussion and decision-making, viewed as an explicitly reflective and critical approach. At least, we should take into account that no knowledge is ahistorical and acontextual.

The point is that no knowledge or scientific enterprise is naïve and innocent in practical terms, just like no practice is deprived of theoretical and ideological foundations. If we seek to overcome the current reduction of knowledge to information and information to data, we should be taking the steps towards pluriperspectivist ("democratic") knowledge—including both scientific and cultural perspectives, both individual and collective subjects of knowledge—instead of monoperspectivist ("authoritarian") knowledge. It does not exclude the structuredness of knowledge, neither does it lead to theoretical and practical relativism. By emphasizing pluriperspectivism, we are pointing to the ways in which knowledge is created and to the aims of knowledge. To recall Ivan Illich once again, it could be seen as the difference between "manipulative" knowledge and institutions, on one hand, and "convivial" knowledge and institutions, on the other hand (Illich 1975).

What is needed in order to think and act differently than usual in relation to life and health is the permanent direction of theory towards practice and of practice towards theory. Second, if we ask for the answer to the question on the role of bioethics within the knowledge landscapes, we should ask: Is the knowledge (unavoidably perceived primarily as the "scientific knowledge") the top of the "knowledge hierarchy"? Some commentators, such as Van Rensselaer Potter, say that it should not be perceived like that. In elaboration of his idea of bioethics, he says: "I take the position that the science of survival must be built on the science of biology and enlarged beyond the traditional boundaries to include the most essential elements of the social sciences and the humanities with emphasis on philosophy in the strict sense, meaning 'love of wisdom'. A science of survival must be more than science alone, and I therefore propose the term *Bioethics* in order to emphasize the two most important ingredients in achieving the new wisdom that is so desperately needed: biological knowledge and human values" (Potter 1971: 1). Moreover, he holds that bioethics is not so much about "knowledge" and the communication of different types of knowledge, but that it is more about a "life wisdom" (Potter 1971: 58). This is what Mittelstraß refers to when differentiating and connecting "instrumental" and "orientational" knowledge, but similar thoughts can be found all across the theory related to the issues of knowledge and knowledge application today, for example, in Russell Ackoff's works. Ackoff, to whom the very authorship of the concept of hierarchy of data/information/knowledge is ascribed, suggests that beneath the knowledge there are understanding and wisdom, as the final goals of science and education (Ackoff 1999: 170–172).

Finally, all of that means that integrative bioethics emphasizes "old-fashioned" connections between power and responsibility ("knowledge as power" and "knowledge as responsibility") and knowledge and morality (Čović 2004).

Anyway, to live and to move within the "knowledge landscapes" today—that is to think and to act within them—is not an easy task, primarily because of the fact that there are still no reliable maps of "knowledge landscapes" and, if we find some maps, they are mostly the maps of limited areas of "knowledge landscapes", approximate descriptions of chaotic data and partial information. In order to create reliable maps of "knowledge landscapes", we should seek integrated knowledge (on the theoretical level), which is not a mere sum of the data and the information, and try to find an appropriate compass and learn how to use it (on the practical and technical level). Practical and technical tasks are not less important than the theoretical tasks. However, they cannot be achieved without a firm theoretical background.

The question on how to orient yourself within knowledge in general should be accompanied by the question on who and how creates and owns knowledge, that is, who is the subject of the knowledge which emerges from the data and information, if they are processed reflectively and critically. If action, responsibility and morality are necessarily connected to knowledge, as we believe, previously mentioned questions are of great importance. In the digital era these questions are becoming more and more complex, because the subjects of the "knowledge" are not anymore only the individual entities (persons) and collective entities (institutions), whose identity can be recognized, described and ethically and politically regulated, but also impersonal, anonymous and elusive entities such as "artificial intelligence". This is why the "physical geography" of knowledge landscapes, that is, data, information and knowledge which create the "landscape" within which we should find a proper orientation, needs the "metaphysical geography" of knowledge landscapes, which means that we should always try to discover and critically assess the presuppositions of visible maps of knowledge landscapes that we are living and acting in, that is, to answer the questions on what actually are the data, information and knowledge, in historical, cultural and social contexts, and what are they for.

We see the knowledge needed to answer the "how-to-act question", in order to achieve orientation in knowledge landscapes, necessarily as a result of education or exposure to some kind of educational processes. Among others, one historically resistant example of such educational practices has been developed as part of the discourse about information education and paradigmatically as becoming literate in relation to the ability to find, select, critically asses and use data, information and knowledge. Concepts such as information literacy, health literacy, etc. have survived long enough to see themselves expanded through different theoretical frameworks. Examples of that would be critical theory and critical pedagogy in the context of concepts such as critical information or data literacy who have by themselves already identified that it is impossible to gain orientation without the critical apprehension of the current economic-political system, that is, biopolitical circumstances (which in turn seeks the understanding and the ability of modification of their underlying systems of knowledge). We emphasize that the orientational act is being metaphorically embodied as navigation in the knowledge landscapes, which we believe implies that (health) data/information/knowledge literacy is a practical act of orientation in a given landscape.

Conclusion

In conclusion, we point out the following points:

1. We perceive bioethics as "an integrative orientative science", that is, as "a pluriperspectival field, in which footholds and measures for orientation in the questions concerning life or the conditions and circumstances of the preservation of life are being created through the interaction of diverse perspectives".
2. We point out the conceptual distinction between (partial) "knowledge about mastering nature and society" and (universal) "knowledge of orientation in nature and society".
3. Being a contrast to *knowledge about mastering nature and society*, orientational knowledge is always based on subjective, to objective prior knowledge. We should use these notions when the questions within our debates relate to orientation, or when it comes to understanding and discerning, instead of reasoning based on techno-scientific reason.
4. We find that to achieve orientation means to be literate in the contemporary sense of the word.
5. We should consider that all information and data-related practices of humans happen in particular contexts and that achieving literacy is also contextual. Rigid structures are bound to stay static and uncritical. This represents the move from the functional to the critical and creative notions of literacy.
6. No knowledge or scientific enterprise is naïve and innocent in practical terms, just like no practice is deprived of theoretical and ideological foundations. Therefore, we have to take into account that biopolitical issues influence the construction of knowledge landscapes and impact our orientational capacities.

We conclude with a proposal that in terms of wider educational policy what is needed is a cultural context through which citizens can cultivate a personal critical attitude towards their practices with information and data, as well as a critical attitude towards the actual creation and characteristics of the information resources they use. Bioethics can play a role in this.

References

Ackoff, R. L. (1999). *Ackoff's best*. New York: Wiley.

Agamben, G. (1998). *Homo Sacer: Sovereign power and bare life*. Stanford: Stanford University Press.

Anders, G. (1962). Theses for the atomic age. *The Massachusetts Review, 3*(3), 493–505.

Beauchamp, T. L., & Childress, J. F. (1979). *Principles of biomedical ethics*. New York: Oxford University Press.

Borš, V. (2016). Istinitost kao bakantski zanos: uloga i važnost pluriperspektivizma u Hegelovoj misli. *Filozofska istraživanja, 36*(4), 775–785.

Čović, A. (2004). *Etika i bioetika: Razmišljanja na pragu bioetičke epohe*. Zagreb: Pergamena.

Čović, A. (2005). Bioethik unter den Bedingungen des Postkommunismus – Fallbeispiel Kroatien. In A. Čović & T. S. Hoffman (Eds.), *Bioethik und kulturelle Pluralität. Die südosteuropäische Perspektive* (pp. 148–172). Sankt Augustin: Academia Verlag.

Čović, Ante Pluralizam i pluriperspektivizam, Filozofska istraživanja, Vol. 26 (2006), 1, pp. 7–12.

Čović, A. (2017). The Europeanization of bioethics: Opportunities for integrative ethical reflection on the basis of intra-cultural differences in Europe. *Facta Universitatis, 15*(2), 111–114.

Čović, A., & Hoffmann, T. S. (2007) Bioethik und kulturelle Pluralitet. *Filozofska istraživanja 107*(3), 738–742.

Foucault, M. (1973). *The birth of the clinic: An archaeology of medical perception*. London/New York: Routledge.

Foucault, M. (1979). *The history of sexuality, volume 1: An introduction*. London: Allen Lane.

Foucault, M. (1988). *Madness and civilization: A history of insanity in the age of reason*. New York: Vintage Books.

Foucault, M. (1990). *The history of sexuality, volume 3: The Care of the Self*. London: Penguin Books.

Foucault, M. (1992). *The history of sexuality, volume 2: The use of pleasure*. London: Penguin Books.
Foucault, M. (2002a). *Archaeology of knowledge*. London/New York: Routledge.
Foucault, M. (2002b). *The order of things: An archaeology of the human sciences*. London/New York: Routledge.
Foucault, M. (2008). *The birth of biopolitics: Lectures at the Collège de France 1978–79*. Basingstoke/New York: Palgrave Macmillan.
Fox Keller, Evelyn. (2003). *Making sense of life: Explaining biological development with models, metaphors, and machines*. London: Harvard University Press.
Gajović, S., & Svalastog, A. L. (2016). When communicating health-related knowledge, beware of the black holes of the knowledge landscapes geography. *Croatian Medical Journal 57*(5), 504–509.
Hardt, M., & Negri, A. (2000). *Empire*. Cambridge/London: Harvard University Press.
Illich, I. (1975). *Tools for conviviality*. Glasgow: Fontana.
Jurić, H. (2012). Multi-disciplinarity, pluri-perspectivity and integrativity in the science and the education. *The Holistic Approach to Environment, 2*(2), 85–90.
Jurić, H. (2017). The footholds of an integrative bioethics in the work of Van Rensselaer Potter. *Facta Universitatis 15*(2), 127–144.
Knoppers, B., & Chadwick, R. (2005). Human genetic research: Emerging trends in ethics. *Nature Review Genetics, 6*(6), 75–79.
Lakoff, G., & Johnson, M. (1980). *Metaphors we live by*. Chicago: University of Chicago Press.
Lloyd, A. (2006). Information literacy landscapes: An emerging picture. *Journal of Documentation, 62*(5), 570–583.
Lloyd, A. (2010). *Information literacy landscape: Information literacy in education, workplace and everyday context*. Oxford: Chandos Publishing.
Lloyd, A., Bonner, A., & Dawson-Rose, C. (2014). The health information practices of people living with chronic health conditions: Implications for health literacy. *Journal of Librarianship and Information Science, 46*(3), 207–216.
Mittelstraß, J. (1982). *Wissenschaft als Lebensform: Reden über philosophische Orientierungen in Wissenschaft und Universität*. Frankfurt a/M: Suhrkamp.
Moran, B. B., Stueart, R. D., & Morner, C. J. (2007). *Library and information center management*. Santa Barbara: Libraries Unlimited.
Pavić, Ž. (2014). 'Pluriperspektivizam' – slučaj jedne natuknice u *Filozofskome leksikonu*. *Filozofska istraživanja, 34*(4), 577–600.

Potter, V. R. (1971). *Bioethics: Bridge to the future*. Englewood Cliffs: Prentice-Hall.

Potter, V. R. (1988). *Global bioethics: Building on the Leopold legacy*. East Lansing: Michigan State University Press.

Potthast, T. (2008). Bioethik als inter- und transdisziplinäre Unternehmung. In C. Brand, E.-M. Engels, A. Ferrari, & L. Kovács (Eds.), *Wie funktioniert Bioethik? Interdisziplinäre Entscheidungsfindung im Spannungsfeld von theoretischem Begründungsanspruch und praktischem Regelungsbedarf* (pp. 255–280). Paderborn: Mentis.

Sass, H. M. (2004). Asian and Western bioethics: Converging, conflicting, competing. *Eubios Journal of Asian and International Bioethics, 14*, 12–22.

Svalastog A. L., Allgaier, J., & Gajović, S. (2015). Navigating knowledge landscapes: on health, science, communication, media, and society. *Croatian Medical Journal 56*(4), 321–323.

Schildknecht, C. (2008). Argument und Einsicht: Orientierungswissen als Begründungswissen. In W. Stegmaier (Ed.), *Orientierung: Philosophische Perspektiven* (pp. 138–152). Frankfurt a/M: Suhrkamp.

Shiva, V. (1997). *Biopiracy: The plunder of nature and knowledge*. Cambridge: South End Press.

Svalastog, A. L., Allgaier, J., Martinelli, L., & Gajović, S. (2014). Distortion, confusion, and impasses: Could a public dialogue within knowledge landscapes contribute to better communication and understanding of innovative knowledge? *Croatian Medical Journal, 55*(1), 54–60.

Svalastog, A. L., Donev, D., Jahren Kristoffersen, N., & Gajović, S. (2017). Concepts and definitions of health and health-related values in the knowledge landscapes of the digital society. *Croatian Medical Journal 58*(6), 431–435.

Taylor, C., & Dewsbury, B. M. (2018). On the problem and promise of metaphor use in science and science communication. *Journal of Microbiology and Biology Education, 19*(1).

5

Exploring the Concept of the Knowledge Landscape Geography: Some Proposals and Reflections

Srećko Gajović

Introduction

Health is increasingly technologized today. The wide array of technologies, many of them digital, are applied in the health field and dedicated to individual diagnostic and therapeutic procedures (WHO 2020). Moreover, the transformation of health caused by digital technologies is highly relevant to individuals and society (Svalastog et al. 2017). This is complemented by the digitalization of health-related data and their processing, curation and analysis. The digital approaches integrate patient-specific and group-associated data creating "big data" collections. These collections claim to represent all-embracing general information with the potential to be reversed and applied to the specific individual providing precisely what each specific patient will need (dubbed as precision, personalized or individual medicine, recently reviewed in Ho et al. 2020).

S. Gajović (✉)
Department of Histology and Embryology, Croatian Institute for Brain Research, University of Zagreb School of Medicine, Zagreb, Croatia
e-mail: srecko.gajovic@hiim.hr

A. L. Svalastog et al. (eds.), *Navigating Digital Health Landscapes*, Health, Technology and Society, https://doi.org/10.1007/978-981-15-8206-6_5

Health-related knowledge is indeed included in the metaphor of knowledge landscapes describing the location, dynamics and interactions of digital and non-digital knowledge representations (Svalastog et al. 2014; Svalastog et al. 2015). The chapters in this book explore the idea of the "digital knowledge landscapes", specifically in regard to the search for health information and how the landscapes are navigated. The broad argument presented here is that navigating, accessing and interpreting the diverse forms of information that are found is never a linear or one-way model wherein expertise is adopted by digital users. Instead, it is more appropriate to frame these processes as a multilateral communication model across different stakeholders using interactive digital capabilities (Gajović and Svalastog 2016), through which information gathering eventually leads to user-generated knowledge.

In this chapter, the notion of "landscape geography" is explored as an analogous model through which we can locate and help understand the dynamics shaping navigation, how perhaps the contours of this landscape might be best understood. The chapter is written primarily from the perspective of a biomedical scholar informed by ideas drawn from the social sciences and concludes with some proposals and reflections. The first section below discusses in brief the shift from conventional "doctor-patient" relationships (as a form of medical paternalism) to multicentric/lateral forms of health engagement and processes and how these are driven by digital health.

Person-Centred Care Versus Medical Paternalism

The synergy of technological and bioethical advances is seen to herald a transformation from medical paternalism towards more person-centred care. Medical paternalism represents a traditional system, where educated and subsequently licensed medical professionals plan and care about the diagnostic and therapeutic procedures needed for patients, affording a clear hierarchy between knowledgeable experts and uninformed users, where users for their own benefit follow the advice of the expert (Murgic et al. 2015).

In contrast to medical paternalism, in person-centred care the users are in the centre entitled to decide on their own care for health. From a bioethical perspective, this allows every individual to be in control of their own body by deciding about any health-related activity, including professionally performed medical procedures, as well as how personal data is handled (Kim et al. 2017; Wildevuur and Simonse 2015).

There is of course a tension here between expert-based medical knowledge and the patient as informed decision-maker drawing on that knowledge and where the boundaries between the two lie: how medical "paternalism" and patient/person-centred care can co-exist is both a practical (therapeutic) and ethical matter. The obvious challenge of the person-centred care is that the one who decides has no professional knowledge about necessary activities to maintain health or cure a disease. Apparently medical knowledge is a necessary resource located in the hands of medical professionals. As the individuals are endorsed to make decisions in the person-centred care, a form of partnership with medical professionals is envisioned that would be developed (Matthews et al. 2018). Through this partnership the medical professionals provide the required knowledge allowing the individual to make an informed decision. Consequently, person-centred care is based on the interpretations made by medical professionals, which represents a rather unbalanced situation where user is dependent on the knowledge of the provider (Gajović 2018). This unbalance is the reason that currently somehow both systems, medical paternalism and person-centred care, co-exist in some way of necessary complementarity. The patients would like to be adequately informed on what to decide and they sometimes expect to hear a clear-cut instruction of what to pursue further (Levinson et al. 2005). On the other hand, the medical professionals are in difficulties to transfer the knowledge and present eventual nuances of situation to the patient (Browne et al. 2019).

Another way to balance the inequality in knowledge between medical professionals and users of person-centred care is to acquire knowledge elsewhere, outside of the formal health system, such as in the digital landscape. Family, friends and books are examples of offline resources available; however, the digital landscape provides a rich, though complex, source of information that can be drawn on (Kopilaš and Gajović 2020). As this has developed over time, considerable effort was put in by those within the healthcare system to capture and mobilize digital information for advice and especially public health purposes, creating a new vehicle for health literacy, so aligning robust health knowledge with patient responsibility (Farmer et al. 2017). This tradition to educate the population has been part of the public health system long before the onset of person-centred care and can be traced back to the nineteenth century (Rosen and Imperato 2015).

The new online environment appeared as a useful vehicle to extend traditional public health strategies for the education of patients. Linear knowledge transfer was eagerly mobilized from the offline to the online sphere. An additional motivation was derived from the importance of health literacy in the establishment of the person-centred care (Goldberg and Crocombe 2017). However, from the biomedical perspective, this approach generated new problems as diverse claims and understandings have circulated across the digital landscape, challenging apparently robust medical programmes, such as regarding vaccination the emergence of a global anti-vaccination culture (Ames et al. 2017). These multicentric, contested domains now characterize the landscape. As such, we need to focus our attention on the processes and patterns found within in, to which we turn now.

Exploring the Geography of the Knowledge Landscapes

We can illustrate this emergent complexity of knowledge landscapes by briefly describing a typical web-based search on a disease. After typing a disease name in a search engine, the first hits would give a fast overview designed to be easy to understand. However, knowledge about the disease would be depicted by multiple sources of various availabilities and various levels of complexity. Moreover, the same knowledge could be present in different forms at different locations. The simplified metaphor here is that a user/navigator collects fragments across the landscape, some new, some repeating themselves, some more complex and subsequently more detailed as the distance travelled increases.

If medical knowledge is taken as an example, the hierarchy of complexity corresponds in part to different types of medical publications. The most detailed would be the original medical research published in the biomedical journals. Many of these are currently open access, which means being freely accessible, with others behind a paywall (Gajović 2020). The original research represents a huge resource dedicated primarily to professional users, though still accessible to lay people. To tap into this resource, there is a continuous effort to organize it in the form of review articles done by experts in the field. This is achieved through various degrees of systematic reviewing, with meta-analysis being the most rigorous. The most active institution in the health field is the Cochrane Collaboration producing systematic reviews with 37,000 contributors from more than 130 countries — "to produce credible, accessible health information that is free from commercial sponsorship and other conflicts of interest" (http://www.cochrane.org/). Another approach to the enormous size of medical knowledge is data mining and data curation. If data would be presented in standardized formats, they could be accessed by algorithms, which enable machine-to-machine communication. The complex analysis of big data can derive, through the application of artificial intelligence, new insights on diseases and their therapies (Meskó et al. 2017).

These research articles and analyses aimed primarily at professionals are further transformed by strategies fostering more informed citizens and an increase in their health literacy. This includes massive open online courses (MOOCs), social networks managed by health professionals and health communication on verified web pages. One way of verification of web pages is through the Health on the Net Foundation, which awards health-related web pages and mobile applications with a HONcode seal (Boyer et al. 2011). The seal is based on providing visible answer to eight questions: who is the author, who is the audience, how collected data are treated, what are the sources of information, if evidence is balanced or biased, is contact information for eventual additional questions provided, where from are the financial sources and what is the advertising policy.

All these approaches use a linear model of knowledge distribution characterized by a hierarchical relation between expert and user. A linear model of knowledge distribution is the intuitive approach learned already during childhood. Children attend school to learn from the teachers. The teachers being experts in their job provide the literacy needed to orient their pupils in a demanding world and foster a growing maturity. The knowledge is transferred linearly from the expert to the user in a hierarchical relationship. At the end, the envisaged result is overwhelmingly positive—the child becoming a respectable citizen, a member of the society.

Subsequently, the model described above is taken as a paradigm on how to provide medical knowledge to the users, being patients or healthy individuals. Following the same line of thought, in order to transfer from medical paternalism towards person-centred care, it is only necessary to increase the literacy of the citizens, so transforming from health-illiterates to health-literates. When citizens reach the literacy level required, they would be capable of playing an informed role in the healthcare system (Ververda and Hauge 2019).

Beyond this linear form of knowledge building, the digital environment allows many other information-seeking and knowledge-generating configurations within the health landscapes (Allgaier and Svalastog 2015). The phenomenon of personalized digital landscapes has been described as digital "filter bubbles", "echo chambers" and "black holes" (Gajović and Svalastog 2016; Sumpter 2018). The filter bubble refers to the feature of search engines to adapt the results of queries to the personal preferences of the searcher (Pariser 2011). The personalization of results reflects the way in which search engines are designed to provide results seen to be as relevant as possible. Consequently, relevance comes before robust knowledge and the concept of the bubble means that the search would refer to what a user wants to hear. However, at the same time it isolates the individual in their own bubble built on the premises of their own expectations. This process of what we can call digital self-isolation is found elsewhere such as the echo chambers occurring in digital social networks, where individuals are surrounded by their like-minded companions (Garrett 2009). The echo chambers of the digital environment share the same opinion and reinforce and influence the individual participants towards a specific way of thinking. The final degree of digital isolation where participants communicate exclusively to like-minded individuals would be represented by what we might call digital black holes, where the landscape geography is ultimately distorted in a closed system (Gajović and Svalastog 2016).

A further complication that needs to be considered here is what we can call the *timing* of information on the web. Here we are not referring to matters of timeliness for the user, but rather to the *temporal positioning* of the information that is found. Often this is quite obscure. In the offline context timing is typically experienced as linear, flowing constantly in one direction from past to the future. However, digital content is normally free from these constraints, so it is reasonable to ask how time is represented in the online environment.

Digital content has rarely an assigned time reference (Quinton and Reynolds 2018). Web pages sometimes provide time information, i.e. they show how recent (and subsequently relevant) is the content. Interactive platforms may provide the time when content is posted; however, this time does not reflect the actual time of the content being produced, nor the time of content being first published. A video posted on YouTube could present an event of yesterday or years ago, without any clue to the user how to determine this. Sometimes the video is original content; sometimes it is a repost, fragment or compilation of already existing videos and sometimes it is a remake of the original content. The web pages dedicated to the person or to the event would rarely present the information in a "timely" order. This could be the case even for the news portals dedicated to the most recent events. A photograph picturing people waiting for a bus on a flooded street was declared on social networks to visualize a recent flood in Croatia; however, it turned out it had already been posted in relation to a previous flood in Italy. Further user comments revealed that the online text in Italian was photoshopped to fit the Italian situation, but the original photograph was taken much before during a flood in Turkey. This is an example of a journey in the digital environment of an interesting story that draws attention regardless of its actual timing(s).

Digital technology as well allows the users to avoid conventional time constraints. The looping of any content (e.g. video or a digital game) allows the viewer to experience the content again and again. The sequence of contents can be freely rearranged. Moreover, the search engines rarely sort the resulting hits according to time (unless specifically requested by the query of the experienced user), and the hits rarely contain the time information.

Timing is important here for the knowledge as it is created through time-dependent layers, with each new layer built on the foundation of the previously created knowledge (Burke 2012). However, if the time sequence of the knowledge in the digital environment is lost, then the arguments for every new layer can be twisted or lost. This phenomenon has been referred to as digital anachronism, that is, that whatever the historical representation or original understanding of a specific health issue, it could be revived as a novelty in the digital environment (Svalastog et al. 2017). Without this time component, the sequence of prior arguments associated with the issue is lost, and previously disapproved arguments can be brought into the discussion again.

This happened in the context of the anti-vaccine debate (e.g. https://www.vaccines.gov/basics). In regard to the geography of knowledge landscapes, this particular time dimension appears circular, where contents reappear again and again. The loss of a time hierarchy influences an overall loss of hierarchy-based linearity (Gajović and Svalastog 2016). The timeless features of the digital environment are in particular exaggerated in interactive environments. YouTube, Facebook, WhatsApp or Reddit are just some of the examples of technological solutions aimed to allow interactivity of users regardless of the content. Although the sequences of the posts seem to preserve the time component, just the opposite occurs. The circularity of the timeless interactions of the digital environment has an impact on offline time linearity. The interactive digital platform represents portals through which a timeless digital environment influences our perception of time in a real-life setting (Firth et al. 2019). Subsequently, the digital society being an online-offline continuum is characterized by time distortions originating from the digital sphere and spreading to the offline environment. The loss of a time hierarchy and the circularity of arguments represent a specific feature of social interaction in the digital society.

Expectations and the Place of Medicine

Earlier in this chapter, two related themes were discussed: the introduction of person-centred care as a dominant healthcare system and the appearance of an interconnected and interactive digital environment. Together these were said to be reshaping the position and status of medical knowledge in the digital society. In some ways, medical knowledge within the digital environment gains a specific appeal not encountered before. In comparison to those medical books primarily aimed at students and practitioners, the digital environment offers the availability and comprehensive coverage of diverse medical topics open to everybody. The digital allure of medical topics is additionally motivated by a rapid pace of innovations and subsequent advances in the field. Biomedical research masters unprecedented technologies like sequencing of the human genome, in vitro fertilization, embryonic stem cells or gene editing. The impression of limitless possibilities of innovative research translated to medical practice fuels citizens' aspirations. This enhances expectations about what medicine can do to maintain health or combat disease (Correia 2017). There is a self-propelling synergy between futuristic features of biomedical research and health-related digital content available online that creates an illusion that the solution for whatever medical issue is already available and just a click away.

The prospect of the potential benefit of life-changing medical advances creates a specific thirst for medical knowledge. Those citizens deciding on their own health within a system based on person-centred care do not expect the routine approach of the average healthcare provided by the local medical institution. Under the influence of global digital technology, they expect nothing less from the medical field than the last and the best treatment for themselves. An imbalance of knowledge between a provider (medical professional) and a user (patient, citizen) is now accentuated by an imbalance between the professional judgement offered by conventional medical institutions and user expectations driven by digitally enhanced medical expectations. The partnership with medical professionals providing knowledge and assuring users autonomy when deciding about treatment comes under strain because of unrealistic expectations of users about what can be achieved for their own health (Vogt et al. 2016; Wensing and Grol 2019; Erikainen and Chan 2019).

Even if the individual is not aware of the concept of person-centred care, still the advances of medicine and the promise of omnipotent cure for everything provide the impression that health is easy to reach, and the relevant knowledge is just a step away to be found and implemented. Those seeking for health would appreciate the new position of person-centred care, as being in the centre one can search, find and apply for one's own benefits the very recent advances of medical research. Subsequently, a situation where citizens can have an individualized approach and decide on their health is additionally enhanced by the universal appeal of the digital resources and online availability of the most recent and innovative health knowledge (Berntsen et al. 2018; Wensing and Grol 2019).

Some Reflections: Digital Circularity and Knowledge

In this chapter on knowledge landscape geography, the discussion has ranged across the changes in the patient/medic relationships with the advent of the digital health system, the arrival of a patient-centred care and enabled travelers through that system and the multiple/multicentric sources of information and their interpretation. This led to some proposals regarding how best to approach the geography of the knowledge landscape, arguing for its three-dimensional topography that is created and changed over time, the latter itself a problematic dynamic in this environment. In addition, tensions between retaining open, transparent forms of access and so more reflexive understanding of health and the tendencies towards (either commercially driven or shared network created) more closed "filter bubbles" were discussed. Managing the expectations of patients/users in regard to the promise of biomedicine circulating on the web raises new challenges for professional practitioners and researchers.

To conclude the chapter, a number of broader concerns can be raised. First, we might describe in broad terms that together with linear information flows, digital landscapes can present as well circular geometries of knowledge where there is no clear locus of authority to distinguish between claims found. Instead, one can become a perpetual navigator in a bewildering subset of landscapes. This circular geometry allows in theory an infinite moving in a finite space. This is especially apparent in the echo chamber phenomena that establish circular pathways for the participants.

Secondly, the level of circularity in the digital environment exceeds any extent of circularity encountered in the offline world, being ubiquitous and widespread. Two novel parameters of circularity emerge in these digital settings, both already mentioned, their synergy being more powerful than ever. The first is the loss of a time component—any content can be approached without any constraints of the time of its production. Endless repetition is possible, or (digital) time can be stopped and started again later, with any combination of orders, fragments or adaptations. The second parameter contributing to the circularity is the loss of an evidential hierarchy, inasmuch as there is no primacy of one digital content compared to another, one digitalized form of knowledge to another. The book of digital knowledge can be read in any direction and in any sequence, and in the same way it can be un-read, or un-reasoned (Carr 2011). When I tried to explain this to my son, he asked me the question, which although pretty obvious hit me with its simplicity. He said: "Do you want to say we cannot learn anything anymore?", and I was caught with the question without an answer at this point.

To answer the question, I want first to argue that indeed we can learn in the digital society. The loss of time and loss of hierarchy resulting with circular geometries of knowledge landscapes do not imply an inability to learn. However, they pinpoint the risk that if we reduce our communication only to linear knowledge transfer and linear geometries of knowledge landscapes, we limit our understanding of the forms of knowledge that are possible and how they are generated. The relation between linear and non-linear forms of understanding and the expectations surrounding both is a key here: circularity in itself does not imply the impossibility of knowledge transfer; rather it implies the need to understand the dynamics associated with this in order to communicate new forms of knowledge in new circumstances.

As a biomedical researcher, my understanding of these dynamics is still rather rudimentary and the fact that I problematize the circular geometry of knowledge landscapes does not mean that I have a simple answer about how to use it. One approach we might take comes from the science fiction field. The movie *Arrival* is based on a short novel, the *Story of Your Life*, by the American writer Ted Chiang (Chiang 2010). The plot is based on aliens coming to Earth, which do not have a concept of time, reflecting as well the absence of the notion of causality. Understanding and learning their language for the main character, a linguist, Dr. Louise Banks, required her experiencing the loss of time sequences, similar to the argument brought here that the digital environment spills over in the offline word by its circular geometries. However, loss of time and causality did not prevent the aliens from being able to communicate. In simplified terms, the language is based on the feature that if there is no time, everything should be said at once. The form embracing the ability to communicate all aspects and details altogether to others was referred to as an ideogram, being a symbol of the completeness of the idea to be communicated. Perhaps ideograms can arise as a form of communication in knowledge landscapes and be used as a tool for knowledge transfer in a way that overcomes the linear/non-linear tensions noted above. The intellectual and practical challenge of the future is in particular at the level of the human mind, embracing and benefiting from the new frontiers open to be explored.

References

Allgaier, J., & Svalastog, A. L. (2015). The communication aspects of the Ebola virus disease outbreak in Western Africa– Do we need to counter one, two, or many epidemics? *Croatian Medical Journal, 56*(5), 496–499.

Ames, H. M., Glenton, C., & Lewin, S. (2017). Parents' and informal caregivers' views and experiences of communication about routine childhood vaccination: A synthesis of qualitative evidence. *Cochrane Database of Systematic Reviews, 2*(2), CD011787.

Berntsen, G., Høyem, A., Lettrem, I., Ruland, C., Rumpsfeld, M., & Gammon, D. (2018). A person-centered integrated care quality framework, based on a qualitative study of patients' evaluation of care in light of chronic care ideals. *BMC Health Services Research, 18*(1), 479.

Boyer, C., Baujard, V., & Geissbuhler, A. (2011). Evolution of health web certification through the HONcode experience. *Studies in Health Technology and Informatics, 169*, 53–57.

Browne, F., Bettles, S., Clift, S., & Walker, T. (2019). Connecting patients, practitioners, and regulators in supporting positive experiences and processes of shared decision making: A progress report. *Journal of Evaluation in Clinical Practice, 25*(6), 1030–1040.

Burke, P. (2012). *A social history of knowledge II: From the Encyclopaedia to Wikipedia*. Cambridge: Polity.

Carr, N. (2011). *The shallows: What the internet is doing to our brains*. New York: W. W. Norton & Company.

Chiang, T. (2010). *Stories of your life and others*. Easthampton: Small Beer Press.

Correia, T. (2017). Revisiting medicalization: A critique of the assumptions of what counts as medical knowledge. *Frontiers in Sociology, 2*, 14.

Erikainen, S., & Chan, S. (2019). Contested futures: Envisioning "personalized," "stratified," and "precision" medicine. *New Genetics and Society, 38*(3), 308–330.

Farmer, A., Williams, V., Velardo, C., et al. (2017). Self-management support using a digital health system compared with usual Care for Chronic Obstructive Pulmonary Disease: Randomized controlled trial. *Journal of Medical Internet Research, 19*(5), e144.

Firth, J., Torous, J., Stubbs, B., et al. (2019). The "online brain": How the internet may be changing our cognition. *World Psychiatry, 18*(2), 119–129.

Gajović, S. (2018). Knowledge-for-data trade at the interface between precision medicine and person-centered care. *Croatian Medical Journal, 59*(3), 132–135.

Gajović, S. (2020 Feb 03). Independent, publicly funded journals adhering to platinum open access are the future of responsible scholarly publishing. *Journal of Korean Medical Science, 35*(4), e13.

Gajović, S., & Svalastog, A. L. (2016). When communicating health-related knowledge, beware of the black holes of the knowledge landscapes geography. *Croatian Medical Journal, 57*(5), 504–509.

Garrett, R. K. (2009). Echo chambers online?: Politically motivated selective exposure among internet news users. *Journal of Computer-Mediated Communication, 14*(2), 265–285.

Goldberg, L. R., & Crocombe, L. A. (2017). Advances in medical education and practice: Role of massive open online courses. *Advances in Medical Education and Practice, 8*, 603–609.

Ho, D., Quake, S. R., McCabe, E. R. B., Chng, W. J., Chow, E. K., Ding, X., Gelb, B. D., Ginsburg, G. S., Hassenstab, J., Ho, C. M., Mobley, W. C., Nolan, G. P., Rosen, S. T., Tan, P., Yen, Y., & Zarrinpar, A. (2020). Enabling Technologies for Personalized and Precision Medicine. *Trends in Biotechnology, 38*(5), 497–518.

Kim, K. K., Sankar, P., Wilson, M. D., & Haynes, S. C. (2017). Factors affecting willingness to share electronic health data among California consumers. *BMC Med Ethics, 18*(1), 25. Published 2017 Apr 4.

Kopilaš, V., & Gajović, S. (2020). Wildfire-like effect of WhatsApp campaign to mobilize predominantly health professionals with a university degree on the health issue: Infodemiology study. *Journal of Medical Internet Research, 22*(8), e17051.

Levinson, W., Kao, A., Kuby, A., & Thisted, R. A. (2005). Not all patients want to participate in decision making. A national study of public preferences. *Journal of General Internal Medicine, 20*(6), 531–535.

Matthews, E. B., Stanhope, V., Choy-Brown, M., & Doherty, M. (2018). Do providers know what they do not know? A correlational study of knowledge acquisition and person-Centered care. *Community Mental Health Journal, 54*(5), 514–520.

Meskó, B., Drobni, Z., Bényei, É., Gergely, B., & Győrffy, Z. (2017). Digital health is a cultural transformation of traditional healthcare. *Mhealth, 3*, 38.

Murgic, L., Hébert, P. C., Sovic, S., & Pavlekovic, G. (2015 Sep 29). Paternalism and autonomy: Views of patients and providers in a transitional (post-communist) country. *BMC Medical Ethics, 16*(1), 65.

Pariser, E. (2011). *The filter bubble: What the internet is hiding from you*. New York: Penguin Press.

Quinton, S., & Reynolds, N. (2018). Temporality in digital research. In *Understanding research in the digital age* (pp. 89–114). London: SAGE Publications Ltd.

Rosen, G., & Imperato, P. J. (2015). *A history of public health*. Baltimore: Johns Hopkins University Press.

Sumpter, D. J. T. (2018). *Outnumbered: From Facebook and Google to fake news and filter-bubbles – Exploring the algorithms that control our lives*. Sigma: Bloomsbury.

Svalastog, A. L., Allgaier, J., Martinelli, L., & Gajović, S. (2014). Distortion, confusion, and impasses: Could a public dialogue within knowledge landscapes contribute to better communication and understanding of innovative knowledge? *Croatian Medical Journal, 55*, 54–60.

Svalastog, A. L., Allgaier, J., & Gajović, S. (2015). Navigating knowledge landscapes: On health, science, communication, media, and society. *Croatian Medical Journal, 56*(4), 321–323.

Svalastog, A. L., Donev, D., Jahren Kristoffersen, N., & Gajović, S. (2017). Concepts and definitions of health and health-related values in the knowledge landscapes of the digital society. *Croatian Medical Journal, 58*(6), 431–435.

Ververda, J., & Hauge, S. (2019). Active care in practice: Long-term experiences from an education programme. *Journal of Multidisciplinary Healthcare, 12*, 871–879.

Vogt, H., Hofmann, B., & Getz, L. (2016). The new holism: P4 systems medicine and the medicalization of health and life itself. *Medicine, Health Care, and Philosophy, 19*(2), 307–323.

Wensing, M., & Grol, R. (2019). Knowledge translation in health: How implementation science could contribute more. *BMC Medicine, 17*(1), 88.

WHO. *WHO guideline: recommendations on digital interventions for health system strengthening*. Geneva: World Health Organization, 2019. Available at https://apps.who.int/iris/bitstream/handle/10665/311941/9789241550505-eng.pdf.Accessed 11 Feb 2020.

Wildevuur, S. E., & Simonse, L. W. (2015). Information and communication technology-enabled person-centered care for the "big five" chronic conditions: Scoping review. *Journal of Medical Internet Research, 17*(3), e77.

Part II

Journeys in the Knowledge Landscapes

The six chapters in this second Part of the book offer a range of empirical cases that explore knowledge landscapes in more detail through rich, qualitative studies of different forms of engagement with digital systems by individuals or groups, making contextual ramifications of agency tangible. The authors are drawn from diverse disciplinary perspectives including science and technology studies, social anthropology and social work.

What is common to all is an interest in the epistemic and ontological dynamics of what we might call the personal/digital nexus, the area where boundaries are created or blurred, where data reifications create and enable movement of not just information about people but their very embodiment in digital systems. In addition, and seen together, the different chapters establish how digitalisation of communication and services can enable and empower, but also reduce and exclude social agency for private life as well as professionals, and reflect how online and offline contexts are intertwined. This is perhaps the overarching meta-theme that the different disciplines contribute towards.

In regard to boundaries, the chapters explore the relationship between offline and online processes, and in some contexts, these are said to be elided through 'digital subjectivity' wherein, as Lamerichs et al. argue, illness and its meaning and experience are actually shaped by engagement with the digital and the affordances it offers, where the ontology of illness is itself co-produced in this way. In contrast, the chapter by Senior and Kriippanon examines the disjunction between a post-colonial online world and the offline knowledge system of an indigenous community in Australia. Here we see a reification of 'health' and so what post-colonial professionals regard as 'best' for indigenous communities, a reification reproduced by a specifically western knowledge landscape. Few, if any, affordances for these communities are enabled here.

Extending this argument, Bister explores the ways in which, in the context of mental healthcare, personal/patient data are translated into 'data objects', and how this form of informational reification then is performative in allowing movement across data spaces and so between professionals and their clients. It asks in short how 'care and policy are performed in material-semiotic practices that include digital systems'. Affordances are clearly made possible here, but where action and practice occur within a specific institutional setting. Outside of such settings, so in a very different knowledge landscape, the chapter by Simenc looks to the ways in which illness networks help patients to make sense on their own terms of the meaning of their illnesses, understood as 'relational' and so as ontologically plastic.

The final two chapters take us into the domain of governance and accountability and where the boundaries of these are to be found. In her chapter on ehealth, Sahinol shows how 'socio-cultural and socio-political norms and practices', and so how ehealth and 'mhealth', vary across different countries and their jurisdictions (e.g. in regard to the provision and oversight of electronic health records, especially, as she shows in her case study of the Turkish system, in regard to data privacy). Boundaries again come to the fore inasmuch as the general benefits to society of integrated ehealth systems have to be balanced against patient rights. The final chapter by Björktomta and Hansen take us down a similar road, here exploring the tensions between social work professionals' use of digital systems for monitoring children's needs and care, and the children's own rights and practice which empower them but also create new vulnerabilities.

6

Fostering "Digital Subjectivity": An Investigation of Digital Health Narratives in Norway, the Netherlands and Czechia

Joyce Lamerichs, Hege Kristin Andreassen, Lucie Klůzová Kráčmarová, and Manna Alma

Introduction: Digital Narratives and "Digital Subjectivity"

The ability to share and access experiential information about health and illness offers a context for people with health and illness concerns to construct a "digital subjectivity" that profoundly affects what living with illness means. In the last two decades and across several countries in the world, digital repositories that carry such experiential information have been developed, as part of an effort to make health and illness narratives available online. The country-specific initiatives are all part of a larger

J. Lamerichs (✉)
Language, Literature and Communication, Vrije Universiteit Amsterdam, Amsterdam, The Netherlands
e-mail: j.m.w.j.lamerichs@vu.nl

A. L. Svalastog et al. (eds.), *Navigating Digital Health Landscapes*, Health, Technology and Society, https://doi.org/10.1007/978-981-15-8206-6_6

effort, grouped together under the header DIPEx (Database of Individual Patients' Experience of Illness: see Ziebland and McPherson 2006), and all make use of a shared research methodology to collect and analyse peoples' illness experiences. The online repositories in each country are co-produced through close collaboration between people experiencing health and illness issues and researchers conducting a narrative interview approach to elicit the stories. Thematically grouped aspects of these narratives, resembling the illness trajectory people experience, are selected for online publication. The aim is thus to produce digital versions of the embodied person experiencing health and illness issues, which are accessible to a wide audience.

We think that approaching the merits of these online repositories from the perspective of "digital subjectivity" can successfully transcend the dualist categories "offline" and "online" and thus enable a more in-depth understanding of what it means to be ill in contemporary society. Both the academic literature and current health policies still fall back on the dual notions of "online" versus "offline" to describe which health information they think patients and carers need and where they would look for it (but see Mazanderani and Powell 2013, also Madianou and Miller 2012 and Ziebland and Wyke 2012). We aim to transcend this binary opposition to consider the online repositories in a society in which the division between online and offline is becoming increasingly blurred.

H. K. Andreassen
Centre for Women's and Gender Research, UiT The Arctic University of Norway, Tromsø, Norway
e-mail: hege.k.andreassen@uit.no

L. K. Kráčmarová
Olomouc University Social Health Institute (OUSHI), Palacky University Olomouc, Olomouc, Czechia
e-mail: lucie.kluzova@oushi.upol.cz

M. Alma
Faculty of Health Sciences, University Medical Center Groningen (UMCG), Groningen, The Netherlands

Our research shows that digital practices are not to be seen as different from, but as an inextricable part of the everyday illness practices that constitute living with an illness for patients and for their carers. Examining the opportunities offered by digital technologies to represent illness experiences allows for a fuller understanding of how people make sense of the ways in which digital technologies and illness experiences can be linked and how they allow for developing particular illness-related identities as co-produced forms of knowledge (cf., Lamerichs and Van Hooijdonk 2019). Our contribution starts from the idea that we need to expand our understanding of how people with health concerns and their carers make use of such digital resources. Digital subjectivity offers us a way to supplement a predominantly informational perspective that concentrates on the way in which online illness experiences fulfil information needs. The concept of digital subjectivity sensitises us for experiences that go beyond the simple act of "collecting" information and helps to expand our scope to include the sense in which digital participation is actually formative of the illness experience itself. It can thus be understood to alter what the illness actually *is*. Our analysis of those who share their illness experiences online and those who visit or access digital platforms where illness repositories are hosted, challenges the point of departure in the literature emphasising how sharing objective, neutral, quantified health information affects the patient's role and the patient's relation to their doctor (Tan and Goonawardene 2017; Karnam and Raghavendra 2017). Our interest is in the (inter)subjective constructions of illness and identity in everyday lives, outside of the consultation room and doctor-patient dialogue. Hence, it is our aim to investigate how the concept of digital subjectivity can illuminate the myriad and interwoven nature of online-offline practices in peoples' experience and understanding of illness.

In what follows we present original empirical findings of interviews with patients and their carers that were held in Norway, the Netherlands and Czechia. To further substantiate the importance of a subjective understanding of the self in the knowledge landscape the World Wide Web poses, we present illustrative interview excerpts of how the interviewees talk about their needs when they try to come to terms with living with a particular illness.

Digitalisation, Digital Subjectivity and "Digital Prosthesis"

Over the last few decades, the interest in the digitalisation of health has grown in many academic disciplines, such as psychology, sociology, organisational studies, informatics and health sciences (Thompson et al. 2011). We explore what illness means as a "construction of digital and subjective formations". Based on our empirical findings, we will discuss if, and if so, how this angle can be of value to explain the complex co-constructions of digitalisation and subjective formations of health and illness in contemporary society, as well as to point to the use of DIPEx platforms as possible resources for such constructive practices.

Digital Subjectivity

Digital subjectivity has not been a much-used concept in studies of health and illness, but is known from other fields such as digital culture studies (Goriunova 2019), work on gaming culture (Charles 2009) and the domain of media studies (Giraud 2015). The concept of subjectivity has a long tradition and is central to both sociological and psychological research. Lately, subjectivity has been introduced as a theoretical angle to understand individuals' relations to digital tools as well as the potential to expand the limits of the self through "digital prostheses" such as mobile phones or personalised medical devices more in general (Rey and Boesel 2014; see also Lynch and Farrington 2018). In what follows we will mainly draw on conceptualisations based on the work of Rey and Boesel (2014) and Giraud (2015).

Rey and Boesel (2014) understand subjectivity as comprised of two equal elements: the body, or an embodied self, and the social conditions of the subject, that is, the historical conditions forming the subjects' social context. There are bodies and there is society. Their point is that both have changed through digitalisation. Embodiment is no longer just a matter of the self that is residing in organic flesh. Rather, today, we are also embodied through our *digital prosthesis*. Digital tools are prolonging the expansion of our selves and can thus be seen as a new element to embodiment (Lynch and Farrington 2018, also Roberts et al. 2019). Further, the societal aspect that is equally central to subjectivity has also changed. The historical social conditions framing the lives of the individuals are no longer the same as for previous generations. Contemporary society is a digital society (Tamminem and Deibel 2018). Central to Rey and Boesel's argument is that the offline social context is neither more real nor more normal than the online context; the latter is just as normal and just as real, only it is new. Hence, both the embodied self and the social conditions of the subject have changed profoundly as we have moved from analogue to digital society. This change in turn causes new and augmented forms of being in the world, of subjectivity. Through this lens, digital subjectivity is not a restricted version nor does it replace subjectivity; rather it opens up new dimensions to it.

Giraud's (2015) approach to "digital subjectivity" stems from critical Internet and media studies. Her approach can be read as a critique of Dean's (2009) somewhat cynical conceptualisation of subjectivity in which users are believed to get trapped in never-ending communicative loops when they go online. This points to the risk that the business models of online information and communication services, based in machine learning, end up restricting and reinforcing the users' knowledge base rather than challenging and expanding it. This is of course an evident ethical and political problem. However, Giraud (2015) argues that there is a need to reconceptualise the digital subject away from such restrictive models and towards a more situated, material analysis of the *affordances* that become available by subjective entanglements with technology (Humphreys 2018). In line with Hutchby (2001) and Gibson (1979), we take the affordance of a technology to be "the possibilities that they offer for action" and acknowledge that these might appear different to different people and in different situations. Giraud (p.131) states that "A burgeoning body of ethnographic work, moreover, has suggested that the affordances of communications media are established through inter-subjective practice (cf., Madianou and Miller 2012; Cammaerts 2014; see also Couldry 2012) and emerge through their broader socio-technical milieu, rather than being intrinsic to the technologies themselves (Ash 2014)."

Subjectivity may be also understood as a perspective in which an individual appraises the world and his/her own self based on their current position in space and time, which is constantly changing or evolving (Gold and De Sousa 2012). The notion of digital subjectivity may also be seen as a way in which individuals approach and interpret their experience with digital media in relation to their position in the world. Neither digital subjectivity nor digital media are stable entities in time and space. Each person makes use of digital technologies or interprets the same information provided by digital spaces in a different way and makes use of these media based on their specific individual needs which might be emotional, social or educational in nature; they may also be driven by personal characteristics, or the abilities to understand and access the information provided in relation to the self (see also Madianou and Miller 2012 for a discussion of media and communicative intent). Furthermore, and similar to other prostheses, affordances of the digital technologies to the users are given by their perception, which will influence their practical usage of these tools. We were interested in how people dealing with specific health conditions make use of digital technologies: what affordances, or possibilities for action, do they realise; is it used as an information source, as a prostheses or as both at the same time?

Methods

In this chapter, we present a secondary analysis of a total of 89 narrative interviews from three national studies concentrated on health and illness experiences. The interviews were selected from a pool of interviews carried out as part of DIPEx research conducted in the three different countries and were concerned with different health concerns: muscular disease; chronic nightmares, complex pregnancies and dementia. We will report on findings found in 5 interviews conducted in Norway, 30 interviews conducted in Czechia and 54 interviews conducted in the Netherlands. The interviews were conducted between 2012 and 2018. The aim of including such a varied selection of narrative interviews on illness experiences is that it enables us to highlight common features in the co-construction of illness and digital participation across countries and health challenges.

Description of the Data

The researchers who shared data and co-authored this chapter all participate in the international research network DIPEx (Ziebland and McPherson 2006). DIPEx International was founded to promote the spread of robust data conveying people's experiences of health and illness (DIPEx International 2020). The members of DIPEx International use the DIPEx methodology which aims to (1) promote excellence of qualitative research into people's experiences of health and illness, (2) advance the use and application of the results of this research to inform and improve health and health care and (3) support cross-cultural comparisons of people's experiences of health and health care and encourage appropriate action of the findings.

Analytical Approach

Our approach intends to pursue whether the empirical findings we present illustrate the notion of digital subjectivity to illustrate that the illness repositories, for both the people who tell their stories and the people who visit them, are not only concerned with gaining information. We propose that a purely informational perspective does not suffice to explain what we see and argue that our empirical data show that "digital subjectivity" is treated as an affordance of the online DIPEx repositories. In line with the work by Lucius-Hoene, Breuning and Helfferich (2018), we present evidence that this affordance is experienced both by the people who share their story in these repositories and for people who access the repositories in different ways. The empirical chapters will be concerned with present findings from three DIPEx repositories in Norway, the Netherlands and Czechia.

For the analysis we scrutinised our data for examples of how narratives shared through health talk websites can represent *digital prosthesis* of the narrators and thus be understood as formative for the participants' digital subjectivity. We will also report some preliminary findings on how people who access online repositories (i.e. secondary users) relate to these narratives and how they include them as part of their lived experiences. We posed the following questions from our data:

1. Can the narratives produced and shared in the different DIPEx repositories be understood as digital prostheses and if so, in which way?
2. How does the extension of the body to also include digital forms, like voice, film or text matter for constructing individual experiences of health and illness?

In sum, we propose that digital subjectivism is an interesting and fruitful lens to the lived practices involved in "accessing" online health experience. We will illustrate this with examples from DIPEx research in three countries. We will now turn to our empirical materials.

The Participants Who Choose to Share Their Narratives: Findings from Three Studies

In this section we present examples from three countries that illustrate our main claim(s) about digital subjectivity and prosthesis.

Embodiment: The Norwegian Account of Muscular Disease

In Norway a small pilot study (five participants) was conducted among people with rare muscular diseases. One of the participants, a 36-year-old man, told us that he had been severely ill since he was 11 years old, but only when he was 30 did he meet a doctor who diagnosed him. Before that he had been in and out of several institutions and met both specialists and general practitioners who had not been able to come to any conclusions about the disease he was suffering from. Our informant had been in a wheelchair for years. Over the last 25 years, he had been ill and he had been experiencing increasing limitations in muscular function in his hands and fingers. When we met with him, he could not write. Another symptom of his illness was hearing loss. In the following quote, he explains about his subjective experience of the illness after he was being diagnosed and discovered there was a patient association for people with muscular disease that he could participate in:

Participant 1: "After I participated in a course (arranged by the Norwegian patient association for muscular disease), I accidently read the participant list and some of the papers and realized that one of the other participants had the same diagnosis as me. I e-mailed her through Facebook. That was the start of our friendship. We have chatted a lot online, sent SMS messages and so on. Most of the communication is online when I talk to my friends. I cannot talk on the phone."

Interviewer: "When you say that you chat online, do you receive help for using the keyboard? Or how do you do that?"

Participant 1: "No, I can do it by myself. That is; I use only my thumb. I can experience it as tiresome, so in fact I always express myself in the short. You could say I use a lot of time for this."

Another informant from the same study was in a wheelchair. She explained her feeling of being an outsider:

Participant 2: "What bothers me most about being ill, is that one cannot mix into society, but is left outside and gets extra notice. You know, sometimes people look a little bit afraid when they see my wheelchair. They are terrified of bumping into me and shy away already one meter away."

Our interpretation is that these two participants experience their illness in and through a digital everyday life, and the characteristics of digital communication must be acknowledged as formative of their subjectivity. These examples show how both elements of subjectivity in

Rey and Boesel's theory (2014), the body and the social conditions, are mediated and given new form by engaging with the digital domain. Embodiment is not only about the organic flesh but also about what the body can perform through digital prosthesis, like a keyboard in the case of informant 1 above. Through this digital prosthesis, the limits of his body and hence its social agency are both confirmed and enabled, conveying a sense of affordance. The Internet, in combination with the keyboard he can operate with his thumb, opens up a new avenue for social participation.

The story of the second participant is a concrete example of how historical and social conditions frame the subjective experience of illness. While not referring to the online domain, our interviewee explains how other people's reactions to her sitting in a wheelchair is a matter of concern for her. Wheelchairs are stigmatised as deviant. As was also referred to by the first participant, the digital domain is described in terms of enabling factors rather than in terms of exclusion and in term of factors that render the social stigma less prominent and less constitutive of the illness experience.

Encountering a Normalising Frame: The Czech Study of Chronic Nightmares

In Czechia, 30 adults were interviewed, of which 22 were female and 8 male. All participants suffered from chronic nightmares and had at least one disturbing dream per week. Interviewees were recruited through various communication outlets and from different parts of the country. In order to create a sample with maximum variation, people with various experiences were involved in the study. In this instance, it involved people who were undergoing different types of therapy, people who varied in frequency and severity of their nightmares and people reporting different causes or accompanying conditions (e.g. sleep paralysis, insomnia, anxiety or depression). The purpose of this study was to explore how individuals with frequent nightmares use the Internet in relation to their chronic nightmares. For the current purpose, we undertook a secondary analysis to relate the interviewees' stories to digital subjectivity.

Out of 30 participants, more than half said they searched the Internet in relation to their nightmares to find information. Participants were typically interested in causes of nightmares, possibilities of treatment, the meaning of their dreams (dream dictionaries) and information on accompanying sleep problems such as night terrors or sleep paralysis. There were also secondary aims involved in what seemed to be a straightforward information need: one of the participants was relieved when the information she found online helped her to find out that symptoms she suffered from (muscle paralysis, hallucinations of demons, etc. before awakening) can be found in sleep paralysis, which is quite common in the general population. She experienced a normalisation of her own symptoms when she realised that other people have the same experience and this even has a name. Such normalisation may not only result in immediate relief but may also have an effect on one's perception of self and how one understands herself or the world:

Participant 3: "I really believed it was there (demon) and I was afraid of looking under my bed. After I found that many people have the same experience and that it is caused by a dream or by a sleep issue, I don't believe it was real anymore."

The power of online information to change the subjective perception of illness and one's self-perception was emphasised by three participants, who rather did not search for information on nightmares on the Internet anymore because they were afraid of worsening their state. They said that some suggestive information might make them feel bad about themselves or they might start to believe there is something wrong with them.

Participant 4: "I don't seek information online anymore because (…) it might make people to start believe they are not alright. Someone online says that something means something and I tell myself 'dang it, it is me! That is terrible!'".

It seems that in comparison to informant 3, who experienced normalisation, informant 4 was worried of experiencing de-normalisation. We may say that digital subjectivity depends on personal interpretations of the information and it is highly contextualised (see also Lynch and Farrington 2018). Individuals' diverse experiences with the illness, symptoms, their own personality, life situation, worries or self-perception influence their interpretations; some of these interpretations help them to cope with their illness and others do not. Importantly, digital subjectivity is not a fixed state, nor does it only pose positive added uses when encountering the digital. The interviewees illustrate this by showing how these sources of information are open to diverse interpretations and discussions of relevance and trustworthiness. One additional example of these multiple interpretations is when interviewees address the topic of "passive digital participation". Interviewees reported to seek stories told by other people with the same concerns which brought them relief. A female participant used social networks to hear about the experiences of other people, but she did not tell the researcher she would share her own experiences. Digital participation may even be formative even if users only listen to experiences of other people with health issues and do not share their own story.

These findings illustrate the broad range of affordances and limiting factors of the Internet for people experiencing frequent nightmares. As an important positive aspect, the online information offered relief in the sense that they are not alone and provide a normalising frame to consider that what they are experiencing is "normal".

A Vocabulary to Convey Subjective Meaning: The Dutch Experience of Living with Dementia

The 48 interviewees who were interviewed for the DIPEx dementia in the Netherlands were all informal carers who cared for a loved one who was experiencing the onset of dementia. In the interviews they point out that they were quite satisfied by the possibilities the Internet offers to search for information about the illness and the many sources that address dementia in particular on different websites. They also point out that they are able to find the information they need and have some sense of discriminating between what is trustworthy information and what is not. A downside they reported on had to do with the use of technical language to describe aspects of the illness, which was considered unclear and limited the accessibility of some information sources.

Participant 5: "[…] You can read a lot and interpret it and well, how do you interpret whatever it says there on the Internet? Often it is medical jargon, terminology that does not speak to me. But what it says, what it means, could still have a big impact."

At the same time, interviewees expressed a clear need for a different type of information they also considered lacking, that is, experiential information on how to live with (someone with) dementia, given that there is no cure for the disease, as participant 6 points out.

Participant 6: (carer for father-in-law)

"Uh yes I find it really horrible that there is no cure. Uh and there is research or something that slows it down the progress of the disease. [-] But it wasn't clear to me at all that was such a hopeless situation. Uh I have, yes wished that I could go somewhere, that I, zap, there is a cure, that can relieve the disease or something. Ehm that was such a blow. And then I have changed my search to uh, to the other side. How can I manage to be with someone who is so seriously ill. How can I help him, emotionally, love him, all those things. Then uh, yes I explored that side, not the medical side but managing to live with the diseased person."

The interviewee below is being asked also to talk to the information she/he thinks is missing in what she is reading on Alzheimer's disease (in addition to recounting her experiences in seeking for help or support for her family member). She states that there is an abundance of technical information available, but that what is missing is the variability in experience and information for friends and relatives on how to be around someone with dementia.

Participant 7: (carer for spouse)
"It is not a uniform package this, so you have to [...) And you can't make any plans for the future because nobody knows exactly how it will go, what will happen and that is true of course for everybody's life [pause 4 sec] But uh I think that for example friends and relatives don't know how to be around someone with Alzheimer's, how you could be around someone [pause 3 sec] because yes there is little information available, in whatever way, for them on how to do that, deal with that."

The Users of Illness Repositories: Findings from Two Studies

To expand our understanding of how patients use the DIPEx narratives, we have been able to explore the experiences of two groups of users of the repositories. This section reports on the findings of a study conducted in Czechia in which 9 of the 30 participants talked about what they would expect from a DIPEx repository on this topic. We also report on a study conducted in the Netherlands involving pupils who learned to become nurses caring for people with dementia. They accessed the online illness repository in an educational setting, in an attempt to close the gap between what pupils learn about dementia in theory and the people they care for in practice, offering a particular contribution to improving communication skills when caring for people with dementia and their families (Lamerichs and Alma 2018).

Availability and Accessibility as Drivers of Awareness

One of the benefits participants speak about is the importance of raising awareness, in multiple ways. For those who do not suffer from nightmares themselves, it can help to understand those who do suffer from frequent nightmares. Participants also stated that people who frequently experience nightmares might open up to other people more and start talking about their experiences. According to another male participant, the website could also help those people, who have no one to talk to about their issues: it may help people who can't or don't want to talk about their problems but still seek support.

Participant 8: "It will help these people to open up and tell what they want or what they needed to say."

Another female participant liked the fact that the repository would contain stories of real people and would therefore not be totally anonymous: "I know that there are others with nightmares. I know what they look like and I can picture them concretely."

If we think about the repository as prostheses, as an enabling technology that helps to understand and manage illness, the very fact that it offers patient experiences in recognisable and therefore accessible language is important because this would enable access and use and an important means to relate to the experiences that are addressed in the repository. Importantly, interviewees consider this to be lacking, currently.

Participant 9: "What I miss is a website with comprehensive information based on fact that would be accessible for a lay public (17)."

Learning the Language of Lived Experience

Online repositories can also offer a vocabulary to talk about the illness, as was shown in the Dutch case (see Lamerichs and Alma 2018 for a full account). The Dutch case illustrated how pupils who were taking courses in dementia care in secondary vocational education in the Netherlands showed that the experiential digital narratives of people who experience the onset of dementia offered them a language to use when communicating with the carers of people with dementia. They also considered it as a unique means to access the lived experience of the person with dementia, as the following excerpts from the educational pilot carried out in the study show:

Participants 10: "It hits closer to home you know to have people—not theory because these people tell it themselves and also you know the lady who told how she felt when her children entered the room they can describe it best you know, what it is like."

The people who experienced the onset of dementia and who were interviewed often made use of vivid anecdotal language and metaphors. Pupils picked up on those metaphors and quickly incorporated them in their own language in class interaction and stressed how useful these metaphors could be to use when talking to relatives, who experienced difficulties understanding that their loved one could experience better days and days in which she felt worse. One woman with dementia used the image of a knotted little ball of wool as a description of how her head felt in the morning and which worked to indicate whether her day would be good or bad, or how it could sometimes also gradually improve, which she compared to finding the beginning of a thread in the ball which would help her untangle it. After hearing about this way of describing this, as an example in the online repository, the pupils discussed with their teacher about its importance in explaining the different states family members sometimes find their loved one in, when entering the care home, without understanding this difference to a full extent: it sometimes even posed problems. To be able to explain to the family members how their mother might be feeling, by using the metaphor she used in her own words, was considered very helpful. It offered them an actual vocabulary to communicate some of these thorny issues and to explain for these apparent differences and learn to read the signs on how their mother might be feeling.

Participant 11: "(..) and next time they might have found a string that runs and then they are able to talk about all kinds of things so then for the family you know for example then they are very well able to talk with their mother about all kinds of things and if it turns into a knot all of a sudden then it is completely different so then when the children enter the room then it is like ah well how is my mother doing today?".

Concluding Remarks

The question of how digital technologies matter for the construction of health and illness in contemporary society needs to be properly addressed. We have entered this discussion in this chapter through the concept of digital subjectivity, to highlight the potential of online participation to expand and alter the performance of illness and health practice in people's everyday practices. Looking at the co-construction of illness and digital participation across countries and health challenges, and through the lens of digital subjectivity, allowed us to illuminate how the particular entanglement of (a) living with health challenges and (b) using tools for digital participation in everyday life, affects the lived experiences of health and illness in contemporary society.

We identified three aspects central to subjectivity formation that are relevant to the production and/or use of digital narratives: embodiment, normality and language. For persons living with illness, these are all integrated into their daily illness practices and thus their subjective construction of illness. For our participants, the distinction between online and offline practices with respect to these three narratives was irrelevant; rather these seem to overlap and are interwoven in their daily lives.

In the literature the objectifying effects of digitalisation have had a strong prominence over the last years (Goriunova 2019; Roberts et al. 2019). Discussions have arisen on how digital tools contribute to the emergence of self-tracking cultures contributing and constituting a "the quantified self" (Lupton 2016; Lynch and Farrington 2018). These studies highlight how computing and digitalisation allows for the monitoring and storing of large quantities of biometric data on individuals, data that in turn can be used by the individuals themselves, or by second or third parties as population statistics. The availability of digital tools increasingly available to health professionals (i.e. the electronic patient record) adds to the same development: the creation of big datasets on population health. The debates that surround these developments exemplify how the digitalisation of health and the construction of the digital subject in terms of data profiles and big data contribute to a strengthened objectification of the individual. A negative side effect of these developments and debates is that it leads to a neglect of individuals' subjective experiences and health practices in the digital domain, which are of central importance for people experiencing illness, their carers as well as people in caring professions.

Our work has attempted to illustrate the importance of supplementing the stories of digitalisation as objectifying statistics and driven by information per se. We have highlighted some of the other stories that can be told about the co-construction of digital society and illness. Digitalisation opens up a resource for individual patients that contains stories about health and illness to be shared in new ways. The digital subject can also be "captured" via objectivisation by commercial interest, as already noted in the introduction to this book, but this has not been the focus of this chapter. We have attempted, as has Giraud (2015, but also see Goriunova 2019: p.127), to examine the digital subject through a micro-level, material analysis of the affordances enabled by digital tools.

We also want to emphasise that we need to go even further when discussing the digital subject. As with other stories, patient's individual narratives can now be stored and travel faster across time and space. They too can have an existence of their own, independent of the storyteller and open for second or third parties to interpret and perhaps exploit. There is a need for more research on how these practices will affect individual experiences of health and illness, as well as how it can be organised to be of benefit to patients, for health care personnel and for quality improvement in the health care sector in general.

References

Ash, J. (2014). Technology and affect: Towards a theory of inorganically organised objects. *Emotion, Space and Society, 14*(1), 84–90.

Cammaerts, B. (2014). Movement media as technologies of self-mediation. In C. Atton (Ed.), *The Routledge companion to alternative and community media*. London: Routledge.

Charles, A. (2009). Playing with one's self: Notions of subjectivity and agency in digital games. Eludamos. *Journal for Computer Game Culture, 3*(2), 281–294.

Couldry, N. (2012). *Media, society, world: Social media and digital media practice.* London: Polity Press.

Dean, J. (2009). *Democracy and other neoliberal fantasies: Communicative capitalism and left politics.* Durham/London: Duke University Press.

DIPEX International. (2020, October 5). About us. Retrieved from https://dipexinternational.org/.

Gibson, J. J. (1979). *The ecological approach to visual perception.* Boston: Houghton Mifflin.

Giraud, E. (2015). Subjectivity 2.0: Digital technologies, participatory media and communicative capitalism. *Subjectivity, 8*(2), 124–146.

Gold, R. A., & De Sousa, P. N. (2012). When does event valence affect unrealistic optimism? *Psychology Health and Medicine, 17*(1), 105–115.

Goriunova, O. (2019). The digital subject: People as data as persons. *Theory, Culture and Society, 36*(6), 125–145. https://doi.org/10.1177/0263276419840409.

Humphreys, L. (2018). *The qualified self.* Cambridge: MIT Press.

Hutchby, I. (2001). Technologies, texts and affordances. *Sociology, 35*(2), 441–456.

Karnam, S., & Raghavendra, P. (2017). Hybrid doctors: The need risen from informed patients. *Journal of Clinical and Diagnostic Research, 11*(2), ZI01.

Lamerichs, J., & Alma, M. (2018). Drawing on narrative accounts of dementia in education and care. In G. Lucius-Hoene, C. Holmberg & T. Meyer (Eds). *Illness Narratives in Practice: Potentials and Challenges of Using Narratives in Health-related Contexts* (pp. 188–199). Oxford, UK: Oxford University Press.

Lamerichs, J., & Van Hooijdonk, C. (2019). Mijn stoma is een #superstoma: Eendiscursieveanalyse van blogs over stoma's. [My ostomy is a #superostomy: A discursive analysis of ostomy blogs]. *Tijdschrift voor Taalbeheersing, 41*(3), 461–484.

Lucius-Hoene, G., Breuning, M., & Helfferich, C. (2018). Illness narratives in practice: which questions do we have to face when collecting and using them? In G. Lucius-Hoene, C. Holmberg & T. Meyer (Eds). *Illness Narratives in Practice: Potentials and Challenges of Using Narratives in Health-related Contexts* (pp. 13–26). Oxford, UK: Oxford University Press.

Lupton, D. (2016). *The quantified self. A sociology of self-tracking.* Cambridge, UK: Polity Press.

Lynch, R., & Farrington, C. (Eds.). (2018). *Quantified lives and vital data.* Basingstoke: Palgrave Macmillan.

Madianou, M., & Miller, D. (2012). Polymedia: Towards a new theory of digital media in interpersonal communication. *International Journal of Cultural Studies, 16*(2), 169–187.

Mazanderani, F., & Powell, J. (2013). Using the Internet as a source of information about patients' experiences. In S. Ziebland, A. Coulter, J. D. Calabrese, & L. Locock (Eds.), *Understanding and using health experiences: Improving patient care*. Oxford: Oxford University Press.

Rey, P. J., & Boesel, W. E. (2014). The web, digital prostheses and augmented subjectivity. In D. L. Kleinmann & K. Moore (Eds.), *Routledge Handbook of Science, Technology and Society* (pp. 173–188). Abingdon: Routledge.

Roberts, C., Mackenzie, A., & Mort, M. (2019). *Living data: Making sense of health biosensing*. Bristol: Bristol University Press.

Tamminem, S., & Deibel, E. (2018). *Recoding life: Information and the biopolitical*. London: Routledge.

Tan, S. S.-L., & Goonawardene, N. (2017). Internet health information seeking and the patient-physician relationship: A systematic review. *Journal of Medical Internet Research, 19*(1), e9.

Thompson, T. L., Parrott, R., & Nussbaum, J. F. (Eds.). (2011). *The Routledge Handbook of Health Communication*. New York: Routledge.

Ziebland, S., & McPherson, A. (2006). Making sense of qualitative data analysis with illustrations from the DIPEx project. *Medical Education, 40*, 405–414.

Ziebland, S., & Wyke, S. (2012). Health and illness in a connected world: How might sharing experiences on the Internet affect people's health. *The Millbank Quarterly, 90*(2), 219–249.

7

Traversing the Online Landscape: A Remote Indigenous Community Perspective

Kishan Kariippanon and Kate Senior

Introduction

This chapter is dedicated to a theoretical appreciation of Aboriginal ways in navigating the Knowledge Landscape (KL) through a case study. With the generous contributions of our study participants from North East Arnhem Land, we map the KL that concerns health and wellbeing. A particular attention is given to the co-existence and a potential dialogue between two distinct epistemologies: the Western biomedical model and traditional health and wellbeing practices of the Indigenous KL.

K. Kariippanon (✉)
School of Health and Society, The University of Wollongong, Wollongong, NSW, Australia
e-mail: kishan@uow.edu.au

K. Senior
School of Humanities and Social Sciences, University of Newcastle, Newcastle, NSW, Australia
e-mail: kate.senior@newcastle.edu.au

A. L. Svalastog et al. (eds.), *Navigating Digital Health Landscapes*, Health, Technology and Society, https://doi.org/10.1007/978-981-15-8206-6_7

KL is defined as a three-dimensional knowledge distribution in both offline and online environments. This chapter begins with a map of the offline context, a region rich in natural and cultural history, with a significant geographical contribution to the political, economic and societal diversity and wealth of the Australian nation. We ask the reader to consider that there are not one but two different landscapes for stakeholders, an Indigenous landscape and that landscape occupied by healthcare professionals, policy makers and health services administrators, but that these two spaces may interact.

The aim of the chapter is to describe this map and draw from it the complexity of Indigenous health and wellbeing (Bodeker and Kariippanon 2020) and to develop strategies that can help health professionals, policy makers and Indigenous users to navigate a commonly relevant landscape with shared meaning and integration.

Point of Departure: What Is the Landscape? Who Are Remote Indigenous Australians? What Is the Health Status of Indigenous People?

A dyadic relationship between the use of the term *Land* and *Landscapes* is conceptualised and used in this chapter and requires clarification. The term Land refers to the breadth and complexity of Indigenous knowledges embedded in the sea, the land and the skies that carry the narratives along with the songlines, the ceremonies and the cultural continuity of Indigenous communities, globally. Landscape then is a term used to describe both the Land and the intercultural subjectivities that co-exist between the non-Indigenous imagination, her structures and Indigenous knowledges as a result of colonisation and globalisation. This landscape includes the way the Aboriginal community in this region use the Internet and social media.

The landscape that forms the backdrop for this chapter is the harsh, often difficult-to-access and extremely remote context of the top end of the Northern Territory of Australia. This landscape is home to communities or towns of mostly Aboriginal Australians, living remotely relative to urban centres. These towns are often separated by great distances and extremely poor roads and are subject to isolation during the wet season, which can extend from November to April. Many of these communities lie within the Arnhem Land Reserve, which is only accessible to non-Aboriginal people through a special permit issued by the Indigenous Land Council or Traditional Owner. Many of the Aboriginal people living in the towns in these regions are close to their traditional lands, and since the 1970s, some families have decided to leave the towns and build small communities on their ancestral lands. These communities, known as outstations (Petersen and Myers 2016), often have very small populations and may lack a range of essential services including electricity, water and sewerage. Access to phone and Internet networks is non-existent. Residents of outstations, however, describe significant health and wellbeing benefits derived from being close to their land and their ancestors and from the opportunity to hunt and gather food (Senior et al. 2018).

The health status of Aboriginal people in the region is poor and characterised by chronic disease and premature adult mortality (Burns et al. 2019). In remote areas, Aboriginal people are more likely to report having heart disease and are twice as likely to have diabetes compared to those living in non-remote areas (28% and 15%, respectively) (Drew et al. 2018). These diseases are often described as 'lifestyle diseases', being influenced by the choices an individual makes regarding such things as diet, exercise and cigarette smoking.

Children suffer from a range of infectious and parasitic diseases, including scabies, and middle ear infections (Burns et al. 2019). These conditions can have long-term effects on an individual's future health and wellbeing. For example, chronic ear infections affect a child's ability to participate at school. However, many positive aspects of community life, including strong social cohesion, and the strength of family groups have a strong influence on the perception of wellbeing based on the collective reflexivity of a given community (Senior et al. 2018).

Service provision to all communities (both towns and outstations) is often extremely difficult and expensive, especially during the wet season. Often, even when communities have health facilities, it can be very difficult to ensure adequate levels of staffing. For example, a purpose-built clinic in one of the larger communities was criticised as failing to respond to emergencies and only providing painkillers due to low staffing levels (Bardon 2018). Under these circumstances, the case for health support and health information, which are accessible digitally, becomes compelling.

In terms of the digital landscape, access is extremely variable. Some of the larger communities, which have been given the status of growth towns with strategic importance by the Northern Territory Government, have very good Internet access, but smaller communities and outstations may have no access at all (Vodic, Senior, Dwyer and Szybiak 2012). People's access to the Internet, however, is also problematic and almost entirely dependent on mobile phones. This is similar to the situation in many Aboriginal communities in the region (Senior, Helmer and Chenhall 2017).

The purpose of this chapter is to describe the potential for, and challenges of, the Indigenous online health landscape. The authors will then discuss the assumptions made about users from a remote digital landscape and the transmission of health information to Indigenous people with the expectation of behaviour change and improvements on their general health status. Finally, we propose a collaborative method, which frames the anthropologist as designer, and argue for the role of design anthropologist for online and mobile technology-driven interventions.

The Use of Technology in the Indigenous Health Landscape

The rapid growth of Internet, mobile technology, wireless connectivity and the ease of use of social media sites such as Facebook, Twitter, Instagram, YouTube and the relatively newer Snapchat and WhatsApp have impacted the way people communicate and consume media (Carlson and Frazer 2018). On these digital platforms, storytelling, knowledge exchange, maintenance of cultural identity and challenging and negotiating mainstream projections of the Indigenous identity are prevalent in communities worldwide (Airhihenbuwa et al. 2013; Carlson and Frazer 2018; Diamond and Starks 2018).

Facebook and YouTube are now ubiquitous in remote Australian communities, and the skills of users continue to develop amongst people who often face difficulties in accessing offline institutional settings for education, health services and social welfare. The success of these forms of social media is due to their ability to be fluid, flexible and adaptable to the changing landscape from both a social and technological standpoint especially on a global scale. The agile nature of social media is bolstered by the power of real-time data and continuous testing. Improvements are made through control systems and feedback loops that gauge engagement and the way users create, consume and share media whilst communicating with each other in the online world (Holsapple et al. 2018).

Social media such as Facebook and YouTube have almost universal adoption, even in the remotest areas of the Northern Territory (Kariippanon and Senior 2017). The utilisation of social media and mobile technology is prefaced by the assumption that technology in general is meaningful to Indigenous people. As a result, many health organisations targeting specific segments of society have often resorted to social media and mobile technology use to engage the hard-to-reach population of Aboriginal and Torres Strait Islanders. The Indigenous people of Australia are among the highest adopters of social media in the country, with about 60% of Facebook users compared to 42% in the non-Indigenous population (Hefler et al. 2019). For example, Hefler et al. (2019) found a range of content from this population with common health-related topics such as nutrition, exercise, mental health and tobacco cessation being discussed. This is more often due to the visually prominent work such as anti-tobacco, nutrition and anti-bullying campaigns by health promotion and social marketing professionals both online and offline.

Reluctance to Engage in Health-Seeking Behaviour: Indigenous Health in Indigenous Hands

In 2003, Senior explored how people in a remote Aboriginal community in Arnhem Land valued health and how willing they were to take responsibility for maintaining or improving their health status. The insights from three years of ethnographic research demonstrate an extremely complex set of beliefs and practices regarding health. These include an abiding belief in health being influenced by factors that are beyond an individual's control, including both diseases brought to the community by Europeans (and sometimes death caused by sorcery) (Senior 2003). Death or illness caused by sorcery could be the result of a ritual transgression, but could also be caused by malicious spirits. A sorcerer's cures could accidentally hit the wrong person or could jump generations. So some forms of illness and even death were often considered arbitrary and impossible to prevent. Under such circumstances, public health advice to eat less fat and sugar or give up smoking appeared to be a waste of time (Senior 2003).

Although some people advocated for the use of the community clinic to maintain health and to control the effects of chronic disease, others were adamant that they did not want to engage with the health system. 'If they find something wrong with you, they will cut you up and then you will be dead', expressed one man echoing the sentiment of many. Screening and diagnosis were considered the first step in a series of undesirable events, which culminated in a person dying in a hospital far from their family and country (Senior 2003).

Another commonly expressed sentiment was that concern about health and longevity were concepts that were considered by Indigenous people as the obsessions of Europeans.

A sense of fatalism, fear of the consequences of engaging with health services and perceptions that a preoccupation with health is a peculiarity to Europeans contributed to an overall reluctance to engage in health-seeking behaviour. Coupled with the nature of sporadic health education by clinical staff, this creates a perception that the clinic staff may 'get cross' or blame an individual for their ill health and the fact that by the time a person entered a clinic, their conditions were so advanced that their fears of dying alone in the hospital were entirely justified.

There is a sense, however, that these attitudes may be changing. People in communities are acutely aware of premature adult mortality, the seemingly endless succession of funerals and the fact that there are very few people over the age of 60 (particularly men) left in remote Aboriginal communities. Such high mortality rates have profound effects on family wellbeing and community cohesion and impacts on the leadership at both religious and non-religious levels.

A health information kiosk in one of the communities was one of the most frequently used booths of its type in the country (Smith et al. 2016). Some communities have also been active in creating their health promotion material, about the importance of drinking water over a soft drink and eating fresh fruit and vegetables with media and film. Other people comment that they are worried about chronic disease, particularly smoking-related illnesses, and that they have used the Internet to find out information to help their families, but that there is so much information available that they don't know where to start (Senior et al. 2018).

A range of online discussions amongst Indigenous social media users in the Northern Territory was studied by Hefler et al. (2019). They covered health-related topics such as mental health, nutrition, exercise and tobacco cessation, a result of the influence of online and offline health promotion and social marketing activities. In addition to this, a broad discussion of the social determinants of health is reflected in discussions and reflections on the importance of preserving and maintaining culture, language, connection to the land and the reinforcement of Indigenous identity (Hefler et al. 2019).

The technology houses the ability to create media, which is then followed by sharing with online social networks. The interactions assessed by Hefler et al. (2019) were mostly gauged with counting 'likes', but online posts may often elicit comments on stories and metaphors related to health that celebrates the Indigenous epistemology and knowledge. According to Torres Strait Islander scholar, Professor Martin Nakata, knowledge construction is embedded in a variety of ways such as 'storytelling, memory making, narrative art and performance; in cultural and social practices, of relating to kin, of socializing children in ways of thinking [and] transmitting knowledge' (Kariippanon and Senior 2018, p. 34). Traditionally, Indigenous people create art and songlines and communicate through ceremonial practice as a traditional method of knowledge construction and dissemination (Morphy 1994, 2009). The use of mobile and Internet technology along with social media accelerates what is already an Indigenous practice of knowledge sharing through a wide variety of media.

In 2013–2014, Kariippanon conducted a study to explore the interactions between a remote Indigenous community and technology in the Northern Territory of Australia (Kariippanon and Senior 2017). This study revealed important insights into how digital public health interventions were perceived. The potential of digital public health interventions was often limited by a lack of dialogue between the health services and the target audience. Health service providers discreetly fear online discussions, as they may provide an uncensored platform for critique, which may in turn hurt their reputation as a leading health service provider (Kariippanon and Senior 2018).

The Use of Social Media in Indigenous Communities as a Familiar and Utilitarian Landscape

The high uptake and adoption of mobile phone among Indigenous Australians were studied across remote communities in the Northern Territory (Brusse et al. 2014; Hefler et al. 2019; Vodic et al. 2012). Mobile phones were the most adopted form of ICT among young people, which, according to Brusse et al. (2014), surpassed television, video games and another form of technological access to the Internet. The novelty and user-friendliness of social media and new-generation smartphones counter language barriers and enable Indigenous people to access the Internet, for recreation, to strengthen familial ties and clan relations and to subsequently engage in the global economy (Kariippanon and Senior 2017). Customarily, all purchased items and objects of ownership were shared amongst close kin and members of the household; in contrast to this rule, however, the mobile phone refused to part from the hands of the owner.

Parents, however, were generally accustomed to sharing their mobile phones and iPads as toys for toddlers and children. The older generation have become fluent with their use of mobile phones and played video games on tiny screens. A new culture of consumerism (Arnould and Thompson 2018) had created a yearning to own mobile phones, to use technology to talk to relatives in another community and to listen to songs and consume various types of media and apps downloaded from an online store (Bronwyn Carlson 2019). The words of Appadurai accurately reflected the context: 'if a global cultural system is emerging, it is filled with ironies and resistance, sometimes camouflaged as passivity and a bottomless appetite, for things Western' (1996, p. 29).

Limited opportunities and employment pathways were compensated with the ownership of things: mobile phone, video games, music and social media. The paucity of life for Indigenous people, in terms of materiality as well as opportunities, stands in stark contrast against the world of the non-Aboriginal residents and demonstrated in the difference of conditions between the geographically close Non-Indigenous and Indigenous towns. The town centre was purpose built for non-Indigenous residents with a BMX track, an 18-hole golf course, an Olympic-size swimming pool, two gymnasiums, a patrolled beach, two squash courts, three tennis courts, a basketball court, a mountain bike track, several parks and playground equipment. Unfortunately, the grand design for the Indigenous community bore no similarity to their non-Indigenous neighbours. Therefore, it seemed that mobile phones and social media were the most convenient and somewhat affordable tools that created engaging social and economic pathways for the Aboriginal community to connect to the global world and to share their stories and promote their identity.

On an individual level, the ownership of a mobile phone conferred an identity that set a person (in this community) apart and enabled them to differentiate themselves in a globalised climate from the traditional communal social structures (Schein 1999). As the acquisition of most material objects for the average person was out of economic reach, the acquisition of mobile phones became a way of constituting selfhood against the communalism that some resisted (Schein 1999). The global consumer culture aimed to cultivate individualism and created an 'aura of individuality by offering tantalizing objects and media products to be manipulated in the production of selves' (Schein 1999, p. 367).

Health Promotion and Online Behaviour Change Efforts

In recent years, the adoption of social media and mobile phones has become a coveted tool by both Indigenous and non-Indigenous, non-governmental and governmental health services (Brusse et al. 2014; B Carlson, Farelly, Frazer, and Borthwick 2015; Kral 2014; Owiny, Mehta and Maretzki 2014; Kate Senior et al. 2017). The assumptions made by service providers on the applicability of their technology are often made on the basis of scant evidence (Kral 2014). For example, Brusse et al. (2014) argue that mobile phones and social media enabled young people's utilisation of new technology to access health information and advocate for their health needs. It has also been assumed that there would be an online movement amongst peers (Kral 2010, 2011), to amplify a stand against bullying and sexting, as well as lateral violence in Aboriginal communities (B Carlson et al. 2015; Langton 2008). In Brusse et al. (2014) mobile technology and social media were claimed to be highly useful in health promotion in remote communities, particularly for engagement and health education. Despite these reports and studies, the typical insight of all these findings are that there hasn't been any change in health outcomes for Aboriginal and Torres Strait Islander in Australia, as mentioned in the recent Closing the Gap Report (Gannon 2018).

Is it possible that technology is not the answer or that engagement measured by Facebook 'likes', for example, is not a suitable proxy for individual or community empowerment? The Ottawa Charter for Health Promotion endorses 'empowerment' as a tool to promote health which was aimed at encouraging people to 'take control' (Thompson et al. 2018) of their lives and foster healthy communities. However, the work of some researchers in Indigenous health explains that the enabling technological features (Christie 2005) of social media and mobile technology are potentially lacking in sensitivity to Aboriginal ways of knowledge construction and communication (Vass et al. 2011) and as such the potential of empowerment through meaningful engagement is reduced. It is the method of delivery and the lack of engagement with the end user's knowledge landscape that pertains to lack of sensitivity and not the technology itself.

Technology-enabled empowerment and self-help formulas came into co-existence in contemporary public health practice with the assumption that certain technologies (i.e. Internet, social media and mobile phones) could break through and intervene directly with individuals and groups in the name of health promotion (Lock and Nguyen 2018). This imagined practice of empowerment took shape through sharing scientific knowledge in simplistic ways utilising different forms of media broadcasted on social media sites, such as YouTube, Facebook and Twitter, and something through the use of mobile health apps (Dingwall et al. 2015).

Those who promoted this process, however, refused to acknowledge the complexity of public health's biomedical viewpoints and assumed that Indigenous people have a similar epistemology to Western culture (Lea 2005). Healthcare professionals often deduced that the absence of healthy behaviours in remote Indigenous community members is due to a lack of *information*, an opinion that frustrated the agency of Indigenous people whose sophisticated *knowledge* of medicine, health and sorcery (Vass et al. 2011) were not included in the conversation.

According to Lea (Lea 2005), new technology was utilised as the 'new microscope', and the premise was that if people could see the germs, they would begin to believe in the Western biomedical model. More than a decade later, this practice of 'showing' equals 'believing' is dominating the online digital knowledge landscape, rationalising with Indigenous people while ignorant to Indigenous knowledge systems. Similarities could be drawn into the idea that if Indigenous people watched their brother rap or talk about healthy lifestyles on social media and mobile phones, the health-promoting messages would be easily accepted and adopted. Variables such as ease of use, perceived relevance and visual appeal were perceived as a proxy for Indigenous people's acceptance of

Western interventions (Dingwall et al. 2015). Dingwall et al. (2015) drew on these variables as part of an evaluation of an e-mental health training course that showed a disconnect between service providers' use of digital tools despite their perceived knowledge and confidence and its deployment in their professional context. This is possibly due to the lack of pull from the consumers for this type of intervention.

This non-technological approach has support from people who have had extensive experience working in communities; for example, Sean, a community development worker for a young parent programme in the region, was an advocate for the face-to-face method of engagement. He acknowledged Indigenous theories of communication (Marika, Ngurruwutthun and White 1992; Marika and Isaacs 1995; Yunupingu and Muller 2009) that prioritised reciprocity, respect, avoidance of conflict and a non-argumentative discussion. He suggested that the best way for the community was the:

> Door to door, sit down, sit in a group, have a cup of tea, talk to people, that's always been the most effective, because it comes back to that relationship building and that trust and you don't get that one through a phone or computer or some automated voice telling a story.

In a global context where non-Indigenous people were more likely to 'Google' their health and wellbeing concerns before consulting a physician (Feinberg et al. 2015), a different scenario is captured in the remote digital Indigenous landscape. Indigenous people did not use technology to identify symptoms or conditions that explained or provided a rigid frame to their health and wellbeing status based on a foreign concept. Instead of being locked down into a discourse of cause and effect, health is reterritorialised into a domain where the collective life of the community places the emphasis on sharing/family/community/material resource/wellbeing (Chenhall and Senior 2018). Having come from a history of colonisation and the loss of kin through disease and premature death, the oppression of some Missionaries who attempted to curtail expression of tradition and Indigenous identity, the celebration of 'being', practicing culture and 'living' together has been reterritorialised as being healthy and well.

The use of mobile technology and online applications as an economic rationale to health services provision is understandable, but the behavioural aspects of Indigenous people towards technology as culturally blank or as an intermediary between the agentic self and Western medicine exclude an equal dialogue between the two distinct knowledge landscapes and ways of being. The push from health promotion to enable Indigenous people to take personal responsibility for their health without much consideration of the barriers and sufficient acknowledgement of a colonial past has resulted in a distrust of the health system (Chenhall and Senior 2018). Against a backdrop of a complex belief in the origins of health and illness which is interwoven with a knowledge of sorcery (Veronese et al. 2019), Indigenous and non-Indigenous knowledge landscapes are at opposite sides of an informal negotiation of validity and rigour (between Western medicine and traditional medicine) instead of a collaborative and empowering dialogue.

The draw-card of visual-based learning and the use of digital technology as a carrier pigeon is still a phenomenon that is poorly understood (Dingwall et al. 2015). We argue that technology is perceived as valuable to Indigenous users, for not only its excellent graphics and user-friendly interface but for its ability to put the user first in the design phase. The product grows and expands around the user, which is a process of engagement and person-centred design that remains challenging to implement in the current health promotion context.

Health service providers perceive that Indigenous people are more receptive to technology-based interventions and have brought a degree of infiltration of digital health promotion programmes into the lives of Indigenous people. As health service providers grasp onto tools which might possibly assist to engage a hard-to-reach population in order to reduce the inequality between Indigenous and non-Indigenous health status, a demarcation between what is valid knowledge (Western biomedical model) and cultural practice becomes unintentionally drawn. This breaches any attempt at reducing the different forms of inequality between Indigenous and non-Indigenous people.

This method of information exchange or health education could be seen as a top-down post-colonial approach. There has been no evidence of the use of person-centred design in the process of app development, nor the creation of feedback loops between users and app programmers to allow the resource to evolve and change to suit the needs of a user. In an online world competing for user attention and engagement, such basic health applications may struggle to compete with other online game applications, or social media platforms such as Facebook, Instagram and YouTube. The design characteristics of mHealth applications tend to replicate offline resources and face-to-face interactions. The process is not holistic. It splices the human experience of health, illness and wellbeing into a disease-based engagement made up of silos. It forces the user to self-diagnose or identify by a label, that is, chronic disease or mental health, before he or she can express their understanding of their world and aspire towards their definition of health and wellbeing.

The Need for Design Anthropology to Engage in the Digital Knowledge Landscape Architecture

The purpose of design anthropology in navigating the digital landscape is to produce and share knowledge that is comprehensible, manageable and meaningful (Fries 2019). Design anthropology aims to bridge two different knowledge landscapes—that of the user and the designer. The general perspective on users is that they do not necessarily have the tools to articulate relationships, values, conflicts or tensions and transactions in their quotidian ways of knowing and being (Gunn and Donovan 2012). The involvement of design anthropologists in the development of digital knowledge artefacts as part of a seamless offline/online landscape primarily pertains to developing the anthropological capacities in people, as users. By doing this, we expect to reframe the relationship between the designer and user, the researcher and the designer or even the organisation with their community of interest—all of whom are somewhat involved in this process. Understanding what different stakeholders want and need through anthropological methods such as ethnography and applying theory to the discourse to map people's perspective, fears and values are part of a process that is cohesive instead of a top-down expert-led approach.

To foster a mutually beneficial and engaging relationship between the many stakeholders and to validate assumptions, ethnographic observations can be a form of engagement and transitional practice. This active practice of ethnography enables a process of mutual learning with a multiplicity of social actors and closes the gap between observation and understanding. The role of the design anthropologist is to capture the sophisticated ways of knowing and doing of the user even though the users are the experts of their knowledge landscape. This process essentially occurs before assisting the user in making their understandings present to the designer (Leach 2010).

Converging Efforts on the Ground

There are three domains where anthropologist and designers converge. The first is where a theoretical contribution rather than design is prominent (dA). The anthropologist dictates the design process by adopting theoretical underpinnings, where design itself becomes the subject of anthropological study.

When the fieldwork of designers dominates the engagement of users (Da), the framing and/or the creation of a meaningful problem is developed with a problem-oriented design approach. Here the user, the community and the diverse stakeholders are not engaged and included in the problem-framing stage of the design journey. The anthropologist, however, is engaged to conduct ethnographic studies for establishing design requirements.

When a project involves both the design and anthropology in equal power structures (DA), each being able to learn from each other (Halse 2008), a different process occurs: a method commonly known in the entrepreneurial technoscape as user persona development, where narratives of the user are co-created in partnership. As a result, instead of a cycle of data gathering, testing and refinement based on functionality and aesthetics (problem-oriented design approaches), an approach to reframing the inter-relationship between the stakeholders, the cultural nuances and the environment occurs. In this type of convergence, the design anthropologist is supported to engage with the landscape (social, cultural, environment, digital) where a problem is not always obvious, recognised or acknowledged. This is a common phenomenon where the design anthropologist is faced with emergent situations, where design is nurtured rather than enacted from a lens of functionality and aesthetics (Kjaersgaard 2011).

Thinking Outside the Prototype Box to Provotypes

The user-centred design process often overlooks the opportunities that prototyping has to offer in establishing a connection between past and current behaviour or perspectives as well as future possibilities in integrating Indigenous health knowledge with Western constructs. Instead of only viewing prototypes as preliminary design solutions, one could think from a standpoint of provoking reflections to encourage reflexive users and designers to question existing practices and examine assumptions. This is termed by Mogensen (1994) as 'provotypes'. As a result of this, the focus shifts from not only making improvements on the physical or visual forms of the prototype to provide future solutions, but the designer with the help of anthropology becomes a conduit or enabler of creative pathways and improvisation (Ingold and Hallam 2007 in Gunn and Donovan 2012).

Engaging users and designers with a design anthropologist requires moving beyond information or data provision about the user to the designer or the developments of appropriate methods to including users in the design process as experts of their 'domain'. This interaction of design anthropology with users and designers is neither one that functions as a mediator—to facilitate competing interests and tensions arising from different world views or to find a compromise. The tools provided by anthropology creates a space to actively deal with the practices, agendas, expectations and contexts of both use and design by 'framing and challenging understandings within and the relations between them' (Kjaersgaard and Otto 2012, p. 187 in Gunn and Donovan 2012).

Reflecting the Indigenous Knowledge Landscapes in a Digital Context

Participatory design is focused on developing methods for Indigenous users to elaborate on their needs in the design process as experts of their own 'world' (Da). Including within this participatory design process an anthropological (DA) approach unravels the whys and the potential use of feedback loops that are meaningful to an Indigenous user. This process allows for the digital landscape to be constructed by framing and challenging understandings between the designer, the user and health services. The design anthropologist in this research area is also aware and has the tools to contextualise health services, the agenda of health promotion programmes and the relations between the designers and users. The framing and challenging happens upstream as well, towards the health services in context of the reality of the user and their priorities in health and wellbeing.

The process of migrating Indigenous knowledge landscape into the online context involves a form of fieldwork that engages differently in order to 'provoke action, elicit insight and challenge assumptions' (Kjaersgaard and Otto 2012 in Gunn and Donovan 2012, p. 187). The examples below unpack the differences between expert-led design, participatory design and design led by anthropology or people-centred design. The following section expands on the elements of these three methods of design and points the reader to the deficiencies in the first two methods and the strengths of the design led by anthropology.

Expert-Led Design

The fieldworker describes the world and practice of users in ethnographic tones. The focus is to provide information to the designer on the user's knowledge and their social interactions and landscape. The outcome of their ethnography is data, representation and requirements (Fig. 7.1).

The user and designer work together by incorporating user skills and knowledge. The focus is to get to a prototype through collaboration and

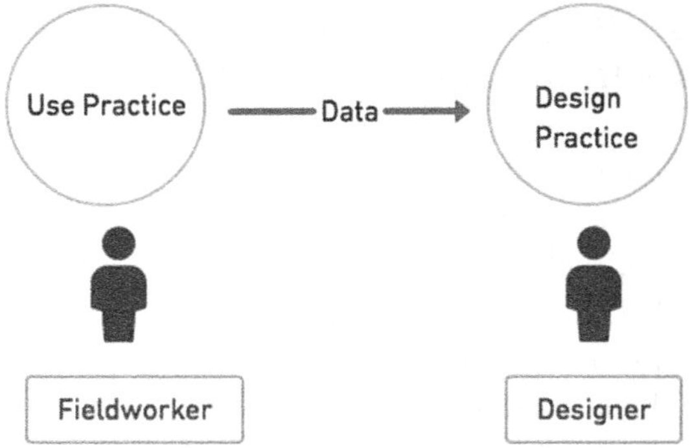

Fig. 7.1 Participatory design. (Source: Mette Kjaersgaard (Gunn and Donovan 2012))

prototyping. The ethnographer may facilitate or mediate the process of interaction but at a mediocre level (Fig. 7.2).

People-Centred Design

The anthropologist reframes relations between use and design as provocateur. The anthropologist understands and maps the intersection of context and practice of the user and the designer facilitates multiple stakeholders' reflections (Fig. 7.3).

In summary, people-centred design does not only engage in this process of online knowledge landscape construction with the lens of the users as its object but includes the health services context and practices through 'conceptualizing and re-conceptualizing relations between these domains' (Kjaersgaard and Otto 2012 in Gunn and Donovan 2012, p. 187). Several limitations to this final method come to mind, as the authors reflect on the many ways anthropology is done on the ground and how kinship relations and project management can be in tension. Stakeholders, contracts and final reports often skew the potential sustainability of a project, and we call on practitioners to apply a critical reflexive approach to both design and implementation. More information of collective reflexivity in health interventions is available in Kariippanon, Gordon, Jayasingle and Gurruwiwi (2020).

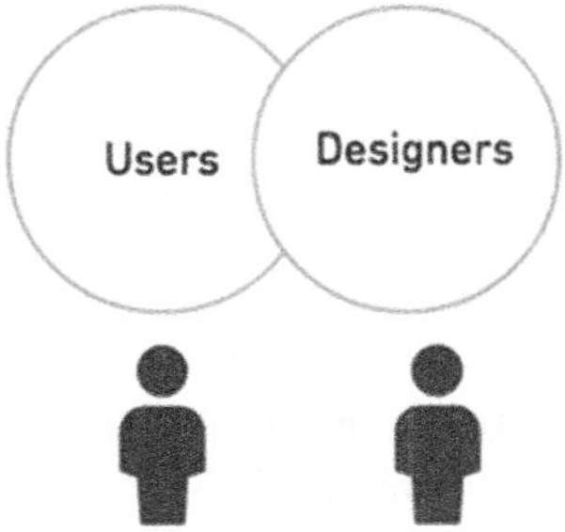

Fig. 7.2 Users and designers. (Source: Mette Kjaersgaard (Gunn and Donovan 2012))

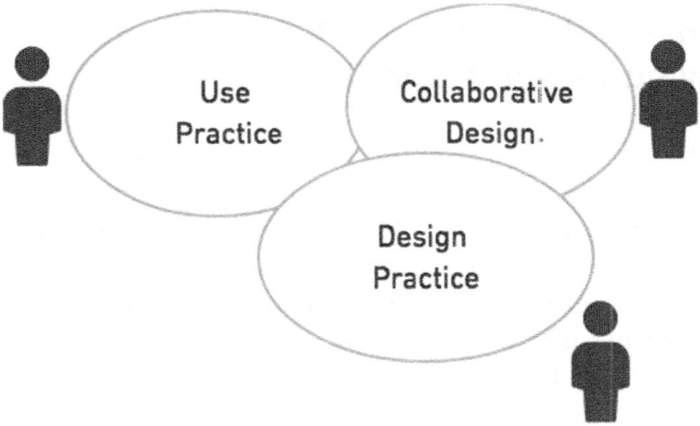

Fig. 7.3 People-centred design. (Source: Mette Kjaersgaard (Gunn and Donovan 2012))

Conclusion

This chapter has explored the problematisation of digital knowledge landscape construction that excludes the perspectives of Indigenous knowledges by focusing only on the potential of mobile technology and social media to transmit a very specific form of 'knowledge' to the user. Both the user and the designer have very little exchange about their experience and their different ways of knowing and being. The current digital knowledge landscape utilises technology with design processes that seek to change behaviour and increase awareness without acknowledging the complex understanding of health and wellbeing from an Indigenous standpoint, pushing the Western biomedical model at the cost of Indigenous pursuit for health and wellbeing.

Although there is an abundance of health information in the online world (Hefler et al. 2019), research has shown that Indigenous users are not able to navigate this maze of information to find the content that speaks to their culture, tradition and priorities of focusing on the wellbeing and solidarity of kin and clan (Kariippanon and Senior 2018), a content that would foster precisely those affordances outlined in Chap. 6.

Recommendations for Online Indigenous Knowledge Landscape Designers

Technology has the potential to overcome the problems of remoteness, distance and an unreliable workforce, but the information contained through such technology must be appropriate and sensitive. Health services designing online engagement platforms must not see technology as the hook to engage people with un-modified Western and biomedical concepts of health; rather there is a need to ensure innovation and deep understanding of both Indigenous knowledges and the Western biomedical model through integration and compromise. The design of future digital knowledge landscapes could benefit from an ethnographically informed process by drawing from local knowledge and opportunities for improving health outcomes and to use social media and mobile technology for reconciliation and co-design through conversation and collective reflexivity.

References

Airhihenbuwa, C. O., Ford, C. L., & Iwelunmor, J. I. (2013). Why culture matters in health interventions. *Health Education & Behavior, 41*(1), 78–84. https://doi.org/10.1177/1090198113487199.

Appadurai, A. (1996). *Modernity at large: Cultural dimensions of globalization*. Minnesota: University of Minnesota Press.

Arnould, E., & Thompson, C. (2018). *Consumer culture theory*. London: SAGE.

Bardon, J. (2018). National indigenous health staffing reaches crisis point as community relies on "Panadol clinic." *Australian Broadcasting Corporation*. Retrieved from https://www.abc.net.au/news/2018-10-28/national-indigenous-clinics-struggling-to-provide-care/10433716. Accessed 28 Oct 2019.

Bodeker, G., & Kariippanon, K. (2020). Traditional medicine: Indigenous health in indigenous hands. In *Oxford Research Encyclopedia of Global Public Health*. Oxford: Oxford University Press.

Brusse, C., Gardner, K., McAullay, D., & Dowden, M. (2014). Social media and mobile apps for health promotion in Australian indigenous populations: Scoping review. *Journal of Medical Internet Research, 16*(12), 280.

Burns, J., Drew, N., Elwell, M., Harford-Mills, M., Hoareau, J., Macrae, A., … Trzesinski, A. (2019). *Overview of aboriginal and Torres Strait islander health status 2015*. ECU Publications. Retrieved from http://www.healthinfonet.ecu.edu.au/uploads/docs/2015-overview.pdf

Carlson, B. (2019). *Love and hate at the cultural interface: Indigenous Australians and dating apps*. https://doi.org/10.1177/1440783319833181.

Carlson, B., & Frazer, R. (2018). *Social media mob: Being indigenous online*. Sydney: Department of Indigenous Studies, Macquarie University.

Carlson, B., Farelly, T., Frazer, R., & Borthwick, F. (2015). Mediating tragedy: Facebook, aboriginal peoples and suicide. *Australian Journal of Information Systems, 19*, 1–15.

Chenhall, R. D., & Senior, K. (2018). Living the social determinants of health: Assemblages in a remote aboriginal community. *Medical Anthropology Quarterly, 32*(2), 177–195. https://doi.org/10.1111/maq.12418.

Christie, M. (2005). Aboriginal knowledge traditions. *The Australian Journal of Indigenous Education, 34*, 61–66.

Diamond, K., & Starks, S. (2018). Social media for health in Nunavik. In H. Exner-Pirot, B. Norbye, & L. Butler (Eds.), *Northern and indigenous health and health care* (pp. 217–219) Retrieved from http://www.northernnursingeducation.com.

Dingwall, K., Puszka, S., Sweet, M., Mills, P., & Nagel, T. (2015). Evaluation of a culturally adapted training course in indigenous e-mental health. *Australian Psychiatry, 23*(6), 630–635. https://doi.org/10.1177/1039856215608282.

Drew, N., Anomie, Burns J., Burrow, S., Elwell, M., Fleay, J., … Trzesinski, A. (2018). *Overview of aboriginal and Torres Strait islander health status 2015*. ECO Publications. Retrieved from http://www.healthinfonet.ecu.edu.au/uploads/docs/2015-overview.pdf

Feinberg, I., Greenberg, D., & Frijters, J. (2015). *Understanding health information seeking behaviours of adults with low literacy, numeracy and problem solving skills: Results from the 2012 US PIAAC study.* Retrieved from https://static1.squarespace.com/static/51bb74b8e4b0139570ddf020/t/54da7889e4b004762df45b52/1423603849970/Feinberg_Greenberg_Frijters_PIAAC.pdf

Fries, C. J. (2020). Healing health care: From sick care towards Salutogenic healing systems. *Social Theory & Health, 18*(1). pp. 16–32.

Gannon, M. (2018). Indigenous health: Closing the gap-10 year review. *Australian Medicine, 30*(3), 25.

Gunn, W., & Donsovan, J. (Eds.). (2012). *Design anthropology*. London: Routledge.

Halse, J. (2008). *Design anthropology: Borderline experiments with participation, performance and situated intervention.* University of Copenhagen.

Hefler, M., Kerrigan, V., Henryks, J., Freeman, B., & Thomas, D. P. (2019). Social media and health information sharing among Australian Indigenous people. *Health Promotion International, 34*(4), 706–715.

Holsapple, C. W., Hsiao, S., & Pakath, R. (2018). Business social media analytics: Characterization and conceptual framework. *Decision Support Systems, 110*(August 2016), 32–45. https://doi.org/10.1016/j.dss.2018.03.004.

Ingold, T., & Hallam, E. (2007). Creativity and cultural improvisation: An introduction. In T. Ingold & E. Hallam (Eds.), *Creativity and cultural improvisation* (pp. 1–24). Oxford: Berg Publishers.

Kariippanon, K., & Senior, K. (2018). Re-thinking knowledge landscapes in the context of grounded aboriginal theory and online health communication. *Croatian Medical Journal, 59*(1), 33–38. https://doi.org/10.3325/cmj.2018.59.33.

Kariippanon, K., Gordon, R., Jayasinghe, L., & Gurruwiwi, G. (2020). Collective reflexivity in social marketing through ethnographic film-making: The Yolngu story of tobacco in Yirrkala, Australia. *Marketing Theory, 20*(1), 123–143.

Kjaersgaard, M. G. (2011). Between the actual and the potential: The challenges of design anthropology. University of Aarhus: Copenhagen.

Kjaersgaard, M., & Otto, T. (2012). Anthropological fieldwork and designing potentials. In W. Gunn & J. Donovan (Eds.), Design and anthropology (pp. 177–191). Routledge. Ashgate, Surrey. UK.

Kral, I. (2010). *Plugged in: Remote Australian indigenous youth and digital culture.* Canberra: The Australian National University.

Kral, I. (2011). Youth media as cultural practice: Remote indigenous youth speaking out loud. *Australian Aboriginal Studies, 1*, 4.

Kral, I. (2014). Shifting perceptions, shifting identities: Communication technologies and the altered social, cultural and linguistic ecology in remote indigenous context. *The Australasian Journal of Anthropology, 25*(2), 171–189.

Langton, M. (2008). The end of big men politics. *Griffith Review, 22*, 48.

Lea, T. (2005). The work of forgetting: Germs, aborigines, and postcolonial expertise in the Northern Territory of Australia. *Social Science and Medicine, 61*(6), 1310–1319.

Leach, J. (2010). Intervening with the social? Ethnographic practice and Tarde's image of relations between subjects. In *The social after gabriele tarde: Debates and assessments* (pp. 191–207). London: Routledge.

Lock, M., & Nguyen, V.-K. (2018). *An anthropology of biomedicine* (2nd ed.). London: Wiley Blackwell.

Marika, W., & Isaacs, J. (1995). *Wandjuk Marika: Life story*. St Lucia: University of Queensland Press.

Marika, R., Ngurruwutthun, D., & White, L. (1992). Always together, YakaGana: Participatory research at Yirrkala as part of the development of a Yolngu education. *Convergence, 25*(1), 23.

Mogensen, P. (1994). *Challenging practice: An approach to cooperative analysis*. Aarhus: University of Aarhus.

Morphy, H. (1994). The interpretation of ritual: Reflections from film on anthropological practice. *Man, 29*(1), 117–146.

Morphy, H. (2009). *From dull to brilliant: The aesthetics of spiritual power*. Canberra: ANU Press.

Owiny, S., Mehta, K., & Maretzki, A. (2014). The use of social media technologies to create, preserve, and disseminate indigenous knowledge and skills to communities in East Africa. *International Journal of Communication, 8*, 14.

Petersen, N., & Myers, F. (2016). Outstations through art: Acrylic painting, self-determination and the history of the homelands movement in the Pintupi-Ngaanyatjarra lands. *Experiments in self-determination: Histories of the outstation movement in Australia*. ANU Press. https://doi.org/10.22459/esd.01.2016.08.

Schein, L. (1999). *Of cargo and satellites: Imagined cosmopolitanism* (Vol. 2). https://doi.org/10.1080/13688799989652.

Senior, K. (2003). *A Gudbala Laif?: Health and wellbeing in a remote aboriginal community – What are the problems and where lies the responsibility?* Canberra Australian National University.

Senior, K., Helmer, J., & Chenhall, R. (2017). 'As long as he's coming home to me': Vulnerability, jealousy and violence in young people's relationships in remote, rural and regional Australia. *Health Sociology Review, 26*(2), 204–218. https://doi.org/10.1080/14461242.2016.1157697.

Senior, K., Chenhall, R., Hall, J., & Daniels, D. (2018). Re-thinking the health benefits of outstations in remote indigenous Australia. *Health and Place, 52*(October 2017), 1–7. https://doi.org/10.1016/j.healthplace.2018.04.007.

Smith, K., Chenhall, R., McQuire, S. and Kowal, E., 2016. Digital Futures in Indigenous Communities: From Health Kiosks to Community Hubs. University of Melbourne.

Thompson, S. R., Watson, M. C., & Tilford, S. (2018). The Ottawa charter 30 years on: Still an important standard for health promotion. *International Journal of Health Promotion and Education, 56*(2), 1–12. https://doi.org/10.1080/14635240.2017.1415765.

Vass, A., Mitchell, A. and Dhurrkay, Y., 2011. Health literacy and Australian Indigenous peoples: an analysis of the role of language and worldview. *Health Promotion Journal of Australia, 22*(1), pp. 33–37.

Veronese, V., Clouse, E., Wirtz, A. L., Thu, K. H., Naing, S., Baral, S. D., et al. (2019). "We are not gays … don't tell me those things": Engaging 'hidden' men who have sex with men and transgender women in HIV prevention in Myanmar. *BMC Public Health, 19*(1), 1–12. https://doi.org/10.1186/s12889-018-6351-3.

Vodic, A., Senior, K., Dwyer, B., & Szybiak, P. (2012). A remote chance? Widening Participation of Remote Indigenous Students in the Northern Territory via ICTEnabled Learning. Charles Darwin University. Darwin. NT.

Yunupingu, D., & Muller, S. (2009). Cross cultural challenges for Indigenous Sea country management in Australia. *Australasian Journal of Environmental Management, 16*(3), 158–167.

8

Minute/s Work: The Participation of Digital Data Objects in the Conjuncture and Disjuncture of Policy and Care

Milena D. Bister

Introduction

It is Thursday morning about 9 a.m. when I accompany Nora, one of the support workers, on her walk through the therapeutic living community bringing a few residents the morning medication. Ms Meyer, a woman in her 70s, is sitting at one corner of the large table in the community's living room, cutting sheets of white paper. Nora approaches her with a small plastic cup filled with a dark liquid.

Nora (N) – Good morning, Ms Meyer! How are you?
Ms Meyer (MM) – Fine, thank you, Ms Konrad!
N – Did you sleep well?
MM – Yes, all fine.
N (while offering the cup) – Look, this is for you!
MM (shouting) – It kills me! I cannot have it!

M. D. Bister (✉)
Institute for European Ethnology, Humboldt University of Berlin, Berlin, Germany
e-mail: milena.bister@staff.hu-berlin.de

A. L. Svalastog et al. (eds.), *Navigating Digital Health Landscapes*, Health, Technology and Society, https://doi.org/10.1007/978-981-15-8206-6_8

N (calm) – Ms Meyer, it is yours.
MM (loud) – This is not for me!
N (insisting) – It is. Ms Meyer, this is your medication. Look, it's just a swig. *(Puts the cup on the table next to Ms Meyer.)*
MM (drinks it up and answers calmly and friendly) – Thank you for the sleeping draught, Ms Konrad.
N (takes the empty cup back) – Welcome. I'll see you later.

Ms Meyer continues slicing the paper. Nora discards the cup and leaves the room, seeking out the next resident on her list.

This chapter, embedded in the anthropology of science and technology, looks at how encounters in public community mental healthcare, such as the one between Nora and Ms Meyer, translate into entries in a digital documentation system, how the entries travel and in which kind of actions they again translate. As such, the chapter deals with particular navigations through the knowledge landscape in an institutional setting. It asks how care and policy are performed in material-semiotic practices that include digital systems. Throughout the analysis the digital documentation system will shape up as a micro-political technology that affects the relationship between agency, moral values and care. As such it is deeply implicated in the ways in which people living with a psychiatric diagnosis are governed.

My usage of the term "translation" emanates from actor-network theory within science and technology studies. A translation is a socio-material process that relates elements irrespective of their kind (be it categories, concepts, numbers, algorithms, people, bodies, things or institutions, for instance) and thereby temporarily ascertains their meaning in the continuous generation of what is made real (Latour 2005). In what follows, I will flesh out the different modes of translation that occur in community mental healthcare through digital documentation practices. My aim is to show how "data journeys" (Bates et al. 2016),[1]

[1] Bates et al. have developed the data journey methodology for the study of "Big Data" practices across different sites. Missing both the component of "Big Data" and the distribution across geographically remote sites in my study, I will show that their conceptual approach still works productively when applied to "small-scale" data practices within narrowly definable places. This emphasizes

here studied as translations from everyday activities into the digital system and onwards, simultaneously produce conjuncture (translations into sameness) and disjuncture (translations into difference) of policy and care in the everyday routines of the services.[2] These translations constitute the knowledge landscape between online and offline practices in community mental healthcare and simultaneously account for the movements and transformations of what counts as data in this very landscape. Through taking advantage of equivocation, we will see how these journeys are largely about workings of and with *minutes* as time values and as short accounts as much as about *minute* work in the sense of a task full of details and taxonomy.

In what follows, I first clarify the theoretical approach to care and policy and then briefly review the context of public community psychiatry in Germany. Next, I analyse the journeys of the digital data from creation to application, thereby highlighting the partiality, tentativeness and contextuality of the knowledge landscape. At the end of the chapter, I will finally discuss in which sense—and for whom—minutes and minuteness work.

Care-Policy

A substantial body of literature in anthropology and science and technology studies has brought out the ongoing, practical, material-semiotic features of care work (Estroff 1981; Desjarlais 1997; Biehl 2005; Pols 2006; Mol 2008; Mol et al. 2010; Pols 2012; Stevenson 2014). In this tradition, care (and so too healthcare) is comprised of emergent, situated and necessarily local knowledge practices which attend to and tackle with the ambivalent flows and relations of bodies, infrastructures, technologies and times. All these contributions deal with the often contradictory and ambivalent impact of policy on care practices. Thereby policy is predominantly treated as a public register of forms and regulations. Only in recent

---

the crucial need of deciding methodologically upon the scaling of the data journeys in the study of digital knowledge landscapes.

[2] Translation in this sense diverges from the usual meaning of the term in policy making. For an overview on different conceptual usages of the term, see Freeman (2009).

years an increasing number of scholars started to interrogate the conceptual boundary that separates policy and care in academic analysis (Levinson 2010; Shore et al. 2011; Freeman and Sturdy 2014; Law and Singleton 2014; Rodriquez 2014; Gill et al. 2017; Lydahl 2019). They foreground that policy and governance as much as care are enacted in practice and that both crisscross in the ways they articulate and perform values and norms, categories and classifications.

In the postscript to a special issue on care and policy practices, political scientist Richard Freeman explains why it is crucial to treat policy and care as strongly aligned practices:

> If care is a good thing, if we want to be sure of it when and where it's needed and not just as it might happen to be available, if we want to mitigate the risk of abuse with which it is associated, then it will require some policy framework or complement, whether formal or informal. Similarly, if policy is to serve any good and useful purpose, if it is to be realized effectively, it will be made and implemented carefully and caringly, painstakingly, with attention to detail and sensitive to relationships and circumstances. … [C]are and policy are enacted together, in sometimes complementary, sometimes contradictory but invariably uncertain ways. They are but different aspects of a single assemblage, something the actor-network theorist might call 'care-policy'. (Freeman 2017: 194)

Freeman, thus, points up the relatedness and interdependence of care and policy in practice. According to him the core distinction should not be drawn between the doing of policy and the doing of care, but between the different ways of knowing "care-policy" from behind a desk or in the field: "Care-policy *in the field* is addressed to the case with which it is immediately confronted; *in the office*, it is to the category or set in which the case must be placed" (Freeman 2017: 196, italics added). Freeman refers to that distinction as the "case/category problem". Documentation practices notably blur the distinction between the lived cases in the field and the (sets of) categories in the office. Documentation itself is a practice that occurs more often than not in office-like configurations that form part of the field. It converts life stories and daily life into (healthcare) cases that speak to the categories predefined by policy documents while codetermining their meaning and relevance in and for practice (Atkinson 1995; Barrett 1996; Berg 1996; Berg and Bowker 1997; Bowker and Star 1999; Hacking 2002).

German Public Community Psychiatry: Doing Presence

Before I explore the involvement of digital documentation in the assemblage of mental health "care-policy" in Berlin, I want to briefly sketch the situation of public community psychiatry in Germany. As demonstrated elsewhere, after the psychiatric reforms in West Germany in the 1970s and the re-unification of the two German states in 1989, community mental healthcare arose as an alternative for people with severe psychiatric diagnosis, who used to be typically referred to large asylums in remote places (Bister 2018). Now, they were classified as mentally disabled and entitled to benefits from the social integration services (*Eingliederungshilfe*) as defined by the German Code of Social Law (Bister forthcoming). In Berlin, this policy move resulted in setting up a public infrastructure of community services in the late 1990s, which slowly developed into a new territory for people classified as "chronically mentally ill" at the last turn of the millennium. In the analytic language of Ian Hacking, I have previously argued that "doing presence" was a central mode of making up the human kind of "the chronically mentally ill" in daily practice (Bister 2018). Doing presence was "all the work that went into making a client present in the services. Professional helpers, clients, their bodies, and biology were as much involved in this process as, for instance, forms, software, medication, and furniture such as chairs" (Bister 2018: 45). This chapter further scrutinizes the shaping of the clients' presence, this time through digital documentation practices and datafication.

My analysis builds on ethnographic research on knowledge practices in mental healthcare in Berlin in the years 2010–2017.[3] It deployed a range

[3] The two ethnographic projects, funded by the German research agency *Deutsche Forschungsgemeinschaft*, were "The Production of Chronicity in Mental Healthcare and Research in Berlin" (2010–2015, BE 3191/3–1) and "Mobilising Clinical Health Care: A Qualitative-

of methods including participant observation in four public community mental healthcare services in Berlin in the year 2013. These were a day care centre, a therapeutic living community, a sheltered workshop and a residential treatment centre. In this chapter I especially mobilize my research in the therapeutic living community (*Therapeutische Wohngemeinschaft* (TWG) in German), where I spent 67 hours over 10 days. The TWG opened in 1997 and was operated by a large German non-profit organization involved in social work for a range of target groups, including people with psychiatric diagnosis. The community was housed in a wing of a multi-storey apartment house in one of Berlin's districts that is known for its poor social structure. Thirteen residents lived here in single apartments. All of them held psychiatric diagnosis and were classified as mentally disabled. A few apartments provided a private kitchen, but most of the clients gathered for meals in the community kitchen next to the common living room. Staff members worked in shifts during day, evening and night. Usually, during a shift, one support worker was responsible for all residents. During day time he/she was supported by a colleague on intermediate duty. Ms Meyer was among the first clients who moved in. The supervisor of the living community[4] introduced Ms Meyer's case to me as prototypic for the deinstitutionalization programme: With the psychiatric diagnosis of paranoid schizophrenia, Ms Meyer had previously spent most of her life in the total institution of an asylum.

In Berlin, now, every district is required to provide a pre-defined variety of public community care facilities, which report to the Senate regularly. In the years of 2000–2019, the so-called Treatment and Rehabilitation Plan (*Behandlungs- und Rehabiliationsplan* (BRP) in German) was the central policy form for organizing, managing and controlling the care-policy in public community services. Developed in the 1990s, the BRP had been introduced as a cornerstone in transforming mental healthcare policy and has become the central technology for

Ethnographic Pilot Study About Health Care Practices in Psychiatric Home Treatment" (2016–2017, BI 1678/1–1). For further information, see www2.hu-berlin.de/sts/bister/

[4] The supervisor functioned as local manager of the TWG. Although her office was located in the same building but outside the facility, she was present all day and, as a professional social worker by training, engaged in some of the direct face-to-face work with residents.

implementing the principles of person-centred care. Person-centred care had been appraised as the most promising alternative to the historical modes of caring for the severely mentally ill in large, remote and closed institutions. (Bister forthcoming) The Federal Act of Participation (*Bundesteilhabegesetz*), which has been adopted in 2016 with regard to the UN Convention on the Rights of Persons with Disabilities, is now on its way to implementation. For community care in Berlin, new administrative arrangements and forms are currently being developed. The BRP will be replaced by a new policy tool in 2020.[5] For care-policy development and the evaluation of the newly introduced measures, it is therefore highly important to understand the small-scale dynamics of classification and digitalization which, although not prescribed by law, impact everyday life in community psychiatry and the ways in which clients are cared for.

Creating Minutes: Translating Action into Digital Data

Organizing (Principles of) Translations

Let us return to the interaction between the resident Ms Meyer and the support worker Nora at the beginning of the chapter. How did the interaction between the two women translate into the digital service documentation? The very short answer is that the support worker Nora pushed the keyboard button with the letter "x" and by that inserted it in a tiny column of a digital grid, which belonged to one of the registers of the electronic documentation record comprising Ms Meyer's case (Fig. 8.1). One line below she keyed in two letters that stood as an acronym for her name. Three lines further she inserted the number 12. The computer that facilitated this translation was located in the administration office on the

[5] These recent developments and transformations in Berlin are subject to the ethnographic research project "The Mobilization of Law Through /as Collectivization? Anti-Discrimination and Equality Law as Institutional and Political Practice" at the Humboldt-Universität zu Berlin, funded by the DFG; see www.euroethno.hu-berlin.de/

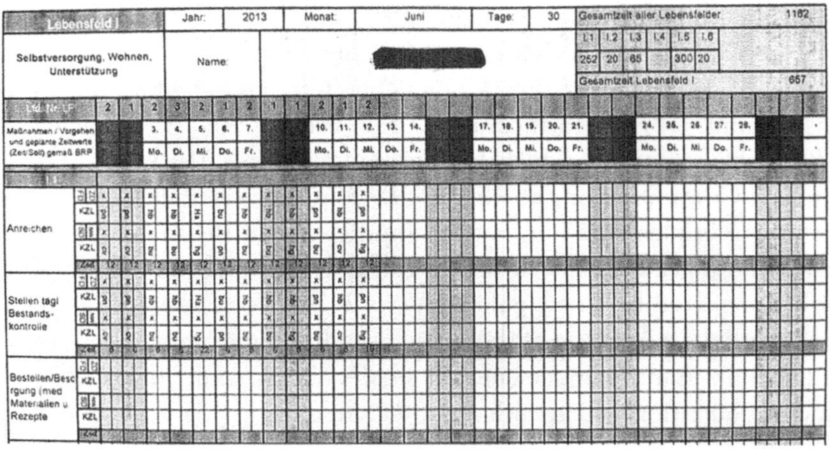

Fig. 8.1 Photo of the print-out of the register "area of life 1" as used in the therapeutic living community (top section)

middle floor of the living community. In this room, staff members coordinated transfers between the work shifts. Also, the binders for each resident were stored here. Whereas personal data of the clients, including their medication plans, were collected and assessed in these binders on paper, service provision and the client's activities were documented and assessed digitally. For this purpose, each client held an electronic record.

Noteworthy, neither electronic documentation nor the software was mandated by the municipality, which was the contracting body and financier of public community psychiatry. Instead, the system is an example of institutional self-governance: The management created it to support uniform documentation and to ensure comprehensible justifications for the scope of support work in the face of recurrent cuts in the budget due to steadily increasing numbers of benefit recipients in the whole municipal area.[6]

Usually, staff members followed the routine to start digital documentation about one or two hours before the end of their work shift. A common habit was to start with the documentation according to the location

[6] For a thoughtful discussion of current challenges within community psychiatry in Berlin, see Bieler and Klausner (2019).

of the residents' apartments, either with the clients who lived on the lowest or upper floor and subsequently moving through the levels. The move through the digital records of the clients hence approximates a passage through the building.

The basic structure of the digital system resembled the major categories of the BRP regarding rehabilitation goals. In the BRP, these goals were split into four "areas of life" (*Lebensfelder*): self-supply/housing (*Selbstversorgung/Wohnen*), recreational activities (*Tages-, Freizeit- und Kontaktgestaltung*), occupation (*Beschäftigung, Arbeit, Ausbildung*) and one residual category named "other impairments due to mental illness" (*Beeinträchtigungen aufgrund der psychischen Erkrankung, welche nicht eindeutig den Lebensfeldern I.-III. zuzuordnen sind*). In the system, a register was dedicated to each one of the areas. The rehabilitation goals of the BRP therefore configured what action had to be considered relevant to standard translation into the documentation system.

Translations into Numbers

Figure 8.1. shows the top of a print-out of the register for area 1. Line one indicates the year, 2013, and month, June, and the numbers of days in the month, 30. Line two gives the name of the register (in this case: self-supply/housing) and the name of the client. Below, two lines present the days of the month in a calendric fashion, numbered from 1 to 30, followed by the days of the week, Monday to Sunday. The columns of the weekends are highlighted. In the chart below, each column of a day is subdivided into two further columns, which give space for tick marks (e.g. of the letter "x") and initials of the different case workers who work in shift schedules. Taken together two columns stand for one day.

One task that has been assigned to area 1 is the administration of medication. In Ms Meyer's case it was subdivided into seven sections: giving meds, filling up the medication cassette, ordering medical material and prescriptions, control and supervision, handover of "When Required" medication,[7] medical consultations and body weight. These subsections

[7] "When Required" medication means that patients may decide upon the intake of the drug according to the circumstances.

were created according to the agreement in the BRP. Correspondingly, for instance, some clients were assisted in taking prescribed medication, while others were not. In Fig. 8.1 the time invested for giving meds (on the form in German *Anreichen*) was recorded with 12 minutes each day, the time for filling up the medication cassette (*Stellen, tägliche Bestandskontrolle*) with 6–22 minutes a day.

"12" was also the number that Nora entered in Ms Meyer's register of area 1. The systematic reappearance of this number as well as of the tick marks and initials conveys that data entry is obviously a highly standardized practice. Indeed, the question arises, how assistance is converted into numbers that represent minutes. How come that the interaction above was indexed by the time value of 12 minutes? How are minutes generated from activities as diverse as meals, medication, excursions, groups, individual meetings, personal hygiene or room maintenance? Let's stay with the example of giving meds. For this task, service managers have assigned 4 minutes. Three times 4 minutes make 12 minutes. In the figure above, staff members assisted the resident in getting his or her medication three times a day. That particular day, during her shift, Nora gave meds to Ms Meyer twice, in the morning, as noted, and again later about noon. Instead of typing in 8, for twice 4 minutes, she directly went for 12. Her colleague from the late shift therefore only had to enter a tick mark and her or his initials. Only if the quotidian routine was disrupted by irregular events such as hospital admissions or overnight stays outside the living community, the number required post hoc re-adjustment. During my participation in five documentation sessions of 13 clients each, this happened with two data entries only. Entering data was thus tantamount to walking the same way through the building every day. Exceptions of the routine required only one or two minor steps off the trail.

This was at least true for a huge number of tasks comprising the services. Excursions, for instance, were depicted with the standard of 30 minutes or waking someone in the morning with 5–15 minutes, irrespective of the actual duration of the events. Participation in therapeutic groups was sometimes also represented by a specified amount of time or, alternatively, calculated by dividing the duration of the group (e.g. 60 minutes) by the number of participants (e.g. 12 minutes in the case of a group of five people). Thus, different conventions and calculations led to the input values for the digital system, with the effects of decontextualizing the translated action and creating comparability of tasks between clients. In practice, the redundancy of data entry and the resulting regular visual pattern supported the experience of monotony that tired support workers in daily life when only little of the clients' capacities and difficulties changed over days and years. At least the daily routine creation of more or less defined minute values, which largely lacked the possibility of attributing residents any agency, conflicted with the support workers' objective of keeping the potential and self-efficacy of clients in focus.

Translations into Notes

Variation in entries was indeed rare. In the case of Ms Meyer the data entries varied most in the section relationship maintenance (*Beziehungspflege*), which was part of area 2, recreational activities. In Ms Meyer's case record, support workers inserted numbers in a range from 10 to 45 (minutes) per day. Instead of a tick mark, here, almost every one keyed in an exclamation mark, which was defined as the symbol to refer to free-text entries on a separate register. At the end of her work shift on the day recalled above, Nora, for example, entered the following minute to this free-text register: "Ms M was sitting in the living room till noon, painting. Largely calm". Familiar with the encounter of the two in the morning, we can speculate that some shouting was rather little, because Nora described Ms Meyer as "largely calm". Still, the message renders no bits of the interactions between her and Ms Meyer available as information and provides minimal indications of Ms Meyer's state, if at all. For example, the minute misses any reference to the cutting of paper with which Ms Meyer was occupied in the morning. The entry of Nora's colleague, who took over the late shift on the same day, reads completely differently:

> Ms M loudly refused to go to the toilet with the employee of the nursing service. I supported the nursing service. Ms M then went to the toilet. When I came to her apartment later, … Ms M seemed much calmer. She was friendly when I spoke to her. I brought her dinner into the apartment

> and hung up the laundered bed linen. It smelled very strong in the room. Anka *[of the nursing service, added]* came to the late shift, put the blanket in the washing machine again and turned it on.

This minute reflects what staff members deemed a major concern with Ms Meyer, mainly her reactions to unknown or less known employees of the nursing service, an additional social welfare service that supported nursing tasks for her. Basically, Ms Meyer did not accept anyone from the nursing service but Anka, a long-term employee whom she knew very well, to carry out activities that were generally considered intimate, such as going to the bathroom or changing incontinence material. After more than 15 years in the living community, Ms Meyer remained true of what she strongly disliked and therefore forcefully and loudly rejected everyone with whom she was not familiar. The minute is the result of a translation of such an occurrence into a short text message. At the same time, it conveys (as does the encounter between Ms Meyer and Nora) the friendly and respectful relationship Ms Meyer cultivated with the staff members of the living community. It also indicates the required effort of keeping Ms Meyer's bed and apartment clean and fresh. The two free-text entries and the number of 35 in the corresponding box in Ms Meyer's digital record were everything of the relationship maintenance with Ms Meyer that went into the digital system on that particular day. Whereas staff paid attention to the digitized numbers only in terms of patterns of regularity, free text entries were routinely reviewed at the beginning of the workshift to get a sense of the current challenges faced by residents. In addition, the effects of measures adopted in dealing with clients were briefly documented and read here. Particularly after longer absences, the employees used the entries to get a first impression of the situation of each individual client and her or his current need for support.

Summing up Minutes: The Algorithmic Creation of Totals of Time

Whereas the software left textual entries unchanged, it further processed the minutes typed in as numbers. In Fig. 8.1, the block highlighted in grey on the top right corner displays the automated calculations using the input values of each day. The value on the top right corner in this grey block stands for the total amount of minutes that has been allocated to the case work of the particular client in the month. The register in Fig. 8.1 shows the number 1162. The next short two lines with six narrow columns show the total amount of minutes charged to the six tasks of area 1, among them the administration of medication in the first column (number 252). The last line displays the sum of minutes that have been entered in the total register of this area (number 657). This way, the software provided basic automated summations that, together with the design of the registers, allow quick evaluation of the ways in which minutes accumulate to totals of time, using a few clicks between the registers and applying skilled views.

In addition, the digital system made the cases and data values easily accessible from any of the supervisors' and managers' computer desks and provided them with the possibility of direct comparison with the rehabilitation goals set in the BRP. As mentioned above, the BRP itself discriminated between the four "areas of life". The form already specified assistance in these areas in minutes per week. In the BRP, the total of minutes across all areas finally determined the required extent of institutional support categorized in 12 distinct support requirement groups. The higher the total of calculated minutes, the higher the support requirement group, the higher the reimbursement by the municipality. Notably, neither documentation nor the amount of performed tasks but the BRP itself delivered the basis for the reimbursement equation. As mentioned above, the digital documentation system was a voluntary measure introduced by the service managers. As we will see now, the time values and totals of time in the digital system were enacted as means for planning and justifying service provision for the period of the upcoming BRP.

Putting Minutes to Work: Translating Data Objects into Arguments

Personal meetings, scheduled by the municipality to review requested support requirement groups, are central to understanding the significance of the created numerical data objects for the everyday pattern of community psychiatry. One such meeting took place between a social welfare officer, a social worker of the municipal health department, the supervisor of the therapeutic living community and Silke, Ms Meyer's primary support worker. The social welfare office was the responsible authority to decide upon the approval of the BRP and endorse public funding. Its officer had initiated the meeting, because she called into question whether the newly requested support requirement group for Ms Meyer was adequate. The health department provided its expertise in judging the need for community mental healthcare interventions from a mental health perspective. Their mental health expertise formed an integral part of the BRP and members of its office regularly participated in meetings that dealt with the details of the form. Silke had asked Ms Meyer to join the meeting in the community living room. Ms Meyer first accompanied Silke, but once she saw the assembled people, she made clear that she was not interested in having a conversation in this setting and went back to her apartment. Lacking Ms Meyer's participation, the hearing was relocated in the office of the supervisor. Everyone was seated around a table, with annotated personal copies of Ms Meyer's newly submitted BRP in hands. The following is an extract of the meeting based on my notes:

> *Officer (social welfare office)* – I wonder whether the goals for Ms Meyer actually comprise individual case support or plain nursing. The support requirement group of 7 is very high compared to the tasks that really relate to individual case support.
>
> *Supervisor (TWG)* – Actually, we have cut the support requirement group from 8 to 7 last year.
>
> *Social worker (health department)* – What is the service really about? You have requested 500 minutes for self-supply.

Supervisor – Well, this entails breakfast, lunch and dinner. 25 minutes each, projected to a week.

Officer – Couldn't this be part of the nursing service?

Supervisor – I don't see the nursing service doing groceries. We are a residential community. We want Ms Meyer be part of our social life.

Social worker – I agree, meals are an important part of the individual case support.

Supervisor – Meals are not everything. We administer the medication, giving meds can take 5 minutes or 20, depending on how well it goes. We do laundry for Ms Meyer. The nursing service fills a washing machine, Silke fills three. Ms Meyer wets herself and we need to react. The nursing service attends Ms Meyer, but we do a lot of work in between. Not to mention that occasionally we need to take over their work, because Ms Meyer refuses to be approached by nursing staff, especially when they send people whom Ms Meyer doesn't know. They have very few permanent employees.

... (The conversation goes on, basically with the social welfare officer doubting the necessity for nursing tasks in regular case support.)

Supervisor (reaches for the calculator) – Okay, let's calculate. The meals make 25 minutes every day, multiplied by 7 make 175 minutes. Medication supply, documentation and control make 20 minutes a week. Giving meds make 18 minutes a day multiplied by 7 make 126 minutes – if Ms Meyer doesn't refuse. Administration of meds make 10 more minutes a week. Laundry – in addition to the nursing service – make 15 minutes. Company and attendance are about 20 minutes every day; make 140 minutes a week. Bringing her to bed plus occasionally changing clothes make 10 more minutes each week. So, we have 496 minutes. And we haven't even calculated communication with the nursing service.

Social worker – You don't see any flexibility in reducing the minutes?

Supervisor – No, not in Ms Meyer's favour.

... (the conversation goes on)

Officer – Well, it's a real problem that nursing tasks have raised, but Ms Meyer does not accept the staff members of the nursing service in the way she accepts you.

Supervisor – You will need to cut 31 minutes to reach the lower support requirement group.

Officer – True.

What might seem an example of an exceptional hearing was an intrinsic and growing part of community work: Requested support requirement groups were made defendable minute by minute. As the BRP was effective for 3 to 12 months, there was a constant need for re-evaluating the situation of the clients and their BRPs (Bister forthcoming). In the meeting, the social welfare officer challenged the existing division between nursing services and integration services. In the German healthcare system, the latter are funded by the municipality, whereas the former are financed by the German long-term care insurance system. Social integration services aimed at supporting the social integration and independence of their clients. Nursing services delivered long-term care and had limited resources for support beyond the provision of basic care services, due to reimbursement restrictions. In individual meetings with the stakeholders of community care provision, such as in the one presented above, social welfare officers were committed to bridging the two tasks of mediating integration services on the one hand and avoiding cost explosion for the municipality on the other. Engaging in calculations of minutes seemed one possible way of doing so. As the discussion of the ways in which minutes are created has conveyed above, life will never fit any of these calculations in a strict sense. Nursing and integration services are not easily separable in daily life. A whole lot depends on social relations of trust. If Ms Meyer only accepted staff members she knew well for nursing, and nursing services typically had a high turnover of staff, shifting services towards the nursing service would not lead to any solution.

As we can see from the calculative exercises of the supervisor in the meeting, she was very familiar with each and every calculation in Ms Meyer's case. A skilful interpretation of the data entries like hers presupposes knowledge of all the calculative conventions and processes involved. Although neither policy nor the social welfare office officially required a breakdown of the temporal units as specified in the BRP, the supervisor applied detailed minute values to defend the totals of time as defined in the BRP. In a staff meeting, the supervisor made clear that she wanted all the work done in the service to be made explicit through conversion in time values. She stated that otherwise she feared their support work would not be remunerated adequately and clients suffered inadequate services. Due to the lack of possibilities to influence the structural framework conditions in any immediate sense, the supervisor reacted to the pressure of the social welfare office by actively dealing with the minute values. While calculations of minutes proved to be an appropriate tool to reconcile policy objectives with planned support measures, they also enabled everyday community life to be kept as far away from negotiations as possible. This was the supervisor's way of balancing demands of neo-liberal accountability with the necessary flexibility of individual support. In the words of the sociologist Jason Rodriquez, who wrote a remarkable ethnography on US nursing homes, she performed "the complex minuet nursing home staff dance between a logic of care and a logic of cost" (Rodriquez 2014: 4). Dealing with the time values and their composition drew attention to the BRP as policy form and normalized structural challenges such as the growing demand for integration services and the resulting increase in municipal budget expenditure, labour shortage in the nursing sector and low social recognition and remuneration of support work. Nevertheless, in the meeting, the supervisor succeeded in making three cases at least: first, a therapeutic case as Ms Meyer should not be left to the nursing services, which was expected to result in a mental healthcare neglect; next, a political case as Ms Meyer had the legal right to integration service; and finally, a material case as the quality of care was related to the amount of allocated public funding.

Discussion

This chapter has tackled the anthropological question of what is at stake when digital data objects participate in the professional knowledge landscape of support workers in German community mental healthcare. Above, I have discussed the sense in which the knowledge landscape might be understood as a skilled movement between encounters and representations and vice versa. The concept of translation has proved to be suitable for the analytical examination of these movement processes. It illustrates how components of the landscape, such as practices, standards, concepts, hardware, software, people and objects, are known by relating them in practice. In community psychiatry, digital minutes played a central role in this process. Created through the translation of action into digital data, minutes as time values and short free-text messages crucially impacted the professionals' ways of understanding, evaluating and projecting daily life in the therapeutic community. Staff members, especially the supervisor, also drew on the minutes to stand up for the integration service. In negotiations with the municipal social welfare office and the health department, minute values became co-actors of persuasion and justification. Hence, the digital documentation system provided the "material anchor" (Hutchins 2005) for perceiving and depicting community life, thus indirectly influencing the financial endowment and associated qualitative arrangement of support work. Conventions on the classification of support tasks formed the basis for the applicability of the digital system in everyday care work.

As argued by the sociologist Jack Levinson, documentation technologies contribute to the translation of the ideals of individual case support into everyday work (Levinson 2010). These technologies "organize the work they document" (Levinson 2010: 164). This is not self-evident at all, because standardized numbers do not represent the flow of care in any straightforward way. Nevertheless, the practice of documenting one's work through applying the same time values at the end of every workday constantly reproduces awareness of how long tasks should take in practice and on which tasks emphasis should be placed. Similarly, the anthropologist Jeannette Pols stresses that "[a]ccounting is not merely a way of legitimating care, but it also structures care on a practical level" (Pols 2006: 418). As such, documentation does not only drain on the resources of a work shift but substantially impacts on the content, temporalities and attentiveness of care practices.

Hence, the digital system operates as a micro-political technology that situates human beings in relation to mental healthcare policy.[8] The system fostered the conjuncture of policy and care, as in practice it translated care work and the presence of the residents into data objects that corresponded with the categories of policy. But then, for the very same reasons, the system also supported a disjuncture of care and policy: the datafication of everyday life in the language of policy illustrated how far the daily support work of employees and the agency of residents departed

[8] Cf. the notion of "human device", in Ureta (2015).

from policy classifications. This oscillation between conjuncture and disjuncture of policy and care forms an intrinsic part of the professional knowledge landscape in community psychiatry. Essentially, it enables a steady exploration of potential capacities for action and an ongoing definition of "the local sense of right and wrong" (Fassin 2008: 336).

Digital minutes therefore work well in respect to a community mental healthcare system that occupies itself more than ever with the quantification of services. Minuteness appears as an ambiguous skill that actually frees everyday care work from the ultimate logic of cost while also subjecting it to its principles. Policy therefore cannot be taken as a map for care, nor can care be adequately mapped to policy. Rather, mapping current non-coherent assemblages of care-policy requires an investigation of the translations into and from minutes that constitute the processes of knowledge landscaping. Finally, this chapter suggests that following the data journeys through the knowledge landscape is a fruitful approach to get hold of the complex and contradictory requirements of healthcare in digital societies.

References

Atkinson, P. A. (1995). *Medical talk and medical work*. London: Sage.

Barrett, R. J. (1996). *The psychiatric team and the social definition of schizophrenia*. Cambridge: Cambridge University Press.

Bates, J., et al. (2016). Data journeys: Capturing the socio-material constitution of data objects and flows. *Big Data & Society, 3*(2), 1–12.

Berg, M. (1996). Practices of reading and writing: The constitutive role of the patient record in medical work. *Sociology of Health & Illness, 18*(4), 499–524.

Berg, M., & Bowker, G. (1997). The multiple bodies of the medical record: Toward a sociology of an artifact. *The Sociological Quarterly, 38*(3), 513–537.

Biehl, J. (2005). *Vita* (Life in a zone of social abandonment). Berkeley: CA, University of California Press.

Bieler, P., & Klausner, M. (2019). Niching in cities under pressure. Tracing the reconfiguration of community psychiatric care and the housing market in Berlin. *Geoforum, 101*, 202–211.

Bister, M. D. (2018). The concept of chronicity in action: Everyday classification practices and the shaping of mental health care. *Sociology of Health & Illness, 40*(1), 38–52.
Bister, M. D. (forthcoming). *Gesundheitliches Gut-achten als sozio-materieller Prozess: Eine Praxeografie der Zuerkennung von gemeindepsychiatrischen Leistungen in Berlin*. Österreichische Zeitschrift für Geschichtswissenschaften.
Bowker, G., & Star, S. L. (1999). *Sorting things out. Classification and its consequences*. London/Cambridge, MA: MIT Press.
Desjarlais, R. (1997). *Shelter blues. Sanity and selfhood among the homeless*. Philadelphia: University of Pennsylvania Press.
Estroff, S. E. (1981). *Making It crazy. An ethnography of psychiatric clients in an American community*. Berkeley: University of California Press.
Fassin, D. (2008). Beyond good and evil? *Anthropological Theory, 8*(4), 333–344.
Freeman, R. (2009). "what is 'translation'?" evidence & policy: A journal of research. *Debate and Practice, 5*(4), 429–447.
Freeman, R. (2017). Care, policy, knowledge: Translating between worlds. *The Sociological Review Monographs, 65*(2), 193–200.
Freeman, R., & Sturdy, S. (Eds.). (2014). *Knowledge in policy: Embodied, inscribed, enacted*. Bristol: Policy Press.
Gill, N., et al. (2017). Care and policy practices [special issue]. *The Sociological Review Monographs, 65*(2): 3–200.
Hacking, I. (2002). *Historical ontology*. Cambridge/London: Harvard University Press.
Hutchins, E. (2005). Material anchors for conceptual blends. *Journal of Pragmatics, 37*, 1555–1577.
Latour, B. (2005). *Reassembling the social. An introduction to actor-network-theory*. Oxford: Oxford University.
Law, J., & Singleton, V. (2014). ANT, multiplicity and policy. *Critical Policy Studies, 8*(4), 379–396.
Levinson, J. (2010). *Making life work: Freedom and disability in a community group home*. Minneapolis: MN, University of Minnesota Press.
Lydahl, D. (2019). Standard tools for non-standard care: The values and scripts of a person-centred assessment protocol. *Health*. London: 1363459319851541.
Mol, A. (2008). *The logic of care. Health and the problem of patient choice*. London/New York: Routledge.
Mol, A., et al. (Eds.). (2010). *Care in practice. On tinkering in clinics, homes and farms*. Transcript Verlag: Bielefeld.

Pols, J. (2006). Accounting and washing: Good care in long-term psychiatry. *Science, Technology & Human Values, 31*(4), 409–430.
Pols, J. (2012). *Care at a distance: On the closeness of technology*. Amsterdam: Amsterdam University Press.
Rodriquez, J. (2014). *Labors of love: Nursing homes and the structures of care work*. New York: New York University Press.
Shore, C., et al. (Eds.). (2011). *Policy worlds: Anthropology and the analysis of contemporary power* (EASA series). Berghahn Books: New York.
Stevenson, L. (2014). *Life beside itself: Imagining care in the Canadian Arctic*. Oakland: University of California Press.
Ureta, S. (2015). *Assembling policy: Transantiago, human devices, and the dream of a world-class society*. Cambridge: MIT Press.

9

'Facebook Is My Guerrilla': On Ways in Which Social Networks Co-create Illness Experiences of Persons with Rare/Atypical Symptoms

Jana Šimenc

Introduction

This chapter draws on my ethnography conducted in Slovenia from January 2016 till December 2017.[1] The analysis focuses on a woman, Eva, and her health narrative and my longer observations of her personal everyday (invisible) struggles and (visible) articulations on Facebook, in the processes of getting a sense of what her symptoms meant, an accurate medical diagnoses and treatment and support in the medical system. In the context of social media, Facebook is, up until now, the most widely used social network in Slovenia.[2] The analysis approaches Eva's narrative

[1] Research 'Health in the Pocket and on the Internet' was financed by the Slovenian research agency.

[2] The use of Facebook in Slovenia is similar to many other countries: despite its controversy and scandals with data manipulations, privacy issues, financial orientations, and so on, this social network remains on the pedestal. Facebook statistics shows that in a country of 2 million population, 960,000 users logged in at least once in June 2019. To obtain as up-to-date data as possible, I used a trick: I started creating a fictive Facebook ad. In the section about potential reach of the 'ad', I saw

J. Šimenc (✉)
Sociomedical Institute, Research Centre of the Slovenian Academy of Sciences and Arts, ZRC SAZU, Ljubljana, Slovenia

A. L. Svalastog et al. (eds.), *Navigating Digital Health Landscapes*, Health, Technology and Society, https://doi.org/10.1007/978-981-15-8206-6_9

within the context of the present Slovenian public health environment and draws on Barth's (2002) understanding of knowledge as an embodied, situated and contextual concept.

Eva is in her 40s. She is a highly curious, caring, thoughtful and reflective person. Her song performances, Facebook posts, writings and small everyday acts[3] talk about her social responsibility and political engagement in the world we live in. As an active citizen, she unquestionably wants to play her part in changing ourselves and the world for the better. It is in this spirit that Eva's engagement is also traceable and noticeable in the health sphere. For over 20 years, she has been suffering from severe, mostly atypical and rare medical conditions that doctors have struggled to diagnose and treat. Over this period of time, she has had more than one opportunity to gain deeper insight into the processes found within the Slovenian medical system, into complementary/holistic medical practices and, indeed, into her body and herself.

Eva has had to reinvent herself many times. With constant recurrence of her disease symptoms and, yet calmer times, physical and emotional ups and downs, she became even more persistent in undertaking an exploration of her body, treatment practices, scientific and holistic etiologies and what might be available to secure better health. Among others, she also formed a Facebook group for persons with a particular autoimmune disease[4] in Slovenia.

In what way is Facebook a social-media arena where Eva acts in diverse ways to render biopower, distress, knowledge hierarchies and uncertainties more manageable? How and why does Eva navigate towards medical knowledge in the online environment? How can feelings of 'knowing the disease' be mobilized and activated on Facebook? How are forms of patient activism, self-care and care for others visible online?

how many users in all age groups are on the platform in Slovenia. Numbers are in line with available, but three-year-old statistics: Facebook in Slovenia has 833,500 users, and 70% of them are daily users (Media+, Valicon 2016).

[3] The name of the artist, 'Eva',cannot be revealed. Full anonymity in the interpretation of the research findings has been assured.

[4] The name of the disease is not stated due to data protection of participants in the research. If the disease had been revealed, the founder of a specific Facebook group could easily be traced down and identified.

These are the main questions I will tackle in this chapter drawing on a range of social science analyses. My main aim is to give a fresh perspective to understand the relational and ontological complexity of contemporary illness experience and the contextualization of knowledge, from a patient/chronic disease point of view. Eva's illustrative case will open up a window towards better understanding of the ambivalent process behind becoming an expert/empowered patient and the dynamics between lay, experiential and professional knowledge. Put otherwise, I will explain how 'traditional' hierarchical/authoritative knowledge structures are challenged during health-seeking behaviour in today's digital society.

Social Media and Health in Theory

Since 2004, the launch of Facebook and other social media, a substantial body of literature on social media's impact, potential and relation to the health domain has emerged. The topic has been explored using a wide array of different methodological approaches and interpretations, where numerous researchers have examined the effects of the growing utilization of social media among patients (for systematic reviews, see Smailhodzic et al. 2016; Kingod et al. 2017; Guistini et al. 2018). Frequent accounts of the sharing of information and patient participation highlight (in many ways the contradictory) participatory nature of new media (Harris et al. 2016). A diverse range of conclusions on the effects of social media on health (especially mental health) can also be observed: on one hand they are to generate new pathologies (e.g. digital addictions, social impairments, etc.), or exacerbate existing ones (e.g. depression, anxiety, etc.) (see Šimenc 2019). Yet, social media also have the potential to alleviate suffering by offering a space for emotional and peer support (Kingod et al. 2017). Still, despite the extensive work on the social media/health relationship, there remains much to be done.

Significant layers of social media have been revealed through critical (predominantly dystopian) literature which pivot on the problematics of hidden power structures behind neoliberal, profit-driven social media platforms. Such literature focuses on the politics of governance, surveillance, transparency, commercialization and the exploitation of personal data (Lupton 2016; Ruckenstein and Dow Schüll 2017; Sharon 2017), free/digital/unwaged/immaterial labour of users (Terranova 2000; Fuchs 2010; Till 2014; Brown 2014) and manipulative, hidden, yet powerful algorithms (Ziewitz 2016; Seaver 2017). These public and academic conversations are of utmost importance. They unquestionably open up and reshape our understanding of the digital (health) landscape and make a contribution towards the reduction of hidden, manipulative and exploitative mechanisms that social media can create (at a political, social and individual level). On the other hand, these discussions leave little room for an exploration of everyday practices of patients or ordinary persons in their struggles with living with disease. What is more, there are some like Eva, who are highly critical of the neoliberal and exploitative aspects of social media. She is thus well aware of the problematic dimensions of social media, yet such concerns do not turn her away from incorporating social networks in her agentive performances as she copes with her health problems. That is why I will intentionally approach Facebook, activism and dynamics in knowledge authorities from a different angle. As Mol (2008) concluded, new technologies should not be interpreted as objects with their own logic, but as actors supporting or extending (personal and other) logics of care.

Alongside critical digital health literature, a loud call for further, more detailed, in-depth and relational exploration of the topic is emerging (Ruckenstein and Dow Schüll 2017). More attention should be given to better understanding of how intersections become enacted in everyday life (Kingod et al. 2017) and which shades and creative ways of online activism with 'tropes of helping and doing good' (Chua 2018: 11) are being developed. Research undertaken within the Navigating Knowledge Landscapes network is important in this regard through its aim to deepen our understanding of the dynamics of information flow and the production of knowledge during a patient's navigation across this landscape (Svalastog et al. 2015, 2018). One useful approach for obtaining a better glimpse into the intersections and dynamics of the small, quotidian micro-circumstances of a patient is ethnography.

That is why, in line with Mol's (2002) relational empirical interpretations, I seek to show how biomedical knowledge is contested, reshaped and enacted by patients' online and offline participation and activism.

Following this orientation, there is no clear (digital) divide between 'online' and 'offline' worlds: I understand the 'online' activities as only a portion, an integrated part of our everyday complex navigation between multiple modalities (for different argumentations that overcome dichotomies of the real and the virtual, see Pols 2012; Hine 2015; Boellstorff 2016; Dow Schüll 2016; Harris et al. 2016; Seaver 2017; Rufas and Hine 2018; Chua 2018). In this sense, I echo the argument advanced earlier by Lamerichs et al. in Chap. 6, especially their arguments in relation to 'digital subjectivities'.

Closed Doors

Since her 20s, Eva has experienced several, mostly atypical medical conditions (from a rare type of cancer to other autoimmune diseases). She has been struggling with unwellness and severe pain that most often remains biomedically unexplained. Due to the low prevalence of certain disease, persons with rare or atypical diseases living in countries with a small population (such as Slovenia with 2 million inhabitants) grapple even harder with obtaining proper diagnosis. Her symptoms and pain did not translate to medical conditions that could define and measure her problem. Through our conversations, she explained how throughout medical encounters she repeatedly went from one disappointment to another, from one sadness to another. She experienced misunderstandings, misdiagnoses, humiliation, unrecognition and de-legitimation of her illness experiences, poor medical explanations and, in her opinion most problematically, a lack of doctors' cooperation.

> *It all started with my first atypical cancer episode. I was very young, a diagnosis was a big shock for me. What happened was, I received my medical results by post and I did not understand it. I tried to get answers from the doctors, but was unsuccessful. That is why I started searching word for word online.*

She not only googled words in medical results she received but also started searching for international experts, who would give answers to her specific questions. She began reading scientific articles on the subject and related material that led to a deep exploration of her condition. Yet still this was inadequate:

> *Still, this online exploration … for me it does not suffice. I need to talk to persons, I really need interpersonal discussion. What I want to say is, from the beginning I was not able to establish good communication with experts. For me, this is the biggest systemic problem: lack of communication between the doctor and a patient like me, who has a lot of questions.*

In her narrative, Eva often mentioned battles in the medical system, when she needed quick specialists' help in an acute state of pain. She went through endless talks on the phone with nurses or administrators and listened to explanations how she needed to wait on a list for a month or, in most cases, even more. In case of payment in a private practice, she would get immediate or quicker help. And if she secured an appointment, according to her experiences, the timeframe for communication and consultation was extremely limited:

> *In most cases, I had about 7 minutes available during one visit, 3 minutes with the doctor, and 4 minutes with the nurse. Quick standardized checks by the doctors, no or limited explanations, no communication. I do not understand, how such generic, protocols health professionals follow are seen as curing. For me, this is not curing; I see such treatment as fordism, similar to assembly lines. This is pure neoliberal fordism. That is why I cannot trust the system. I am not a part of the body, a piece of meat that needs examination.*

Eva might be regarded as a well-informed, engaged, resourceful and emphatic expert patient. Nonetheless, she is one of many who complain over the lack of opportunity to discuss their problems with their doctors. In Slovenia today, professional standards state that a doctor has seven minutes available for each patient visit. This limited provision is highly criticized, not only by patients but in the media and via anecdotal evidence by the medical professionals as well.

Currently, a lack of interpersonal communication, slower access to health specialists, long waiting lists and financial issues are at the forefront of publics' dissatisfaction and disappointment over the Slovenian public healthcare system. These are also the terms that dominate political and media discourse. In the broader context, after gaining independence in 1991, Slovenians were full of hope for a better future. Utopian dreams about becoming economically successful and being a green and beautiful European country, like Switzerland, were widely shared. Similar to other post-socialist states,[5] Slovenia underwent a process of transition to a market economy and reforms in the healthcare system as well. Many authors agree that compared to other countries, Slovenia had a slower, yet more careful and successful implementation of health reforms (Albreht and Klazinga 2010; Bazylevych and Hresanova 2011). It is in keeping with the public health tradition, based on (Bismarck's) solidarity-based public healthcare system, that is founded upon compulsory health insurance. The Law on Health Care and Health Insurance laid the basis for the present system of compulsory and voluntary health insurance, permitted privatization of healthcare and transferred some administrative functions to professional chambers (Albreht et al. 2002).

Still, after 18 years of transition, many desired visions for healthcare failed to materialize. For many people, the healthcare sector is one of principal disappointments in this young country. (Mostly incompetent) ministers are constantly changing, while ineffective bureaucratic demands are increasing, causing burdens in everyday medical practice. In addition, the poorly managed introduction of eHealth solutions is generating further criticism of healthcare among health professionals and patients (see Šimenc 2017). Debates about assuring finances for increasing healthcare costs, long waiting lists and additional work regulations dominate political and media debates.

One can observe traces of a highly idealized Yugo-nostalgic view over the healthcare services of the past which continue to influence health-seeking behaviour: a conflict between the high inherited expectations of the people and the current limited resources of the public system is evident (Albreht et al. 2002). Much of the public discontent over the current system arises out of access to healthcare, which today is not the same as under the previous communist system. The introduction of private

[5] See Petrović-Šteger (2016) for insight into some aspects of Serbian contemporary healthcare sphere.

healthcare providers and co-payments for certain services is creating a gap between those who can afford immediate care and the best specialists and those who cannot afford to pay for such services and are put on long waiting lists. Private healthcare services remain limited, though commercial and business models are increasingly entering this sphere. In the media and politics, polarized tensions between further privatization and stronger public healthcare continue to mark the current debates and future orientations of the healthcare system in Slovenia.

Facebook: From Transcending Loneliness to Care for Others

Referring back to Eva, she experienced many uncertainties and tensions within the medical system. She felt she lost her autonomy and body integrity, and the system had failed her. A number of unfortunate events and unpleasant circumstances contributed to her loss of institutional and interpersonal trust. In her narrative and frequent Facebook posts, it is noticeable that through the processes of diagnoses and treatments she experienced multiple layers of uncertainty and (structural) invisibility (for more on patient's uncertainty and invisibility, see Dumit 2006; Masana 2011; Phillips and Rees 2018). Even today, she frequently feels like she is completely alone with the disease. But her social supports have played an important role in easing the suffering and overcoming a feeling of loneliness.

> *"I have many friends, a partner, and live a relatively prosperous social life. But in your pain, you are extremely alone. It is a state of endless loneliness, even when you have people around you. I cannot talk to my partner, nor with my close friends about my suffering. This is one of the hardest aspects of being sick. That loneliness and inability for my friends, even my partner to grasp the dimensions of my pain ... That is why I post my deepest reflections on Facebook and communicate with people who are experiencing similar pain. I know how it feels, and share the feelings. After writing and posting, I do not feel that alone anymore," she explained during one of our long conversations in the spring in 2017.*

Phillips and Rees (2018), who studied people with sensitivity to everyday chemicals (so-called multiple chemical sensitivity), write how similar experiences echoed among their respondents. They showed how only people with the same disease, their peers, are able to understand what they are going through. Regrettably, most friends, family and medical professionals can't. Authors further draw on similar cases of atypical or multidimensional complex chronic diseases, where patients recognize the online sphere as the rare 'place' for actual emotional support, where feelings of mutual understanding and not being alone develop (Phillips and Rees 2018). Likewise in Eva's case, Facebook plays an important part in the process of constructing, living with and easing a disease. With activities on social network, she is not only practising self-care but also care for others:

> *I see that I help others feeling less lonely as well. It is comforting for me and others. That is why I post on Facebook.*

The observation about the socio-emotional support that social networks provide to patients is nothing new nor original (see Kingod et al. 2017; Phillips and Rees 2018). That is why it is important to highlight another aspect of Eva's online actions. I draw attention to the individual and relational scope behind it: how did she become an expert on her disease, the 'knower' of the disease? What motivates her to bring her understanding of her condition into the public domain and socially distribute it on Facebook?

To exploit the analytical possibility for understanding the knowledge of the symptoms and the disease, I will refer to Barth's (2002) lecture on 'An Anthropology of Knowledge'. He understands knowledge as 'what a person employs to interpret and act on the world'. Under this framing he includes 'feelings as well as information, embodied skills, verbal taxonomies and concepts: all the ways of understanding that people use to make up their experienced, grasped reality' (2002: 1). For Barth, knowledge is thus an embodied, situated and contextual concept (rather than the encyclopaedic, formalized version of knowledge). He suggests that an anthropology of knowledge gives attention to the 'knowers and to the acts of knowers – the people who hold, learn, produce, and apply knowledge in their various activities and lives' (2002: 3).

A 'Manager' of Knowledge and a Rebel

In Eva's case, through years of exploration of the disease and herself, she put an enormous effort and time into her search for information, scientific literature, popular articles, video material and other available sources of information. She managed to gather an impressive collection of scientific literature on her specific disease, useful links, medical and holistic practitioners' advice, diverse explanations of disease aetiology, artistic articulations and visualizations of pain and practical lifestyle suggestions for easing the disease, through diet, exercises and so on. She expressed that gathering and understanding this material was never easy:

> *You know, searching for information is quite a tough task. The right information is not easy to find, absolutely not. One needs to know foreign languages, be skilled in online searching, and needs to have certain filters engraved to separate fake or commercial staff from something that seems credible, relevant, and trustworthy. I did not study medicine, so for me it is even harder to differentiate sponsored articles from scientific findings.*

Eva believes she knows the mechanisms and has digital literacy and other qualifications needed to differentiate and filter miscellaneous online information (e.g. the ones that are spreading medical mistrust or are part of larger political ideologies, pharmaceutical agendas and similar). She does not accept all information as a given fact; she constantly cross-checks the material from diverse sources. In these endeavours, she is combining available online and offline resources and options. Over the years, she gained a stock of information. By now she felt she had become a proper expert on the subject. She knows the disease in all its spectres, darkness and unpredictable expressions. But it is not only the acquisition of online information that outlines the foundation of her feeling of being knowledgeable. She highlighted her embodied dimensions of knowledge. All rich experiences in her long-term relationship with the disease made her an expert: her body talk, the shades of pain and non-movement she is going through every day are constantly widening her expertise. Both interrelatedness of lived experience and online self-learning and communication validate her as a knower of the disease. What is more, knowing the disease as much as possible gives her comfort and supports her when dealing with everyday unwellness. But even more importantly, her sense of having knowledge gives her power and the basis for further actions she sees as of considerable importance at a societal level. Eva is not, therefore, a passive information 'receiver' and an individual 'expert patient'; she is an active mediator of knowledge that she has embodied and accumulated.

In Eva's case, the knowledge can be also interpreted as an abstract resource, to which individuals have selective access. Not all patients are as active, resourceful and curious as she is. Through encounters with peers, she was astonished by the difference in the stock of knowledge between her and them.

> *When talking to other patients in rehabilitation center, I found out, they know almost nothing about our disease. Most of them cannot even pronounce the name of it. That genuinely surprised me.*

Such obliviousness and passiveness among her peers raised serious concerns for Eva and called her to action. She was determined to do something about it. She said that more information and knowledge open up more options for coping with the disease and make one more prepared for the unexpected turns. Thus, to make her contribution towards a change of the situation, she opened a Facebook group for people with the specific autoimmune disease in Slovenia.

> *I made a decision, and opened a Facebook group. I started sharing everything I know, all material and information I have. It is available all in one place now.*

With posts on her Facebook group, she is bringing knowledge into existence and making it mobile, making it visible to others. As the advanced knower of the disease, she felt socially obliged to share the knowledge. Put otherwise, as the 'manager' and the holder of the knowledge, she felt obligated to share it among less knowledgeable and less informed patients. And what motivated her?

> *You know Jana, this is my guerilla. My guerilla action. It is my way of helping me and others.*

Letting others know everything she knows and sharing all the resources is her small act, a contribution to doing something good for the society. Eva continued our conversation explaining that her rebellion and active coping with the disease has roots in her childhood.

> *I observed my parents, struggling with the same condition. They were passive, according to my opinion, they did not do enough to get better. They were so inert in their pain. I had extremelly hard time watching them. That is why I want to be all the opposite. I do everything and beyond the possible to make me and others feel better. And searching online, asking international experts for advice, being and communication on Facebook are some of the available options, I have to achieve my mission.*

Contemporary 'Expert Patient'

Gaining and mediating knowledge is Eva's way of living easier, managing the disease and doing something good. At first glance she seems like the perfect 'expert patient' (see Fox et al. 2005) that policy makers and those in public health are anticipating: knowledgeable, empowered, with high self-esteem, in control of a chronic condition and manager of the disease. She has the competences and is capable of making decisions and taking actions concerning treatment. She is also taking a holistic approach, making constant adjustments to the disease in her lifestyle. But in medical practice and everyday social relations, such patient's expertise raises new challenges.

According to Eva, the mediation of knowledge between peers is important, but intercommunication with doctors is essential during the disease experience. She is confident that, for a good doctor-patient relationship, it is crucial, almost obligatory, to let each other know everything they know. Only honest, direct, concise communication based on 'knowing the disease' can lead to desired goals: a proper diagnosis and support through curing and towards better health.

In reality one vital link in the mediation and trajectory of expert knowledge for disease management and treatment was missing: medical doctors. Eva did not experience much needed connections with experts in the system. When living with the disease, she wished to know and to understand what was going on in her body. She sought to see the medical visualizations of the symptoms and to talk about the situation in detail. She hoped that doctors would have theorized and explained her condition, those feral symptoms and pain, and provided answers to her questions, even if their response would have been 'I do not know'. Instead, they would be either overloaded with work or uninterested or would underestimate the relevance of her questions. On many occasions, Eva felt frustrated and humiliated; she could not get explanations nor any communication about questions she had prepared in advance:

In such a rush and in the limited time I had with the doctors, either at regular check-ups or in the hospital, there was no chance I could have asked questions.

Still, for Eva medical doctors are knowledgeable authorities. It was never her intention to challenge them, to compete with them. Moreover, she never underestimated their extensive cultivation and possession of a body of medical knowledge and was aware of her limits in interpretation of material and information. In fact, she recognized their expertise and wanted to rely on them, to cooperate, to have discussions and to listen to their interpretations:

I am aware of years of the study they went through and the experiences they have gained through practice. That is why I always want to talk to the doctor, not a nurse. I want to talk to the specialist in the field of my disease, with people, who have a lot of knowledge on the subject, who are authorities in the field. I do not need some generic explanations and answers, I seek specific discussion about my condition.

However, the desired balance in sharing and distribution of knowledge in doctor-patient relationship was never established. In her opinion, doctors saw her as a threat, as someone who intruded herself into their domain without proper knowledge and professional background. They were not supportive in her exploration of the disease. In a way, she disrupted and destabilized existing power relations in the doctor-patient communication. With her acts in seeking responses, exploring available sources and yearning for communication, she rapidly became labelled as an undesired patient in the system.

I noticed many medical doctors saw me as a difficult patient, but I think medicine should become more aware of the fact that a number of patients who, for diverse reasons, inform and educate them self about certain condition is growing.

The absence of communication with knowledge authorities in the system led to her personal and solitary actions of developing self-authority in knowledge, becoming an expert.

At least with the support of the internet you can actually turn the situation around: from being the subject of medical study or docile patient to being a researcher of your condition and an active controller of the situation.

Precisely because of the lack of reciprocity between herself and her doctors, she created her own criterion and principles of valid, accurate and authoritative knowledge. The wider healthcare system had failed too:

It seems to me like we are stuck in 19th century. This ideology about docile, quite, uninformed, passive, unknowledgeable patient should be passé. Obviously, in our country it is not.

It is widely acknowledged that patient's expectations and roles in the patient-doctor relationship are changing. Murgić et al. (2015) write about the problem of paternalism and patient autonomy in Croatia, a country with whom we had a joint public health system in former Yugoslavia. I agree with their observation that it 'is somewhat confusing when, on the one hand, medical paternalism appears to be trumped by autonomy, while on the other hand, many individual patients still expect, hope for, and even urge (in both subtle and outright ways) the doctor to be paternalistic' (2015: 1). The tensions here are similar in all post-socialistic countries—reorganizations of the powers of the state are placing increased emphasis on the responsibility of individuals. Authors moreover argue, in healthcare transitional or post-communist countries, they face more challenges in acceptance of active, knowledgeable patients in the treatment process, as 'paternalistic attitudes have been interwoven into all relationships, including medical ones' (2015: 1).

I would not like to make a generalization based on one case. There are many variations in doctors' opinions, medical performances and relationships.[6] Yet, based on my longer observations and experiences in Slovenian medical system, I would argue that medical doctors predominantly still hold the authority to translate untamed symptoms into disease. They continue seeking to monopolize the tradition of medical knowledge, relying on conventional, so-called objective and scientific body of knowledge, while largely ignoring experiential, embodied knowledge of the patients.

In line with the modern participatory medical paradigm (see Cordier 2014), Eva is calling for inclusion of experiential knowledge into conventional medical research protocols. She proposed different ways of relating and better futures:

> *For changes and advances in medical treatment, especially of autoimmune diseases, where many remain incurable or unknown, a more egalitarian, horizontal and reciprocal cooperation between the patients and medical doctors is needed. At the end of the day, it is us, the patients, who with diagnoses, our symptoms, and understandings of disease make crucial contributions towards new discoveries in medicine.*

---

[6] Despite a series of, mildly said, unfortunate events in the medical system, Eva articulated some optimism and positive episodes as well. 'Today, I am much more experienced as I was at my first cancer episode. I do not expect any emotional comfort, nor answers to my questions by the medical doctors anymore... On the other hand, there is always somebody in the medical system, usually a woman, a nurse, a cleaner, never mail doctor, who comforts me, gives me courage and emotional support. These are extremely beautiful moments. What I want to say is, the situation is never completely hopeless. And I know there are different medical doctors in the system, Maybe it is only my shitty luck I always get the bad ones'.

Conclusions

In this excursion into a specific case, I wanted to make meaningful sense of everyday practices and motivations that shape the emergence of the expert patient today. I have discussed the context within which acquiring knowledge in contemporary healthcare systems via social media is characterized by vulnerability and disruption in communication and information seeking. In many aspects, Eva is not an isolated case. She is one of the loud voices, pioneers and examiners of a different future. She is loudly disrupting established medical authorities, calling for paradigmatic shifts in medical practice and research. In her case, Facebook is an important public arena that enables her to perform the actions and to follow her mission.

Too often, workers in the medical system are not supportive of advanced and experienced knowers of the disease, who too easily and quickly become abandoned in the system, labelled as problematic and difficult. Eva clearly experienced how no or too little room is given for patients' knowledge distribution and representation in the medical system. That is why she turned to other available options, outside the medical system. She interprets her regular Facebook posts and patients' group formation as a form of activism, as a chance to resist to established power relations in biomedicine and as a call for more inclusion of experiential patients' knowledge into medical practice and research. Rabeharisoa, Moreira and Akrich (2014) propose the notion of 'evidence-based activism' to capture patients' and health activists' groups' focus on experiential knowledge production and knowledge mobilization. Current social science research is thus opening the focus to a broader spectrum of knowledge-related activities, where search for cure is not the exclusive motive that drives patients and activists to engage with knowledge.

Similarly Eva sees her actions not only as a patient quest for cure and improved treatment of her autoimmune disease but as one of the options through which to have a wider beneficial impact at the broader societal level as well. In resonance with Robins' (2013) call for an anthropology of 'the good', I believe we should not be dismissing individual ideals as unimportant or trivial. It is important here to give more attention to the ways in which people 'strive to create something good in their lives' and 'how people organize their personal and collective lives in order to foster what they think of as good' (Robins 2013: 457). Here we see quite directly the connection between the 'relational and the 'ontological' dimensions of health and disease. Navigating knowledge landscapes online helped Eva to build a sense of her (ontologically defined) disease and disorder, but precisely through her relational engagement with diverse social actors. This involved at times being disruptive—her guerrilla practices—yet being so in order to be constructive.

Acknowledgement I would like to express my deepest gratitude to 'Eva'. Her cooperation and straightforward narrative made this article possible.

References

Albreht, T. & M. Česen & D. Hindle & E- Jakubowski & B. Kramberger & V. Kerstin Petric & M. Premik (2002). Slovenia. *Health Care Systems in Transition, 4*(2). WHO: European Observatory on Health Care System.

Albreht, T., & Klazinga, N. S. (2010). Balancing equity and efficiency through health care policies in Slovenia during the period 1990–2008. *Zdravstveno Varstvo, 49*(2), 49–60.

Barth, F. (2002). An anthropology of knowledge. *Current Anthropology, 43*(1), 1–18.

Bazylevych, M. Y., & Hresanova, E. (2011). Introduction: Health and care work in postsocialist Eastern Europe and the former Soviet Union. *Anthropology of East Europe Review, 29*(1), 1–7.

Boellstorff, T. (2016). For whom the ontology turns: Theorizing the digital real. *Current Anthropology, 57*(4), 387–407.

Brown, A. B. (2014). Will work for free: The biopolitics of unwaged digital labour. *TripleC, 12*(2), 694–712. Available at: https://www.triple-c.at/index.php/tripleC/article/view/538/620. Accessed 21 Aug 2019.

Chua, L. (2018). Small acts and personal politics: On helping to save the orangutan via social media. *Anthropology Today, 34*(3), 7–11. Available at: https://rai.onlinelibrary.wiley.com/doi/full/10.1111/1467-8322.12432. Accessed 3 Aug 2019.

Cordier, J. (2014). The expert patient: Towards a novel definition. *European Respiratory Journal, 44*, 853–857. Available at: https://erj.ersjournals.com/content/44/4/853#ref-28. Accessed 10 Sept 2019.

Dow Schüll, N. (2016). Abiding chance: Online poker and the software of self-discipline. *Public Culture, 28*(3), 563–592.

Dumit, J. (2006). Illnesses you have to fight to get: Facts as forces in uncertain, emergent illnesses. *Social Science & Medicine, 62*(3), 577–590.

Fox, N. J., Ward, K. J., & O'Rourke, A. J. (2005). The "expert patient": Empowerment or medical dominance? The case of weight loss, pharmaceutical drugs and the Internet. *Social Science & Medicine, 60*, 1299–1309.

Fuchs, C. (2010). Labour in informational capitalism. *The Information Society, 26*(3), 176–196.

Guistini, D., Ali, M. S., Frazer, M., & Kamel Boulus, N. M. (2018). Effective uses of social media in public health and medicine: A systematic review of systematic reviews. *Online Journal of Public Health Informatics*, (2), 10, 215. Available at: https://www.ncbi.nlm.nih.gov/pmc/articles/PMC6194097/. Accessed 27 June 2019.

Harris, A., Kelly, S., & Wyatt, S. (2016). *CyberGenetics: Health genetics and new media*. London/New York: Routledge.

Hine, C. (2015). *Ethnography for the Internet: Embedded, embodied and everyday*. London/New York: Bloomsbury.

Kingod, N., Cleal, B., Wahlberg, A., & Husted, G. (2017). Online peer-to-peer communities in the daily lives of people with chronic illness. *Qualitative Health Research, 27*(1), 89–99.

Lupton, D. (2016). *The quantified self: A sociology of self-tracking*. Cambridge: Polity Press.

Masana, L. (2011). Invisible chronic illnesses inside apparently healthy bodies. In S. Fainzang & C. Hexaire (Eds.), *Of bodies and symptoms* (pp. 127–149). Tarragona: Publication URV.

Media+, Valicon. (2016). *Media+ research on the use of social networks in Slovenia, n=9.798*. Available at: http://www.valicon.net/files/Sporocilo%20za%20javnost%202016-06-23%20(1).pdf. Accessed 10 Aug 2019.

Mol, A. (2002). *The body multiple: Ontology in medical practice*. Durham: Duke University Press.

Mol, A. (2008). *The logic of care: Health and the problem of patient choice*. New York: Routledge.

Murgić, L., Hébert, P. C., Sović, S., & Pavleković, G. (2015). Paternalism and autonomy: Views of patients and providers in a transitional country. *BMC Medical Ethics, 16*, 1–9.

Petrović-Šteger, M. (2016). Understanding self-care: Passing and healing in contemporary Serbia. In P. Bjerregaard et al. (Eds.), *Materialities of passing. Explorations in transformation, transition and transience*. New York: Routledge.

Phillips, T., & Rees, T. (2018). (In)Visibility online: The benefits of online patient forums for people with a hidden illness: The case of multiple chemical sensitivity (MCS). *Medical Anthropology Quarterly, 32*(2), 214–232.

Pols, J. (2012). *Care at Distance: On the closeness of technology*. Amsterdam: Amsterdam University Press.

Rabeharisoa, V., Moreira, T., & Akrich, M. (2014). Evidence based activism: Patients', users' and activists' groups in knowledge society. *BioSocieties, 9*(2), 111–128.

Robins, J. (2013). Beyond the suffering subject: Toward an anthropology of the good. *Journal of the Royal Anthropological Institute, 19*, 447–462.

Ruckenstein, M. & Dow Schüll, N. (2017). The datafication of health. *Annual review of anthropology, 46*, 261–278.

Rufas, A., & Hine, C. (2018). Everyday connections between online and offline: Imagining others and constructing community through local online initiatives. *New Media and Society, 20*(10), 3879–3897.

Seaver, N. (2017). Algorithms as culture: Some tactics for the ethnography of algorithmic systems. *Big Data & Society, 4*(2), 1–12.

Sharon, T. (2017). Self-tracking for health and quantified self: Re-articulating autonomy, solidarity, and authenticity in the age of personalized medicine. *Philosophy & Technology, 30*(1), 93–121.

Šimenc, J. (2017). Sinhronizacija digitalnosti v medicinski praksi. *Glasnik Slovenskega etnološkega društva, 57*(1–2), 45–53. Available at: https://www.sed-drustvo.si/domains/sed-drustvo.si/modules/Domino/Files/glasnik-sed-57-12-2017-low.pdf. Accessed 3 May 2019.

Šimenc, J. (2019). Umeščanje duševnega zdravja na družabna omrežja – primer program OMRA. In L. Šprah (Ed.), *Z več znanja o motnjah razpoloženja do izhodov iz labirintov: Izkušnje in razmisleki* (pp. 113–127). Ljubljana: ZRC SAZU.

Smailhodzic, E., Hooijsma, W., Boonstra, A., & Langley, J. D. (2016). Social media use in healthcare: A systematic review of effects on patients and on their relationship with healthcare professionals. *BMC Health Services Research,*

16(442). Available at: https://www.rug.nl/research/portal/files/49772771/Social_media_use_in_healthcare.pdf. Accessed 10 Aug 2019.

Svalastog, A. L., Allgaier, J., & Gajović, S. (2015). Navigating knowledge landscapes: On health, science, communication, media, and society. *Croatian Medical Journal, 56*(4), 321–321. Available at: http://www.cmj.hr/2015/56/4/26321023.htm. Accessed 7 July 2019.

Svalastog, A. L., Allgaier, J., & Gajović, S. (2018). Navigating knowledge landscapes in the digital society: A look back and visions for the future. *Croatian Medical Journal, 59*(5), 274–278. Available at: http://www.cmj.hr/default.aspx?id=12904&issue=yes. Accessed 20 Sept 2019.

Terranova, T. (2000). Free labor: Producing culture for the digital economy. *Social Text, 18*(2), 33–58. Available at: http://web.mit.edu/schock/www/docs/18.2terranova.pdf. Accessed 16 Aug 2019.

Till, C. (2014). Exercise as labour: Quantified self and the transformation of exercise into labour. *Societies, 4*, 446–462.

Ziewitz, M. (2016). Governing algorithms: Myth, mess and methods. *Science, Technology, & Human Values, 41*(1), 3–16.

10

eHealth Applications in Knowledge Landscapes

Melike Şahinol

Introduction

I define health as the overall concept of well-being in all known forms. In doing so, I align my understanding of health with the definition offered by the World Health Organization (WHO) that "health is a state of complete physical, mental and social well-being and not merely the absence of disease or infirmity" (Official Records of WHO, no. 2, p. 100). Health as such is striving to prevent as well as to recover from any form of illness. In order to do so and in an ideal setting, information shapes knowledge that passes on new and/or improved information that in return shapes new and/or improved knowledge and so on. A knowledge landscape is formed. As the name implies, knowledge landscapes are metaphoric landscapes shaped by the various environmental factors impacting on them. Environmental, here, refers to socio-cultural, socio-political and socio-technical environments that all directly or indirectly impact the personal

M. Şahinol (✉)
Human, Medicine and Society, Orient-Institut Istanbul, Istanbul, Turkey
e-mail: sahinol@oiist.org

A. L. Svalastog et al. (eds.), *Navigating Digital Health Landscapes*, Health, Technology and Society, https://doi.org/10.1007/978-981-15-8206-6_10

shaping of knowledge landscapes. They are continuously transforming taking on new shapes as the knowledge that feeds them grows and changes too. Technology can assist in storing and organizing as well as analysing and further improving this flow, exchange and transformation of information into forms of knowledge, so it can be accessed easily, readily, effectively and practically anywhere. Knowledge landscapes are personal and continuously evolving.

Lately, digital transformation trends in healthcare services have enjoyed a remarkable degree of interest across the world. The adoption of information and communications technologies (ICT) into healthcare systems is not a new topic as such, but eHealth applications considered as socio-(bio-)technical systems are a relatively new perspective. Socio-technical constellations consist of interactions ("Interaktion") between human actors, the intra-action of technical objects ("Intra-Aktion") as well as the interactions ("Interaktivität") between humans and technical objects and ultimately "physical routines, factual designs and symbolic control dispositions" (Rammert 2007, p. 35). This definition implies the importance of human actions as well as designs, software programs and ICT and is, therefore, linked to mHealth (mobile health) in knowledge landscapes and their individual/societal implications. mHealth is the delivery of healthcare and health information based on all applications of telecommunications and multimedia technologies for all forms of mobile devices. Şahinol (2016) expanded the concept of socio-technical constellations insofar as self-recursive bio-technical assemblages play a significant role. This is because technologies used in the health sector have an impact on the physiological, biological, psychological and social health of the individual and of society at large. Against the background of this theoretical foil, itself anchored in science and technology studies, the chapter gives an overview of eHealth applications in knowledge landscapes.

As a growing number of eHealth systems, applications and landscapes gradually appeared, eHealth became part of our daily lives. The next section gives an overview of eHealth and its development in the advent of ICT and as encouraged by the WHO at a global level since 2005, followed by an outline of the systems used and their purposes installed, pointing out key factors and values.

Concerning eHealth in Knowledge Landscapes

Since the 1990s, with the widespread use of computers and the Internet, paper-based health records have been digitized, then made remote (telehealth, eHealth) and, lastly, expanded to mobile units (Costa et al. 2012).

> Telehealth involves the use of telecommunications and virtual technology to deliver health care outside of traditional health-care facilities. Telehealth, which requires access only to telecommunications, is the most basic element of 'eHealth,' which uses a wider range of information and communication technologies. (WHO 2018)

The use of ICT for the benefit of a globally healthy future (Healy 2007) is associated with eHealth. The term eHealth has been frequently used, since 1999 (Della Mea 2001; Eysenbach 2001), but there is no agreed, precise definition of this term in the literature. Oh et al. (2005) obtained 51 unique definitions of eHealth (or e-health) from their searches through databases, dictionaries and an Internet search engine. As a summary, they identified health and technology as universal themes and six less general (commerce, activities, stakeholders, outcomes, place and perspectives). Almost all the definitions include positive terms such as benefit, efficiency, enhancing, and so on and contain no negative words or do not point to disadvantages (ibid.).

According to the results (Oh et al. 2005), the term

> eHealth encompasses a set of disparate concepts, including health, technology, and commerce. (…) Health, as used in these definitions, usually referred explicitly to health care as a process, rather than to health as an outcome. (...) In the definitions of eHealth … technology was viewed both as a tool to enable a process/function/service and as the embodiment of eHealth itself. (ibid.)

Looking at developments of eHealth in the context of global efforts, process and service-oriented improvement are important features of eHealth enlargement. In 2005, at the 58th World Health Assembly (WHA) in Geneva, the importance of eHealth was also stressed by the

WHA, which approved an "eHealth resolution" (WHA 58.28), where the importance of eHealth is stressed and the target was defined as "cost-effective and secure use of … ICT in support of health and health-related fields, including health-care services, health surveillance, health literature, and health education, knowledge and research" (WHO 2005). In the resolution the WHO was called to be supportive to countries in adapting eHealth into their health systems and services (WHO 2005). Until today, the WHA has passed a series of resolutions adopted by three of the six WHO Regional Committees. The implementation of these resolutions is closely linked to the achievement of the Millennium Development Goals (MDGs). For WHO, eHealth (still) holds the promise for reducing healthcare costs and improving quality and equitable access to healthcare and healthcare services (Al-Shorbaji 2013).

According to the report of the third global survey on eHealth of WHO (2016b), wherein 125 of the 194 WHO member states were surveyed, 58% reported having national eHealth policies in place. The participants were also asked about the year of adoption of policies on Universal Health Coverage (UHC), eHealth, Health Information System (HIS) and telehealth. The data show a substantially increasing number of UHC, eHealth, HIS and telehealth policies since 1990. The report explains the lower rates for telehealth by the fact that many eHealth policies also include reference to telehealth itself (Fig. 10.1).

The next figure (Fig. 10.2) shows the increase in numbers each year and also the adoption of eHealth strategies in the different countries, which indicated the year of adoption of their policies.

Later Turkey, Bermuda, Equatorial Guinea, São Tomé and Principe, Indonesia and Malawi were added to these countries by changing their eHealth policies (Greenleaf 2017). Other key findings of the study are that three "quarters of countries have institutions that offer pre-service training or continuing education training on … ICT for health for health sciences professionals; 25% of countries offer in-service training on social media for health" (WHO 2016b, p. 11).

The development of country-specific eHealth policies and education goes hand in hand with the "emerging mobile communications and network technologies for healthcare" (Istepanian et al. 2006, p. 3; see also Kay et al. 2011; for empirical studies on the usability of mHealth apps,

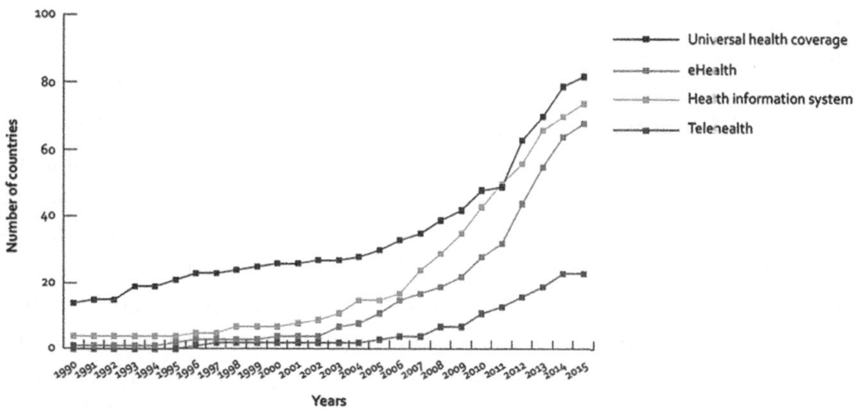

Fig. 10.1 "Number of countries with UHC, eHealth, HIS and telehealth policies or strategies cumulatively by year of adoption (1990–2015)". (Source: WHO 2016b, p. 14)

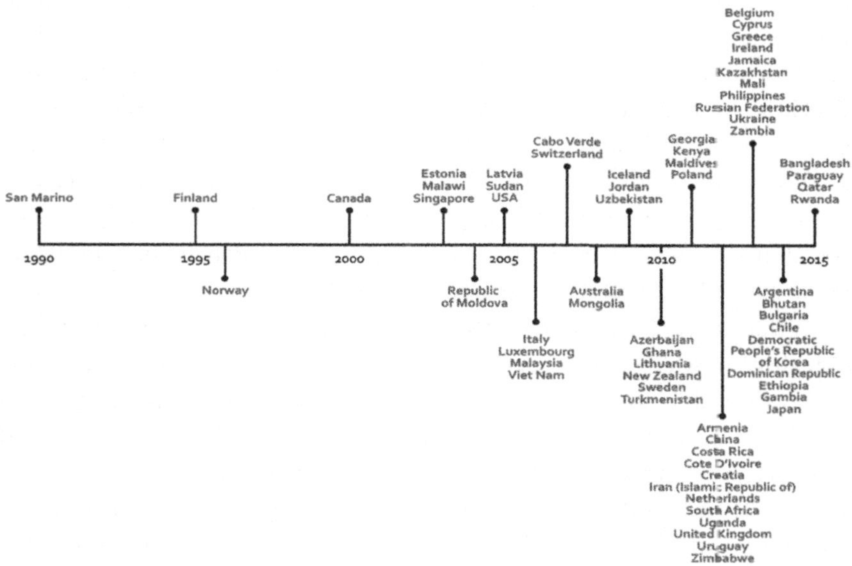

Note: Of the 73 reporting countries, 68 are shown (5 did not report the year of eHealth adoption and were omitted).

Fig. 10.2 "Timeline of country adoption of eHealth policies or strategies, 1990–2015". (Source: WHO 2016b, p. 14)

see Zapata et al. 2015), summed up as mobile health (mHealth), which indicates the mobility of health-related applications. As a part of the term eHealth, issues on mHealth have also been surveyed by the WHO. "In the GOe 2015 survey, mHealth was defined as the use of mobile devices—such as mobile phones, patient monitoring devices, personal digital assistants (PDAs) and wireless devices—for medical and public health practice" (WHO 2016b, p. 27). The key findings with regard to mHealth are that 87% of the responding member states specified to have at least one mHealth programme in their country. 91% of high-income countries (n=40) whereas 80% of the responding low-income countries (n=16) have at least one mHealth programme. Since 2010 there is an increase of the number of programmes reported as being launched. Only 14% (n=16) of the countries have evaluated a government-sponsored mHealth programme (WHO 2016b, p. 27). The most common group of programmes include community mobilization/health promotion campaigns, access to health information and databases, mobile telehealth consultations, emergency and disaster response and management, access to patient records, mLearning online education resources, data capture and transmission for patient monitoring and data collection for health surveys shown in the next figure.

Internet-delivered health intervention methods like websites (Massicotte 2015) or mobile applications (Carroll et al. 2017) or even social media (Merolli et al. 2013) have been used widely by people (Baker et al. 2003; McIntosh et al. 2017).

In that respect, the characteristics of digital technology and, therefore, eHealth knowledge landscapes are perceived as positive, "improving the prevention, diagnosis, treatment, monitoring and management of health and lifestyle. Digital health and care have the potential to innovate and improve access to care, quality of care, and to increase the overall efficiency of the health sector" (European Commission 2019). As one can see in the variety of the mHealth programmes in Fig. 10.3, the multidisciplinary character of mHealth is not to be underestimated, but on the other hand it leads to coordination difficulties, as for instance technical developments within the health sector are faster than legal regulations (see next section). Nevertheless, the digitization of health is associated with mostly positive aspects as it is linked "to deliver better value healthcare against a backdrop of increasing levels of chronic disease, ageing

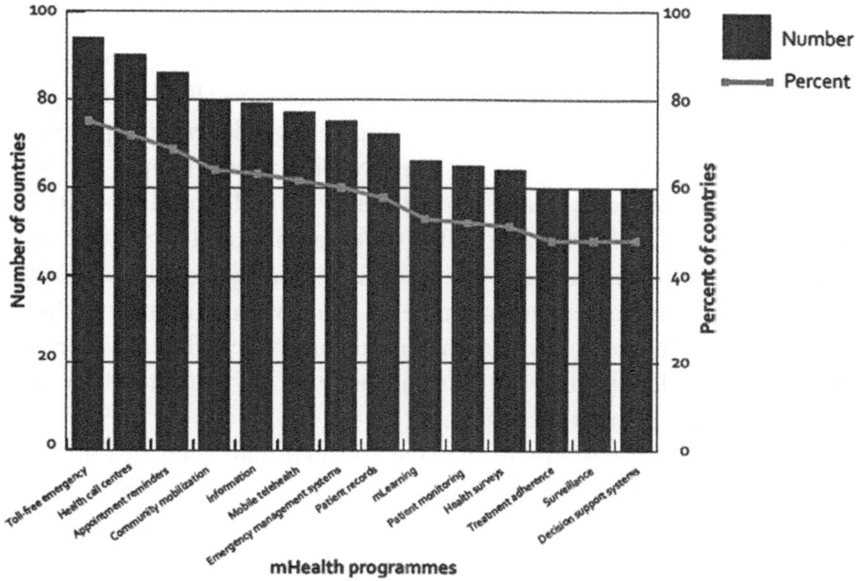

Fig. 10.3 "Number and percentage of countries that reported employing an mHealth programme, by type". (Source: WHO 2016b, p. 31)

populations, global financial crises and reduced public spending, and digital health tools and services are widely touted as being part of the answer, offering low-cost and patient-centred solutions" (Powell et al. 2016, p. 1). On a more individual level, mHealth provides information to lay people regarding their own healthcare, helping them "share their experiences of health and illness, training and educating healthcare professionals, helping people with chronic illnesses to engage in self- care and encouraging others to engage in activities to promote their health and wellbeing and avoid illness" (Lupton 2018, p. 1).

Electronic Health Record Systems, Mobile Health Applications and Governing eHealth

Expectations of improving health and healthcare systems via ICT are associated with the developments outlined above; hence, governments and public health organizations are constructing webpages, mobile applications, and so on for tracking and/or promoting and protecting public health (Tucker 2011). On the other hand, there are countless self-based-regulation eHealth applications on the markets (Pohl 2017). Even though many of these apps were developed by independent people or organizations, there are some online libraries where people can find government-approved eHealth apps, such as United Kingdom National Health Service (NHS) (Kwong 2015). These self-based-regulation apps seem to promote healthy lifestyle, while at the same time they stress the need for self-management and an increase in individual and social responsibility of their usage. This makes the discussion of the differences between these formal eHealth interventions and patients' own attempts for their healthcare management inevitable.

A possibility for patients to manage and maintain their health information is given through Electronic Health Record (EHR)/Personal Health Record (PHR)[1] systems (for a historical overview and trends of PHR, see Kim et al. 2011). In the WHO survey, EHR is defined as

> real-time, patient-centred records that provide immediate and secure information to authorized users. EHRs typically contain a patient's medical history, diagnoses and treatment, medications, allergies, immunizations, as well as radiology images and laboratory results. (WHO 2016b, p. 94)

EHR systems are associated with many promises. On the one hand, EHR systems promise medical information in paper form to be processed effectively—for all parties and processes involved. This includes caretakers, care and support of patients, processes, financial and other administrative processes. The EHR is connected with the hope to prevent medical errors and a better administration of medication (e.g. for allergy sufferers) (Ambinder 2005). Of particular importance is the self-administration of the patient. In this connection, the concept of "patient empowerment" (Bravo et al. 2015; Reichardt and Gastmeier 2013) should be noted as a

[1] "The specific area that PHR refers to has become conflated by continued mixed usage with phrases such as EMR/EHR. In other words, the term PHR started to be accepted as a separate concept from EMR with the use of phrases like personal medical record (1995) and computer-generated patient-held medical record (1996). This separation from digitized and paper records occurred when computerized records became the standard, and the word 'electronic' was added to PHR in order to distinguish it from past paper records" (Kim et al. 2011).

relatively new movement with the aim to improve the patient's position through information and participation—also in the decision processes regarding medical treatment (especially in chronic diseases). This concept has been implemented in recent years, especially in the treatment of chronic diseases (see Rossi et al. 2015 or te Boveldt et al. 2015). More recently, the patient's active involvement in patient safety initiatives has become more prominent (WHO 2016a). Thus, on the one hand, there are several advantages associated with EHR systems; on the other hand, the greater involvement of patients does not always have to be the preference of patients and members of voluntary groups—since this entails more responsibility (Thompson 2007).

> A National Electronic Health Records system is most often implemented under the responsibility of the national health authority and will typically make a patient's medical history available to health professionals in health care institutions and provide linkages to related services such as pharmacies, laboratories, specialists, and emergency and medical imaging facilities. (WHO 2016b, p. 94)

In the WHO survey, 47% of the responding countries reported to have an EHR system, whereby the number of countries with regard to the adoption of national EHR systems constantly increased since 2000. The integration of EHR systems with laboratory information systems was reported by 77%, with pharmacy information systems by 72%, and 56% reported an integration of EHR with picture archiving and communications systems (PACS).

Lack of funding, infrastructure and capacity are important barriers for the implementation of EHR (WHO 2016b).

> Legal issues were also considered to be a significant barrier (44%; n=53). Protecting the privacy and security of patients' health data must be a high priority for all countries. Chapter 6 [WHO 2016b, MŞ] reports reports that just over half of the responding countries (n=68; 55%) have legislation to protect the privacy of individuals' health-related data in EHRs; this indicates that a large proportion of countries have still not taken action. (WHO 2016b, p. 99)

Accordingly, global data protection of health data is not achieved across national borders. Even privacy of individuals' health-related data seems to be problematic at a single governmental, legal and societal level (Anderson 2007). Despite this, different studies show that eHealth mobile applications are very common (Kay et al. 2011) mostly for improving health, having healthy diets and controlling weights (Carroll et al. 2017; Ernsting et al. 2017; for the acceptance of HIT and mHealth, see Garavand et al. 2017; for the factors of the consumers' eHealth acceptance, see Scholz and Roth 2017). For this reason, it is worthwhile to consider user statistics.

In their national survey, Krebs and Duncan (2015) studied the usage of health apps among US mobile phone owners (*n*=1604). More than half (58%) had downloaded a health-related mobile app, where apps concerned with fitness and nutrition were the most popular and also used at least on a daily basis. "Interestingly, among those who had downloaded health apps, trust in their accuracy and data safety was quite high, and most felt that the apps had improved their health" (Krebs and Duncan 2015).

Houdek Von Holtz et al. (2015) showed in their study (*n*=300, 71% smartphone users) that 44% of smartphone users had health apps. "While participants most often shared information about health apps within their social networks, information was less frequently shared with providers, and physician recommendation played a small role in influencing patient use of health apps" (Houdek Von Holtz et al. 2015). These findings correlate with other region-specific studies.

55.2% of the population of Turkey are smartphone users. United Arab Emirates is the first country of the list with 82.2% (Newzoo 2018). Turkish revenue in the "eHealth" market is $152 m in 2018. This number is $3821 m for USA and $652 m for Germany (Statista 2018b). According to a survey of Statista with 1042 Turkish participants (age group: 18 to 64), most of the people (33%) used health-related applications or smart health devices (i.e. medication reminders, symptom checker, etc.). Fitness-related apps were the second biggest percentage with 32% (Statista 2017b). However, in literature, there are no statistics for Turkey on the number of health applications released and the number of users.

A representative survey carried out by bitkom research (n=1003, including 798 Internet users and 698 smartphone users) showed that nearly every second a smartphone user in Germany (45%) already uses a health app. Apps that record only body and fitness data, such as heart rate, blood pressure or steps, are the most popular ones. A quarter of all smartphone users (27%) are already using these digital healthcare providers. 74% are motivated in using these apps to improve their overall health. More than a half enjoys checking their own fitness data and nearly half say that they want to know more about their health status. Data protection reasons, such as the fear that the health data could be misused, are a reason for 25% of non-users not to use health apps (bitkom 2017).

As a result of their study on the impact of patient-centred eHealth applications on patient outcomes, Wildenbos et al. (2016) point out that "the content and design of eHealth solutions [should be tailored,] according to patient user profiles, so as to enhance eHealth interventions' impact on patient behaviour, self-efficacy, and health-related outcomes" (ibid.). An important factor could be the safety of patients' health data and data protection in general. Yet still, eHealth interventions are becoming increasingly popular (Elbert et al. 2014; McIntosh et al. 2017). This could be due to the high technology push into the market: according to the mHealth App Economics Report 2017/2018 (research2guidance 2017), in 2017, there were 325,000 health apps, which were released by 84,000 different publishers, available in the popular markets and this number was increased by 78,000 from the previous year. Moreover, it is estimated that the global revenue of mobile health devices and services will be around 35.8 billion dollars by 2020 (Statista 2017a).

The US Food and Drug Administration (FDA) encourages the development of mHealth, as mobile apps support self-managed health and wellness of their user and access to useful health information.

> According to industry estimates, 500 million smartphone users worldwide will be using a health care application by 2015, and by 2018, 50 percent of the more than 3.4 billion smartphone and tablet users will have downloaded mobile health applications.[2] These users include health care professionals, consumers, and patients. (FDA 2018)

[2] http://www.research2guidance.com/500m-people-will -be-using-healthcare-mobile-applications-in-2015/

Hence, such governmental regulations and organizational guidelines on health apps could foster a more responsible health landscape and its structures of communication (for the regulatory controls that apply in the USA and Europe, see, e.g. Boulos et al. 2014). Surely, legal regulations and guidelines could help in assessing and navigating eHealth knowledge landscapes. Nevertheless, NGOs could play a key role in testing health apps, showing certain eHealth trends and innovations and creating market analysis for healthcare decision makers (see "The Health App e-Nabız"). This could be a chance for the responsible use of the possibilities of digitization in order to make healthcare patient-oriented. A cooperation with representatives of patients, consumers, clinicians, nurses, health insurers and healthcare companies would be beneficial for all parties.

The results of the development of country-specific eHealth policies in general and eHealth applications in particular offer evidence for eHealth being embedded in digitization processes dependent on socio-economic infrastructure policies (communication and network technologies for healthcare, pharmacies, laboratories, etc.) and socio-political (health policy, legal issues) landscapes of the respective country. Consequently, social factors shape the knowledge landscape, as patient-specific mHealth programmes might be used, but also technical possibilities shape individuals' health-related practices.

Information: Transparency—Data Protection

Nowadays, data privacy and security rules are being established in many countries at a great pace, with some countries enacting new laws and others updating existing ones. Historically, Germany was one of the first countries in preventing uncontrolled use of personal data enforcing legal actions on those violating these laws (Schriver 2001). Germany adopted the first data processing regulation in 1970. Then, Sweden released the first national data protection law in 1973 and, in 1978, France took a step in the same direction (Schriver 2001).

Only two years after the establishment of the European Union in 1993, the Data Privacy Directive was created. The directive came into force in 1998 (Andrews 1998) and stated that privacy is a "fundamental human right" and with Article 25 (1) regulated that the transfer of personal information to countries outside the EU can only be possible if that country guarantees adequate protection for the data:

> The Member States shall provide that the transfer to a third country of personal data which are undergoing processing or are intended for processing after transfer may take place only if, without prejudice to compliance with the national provisions adopted pursuant to the other provisions of this Directive, the third country in question ensures an adequate level of protection. (ibid.)

Hence, the EU has a big influence on data protection regulations and data privacy practices in the global context (Sherman et al. 2016). This is one of the main reasons why many other countries are establishing new laws and regulations, in order to be able to establish, maintain or intensify business relations with EU member states. With respect to data protection, the Data Protection Directive 95/46/EC was replaced with the EU General Data Protection Regulation (GDPR) on 25 May 2018. The regulatory policies of the new directive have, as written on the website, changed a lot, since the world is now "vastly different from the time in which the 1995 directive was established" (EU GDPR Portal 2017).

The main reason for the avoidance of establishing certain laws and regulations is probably the economic and social costs that privacy brings to governments, industry groups or companies (Diamond et al. 2009; Fromholz 2000), although the aim of the principles of personal data protection is neither to establish barriers in front of technological developments nor prohibiting data processing that may be useful or necessary (Küzeci 2010).

Today, personal data is under protection by certain laws in 120 countries (Greenleaf 2017) and Turkey is the newest country among them. The first Personal Data Protection (PDP) Law of Turkey was published on 24 March 2016 ("Kişisel verilerin korunması kanunu" 2016).[3]

[3] However, since the law came into effect, there have been many debates on its articles, and even the biggest opposition party (CHP) appealed to the Constitutional Court for the cancellation of the provisions of the law on 3 June 2016 ("CHP kişisel verilerin korunması kanunun iptali için

With the diffusion of ICT and a growing number of eHealth systems and landscapes, the penetration of eHealth is also closely linked into privacy in daily life. Many data scandals in recent years underline the importance of implementing legal regulations as there seems to be a discrepancy in legal regulations and in practice. For instance, following the Cambridge Analytica scandal (Confessore 2018), Facebook was accused of collecting anonymous patient data and matching them with patients' Facebook profiles (Farr 2018; Geib 2018). According to news agency CNBC (Farr 2018), Facebook was asking some major American hospitals for anonymized patient data (i.e. diseases, medicines info) on March 2018. Despite Facebook's announcement that this situation does not go beyond a project stage and that they have not bought any health data yet, this recent development raised public concerns, which were already at high level.

Gemalto's 2017 annual report on data breaches showed that the highest number of breach incidents occurred in the healthcare industry. Parallel with the increasing number of these scandals and the breach news in the media (Statista 2018a), the number of people concerned about their data privacy is rising continuously (Madden and Rainie 2015). If it is about sensitive data, such as health-related ones, the greater the risk or the danger that is perceived. Nevertheless, experts indicate that with the help of the technical developments and stronger regulations, concerns about security and privacy can easily be eliminated in the near future (Rainie and Anderson 2017).

A meta-study (Sankar et al. 2003) examined 110 articles about people's attitudes and opinions on privacy and confidentiality of their medical data. The study reported that people tend to postpone or do not seek treatment, hiding or altering medical history due to worries about their privacy. These results were renewed by the survey conducted in 2011 in Turkey. According to the results of the Turkish survey (Özkan 2011), people have similar tendencies about not seeking/postponing the

AYM'ye başvurdu", 2016). The case was concluded on 28 September 2017 and Constitutional Court rejected all cancellation requests of CHP on the cancellation of certain articles of the law (TC Resmi Gazete, 2018). Although the Constitutional Court finalized the case in the opposite direction and the law was written based on EU Directive numbered 95/46/EC, the PDP law also criticized and stated that "it is not yet in line with European standards" in the recent EU Commission Turkey report (European Commission 2018).

treatments and hiding/altering data about their conditions. These results showed the vital importance of data privacy in healthcare.

In the case of informational privacy, it can be understood as the right to retain personal information or the right to have control about who should or should not receive which information (Rössler 2001; Schaar 2014). From a legal point of view, it is a protective good that is a conglomerate of various individual rights and (basic) laws (Wiederin 2003). From a sociological and cultural perspective, it is a cultural value, which is also secured by non-legal values and societal norms (such as discretion) that are inscribed in the body[4] (Heyl 2004). Even though every modern democratic society must set up a (political) public sphere and a protected area of privacy accessible to all citizens (Peters 2007), the information or data to be subject to the protection of privacy or considered sensitive can (and must) constantly (publicly) be negotiated (and legitimized). It shows that the conceptions of what is or should be private vary between the legal systems of different states and different (national) cultures and possibly evolve in different directions (Şahinol and Kirschsieper 2016).

Freedom of information, the right to transparency and data protection are all crucial for a responsible eHealth knowledge landscape; indeed, their intermutual relationship shapes the structures of communication within health systems. The relationship between transparency and data protection in a given society, however, is culturally specific, with practices embedded in specific historical, ethical, legal and cultural contexts and practices (Freude and Freude 2017). In their discursive approach, Şahinol and Kirschsieper (2016) compared the privacy culture in Germany and Turkey within the field of medicine. Since health information are traditionally and largely cross-culturally considered as particularly "intimate" due to their physical reference, they focused on health apps. Some of these apps collect and evaluate personal information on a large scale. There is not only the risk that these data could be delivered to unintended recipients. There is also the risk that the recipients of this data and/or the apps themselves comment on and evaluate the user's private life based on the private information they collect and thereby limit the user's autonomy (Şahinol and Kirschsieper 2016). Thus, not only informational

[4] Social issues and social practices and, as a result, social norms become an integral part of the body.

privacy is threatened but also, as related to it, decentralized privacy, which is the right to make self-determined decisions without interference by public authorities or by other persons (Rössler 2001).

Therefore, data protection in general and in specific health-related data protection should be a key issue for the implementation of eHealth systems and programmes. Recently, the need and urgency of protecting health-related data is also reflected by the subject "big healthcare data", as big healthcare data rises questions with regard to anonymization, encryption (Abouelmehdi et al. 2018) and pseudonymization. These terms have very close meanings to each other but they are not synonyms. Anonymization is the irreversible action of removing identifiable parts from the data, so there is no link back to the original version. On the other hand, encrypted data can be read with a secret key by a system or person. Pseudonymization uses also secret keys—a personal identifier is kept in a separate location, for reaching the data; however, unlike encryption, pseudonymization uses the same strings for the same inputs (Stevovic 2017). Pseudonymization is newly added and highly recommended by the GDPR (EU GDPR Portal 2017).

The case of Turkey is particularly interesting because, since May 2015, the health app "e-Nabiz" developed by the Turkish Ministry of Health is in use even though a lot of concerns about privacy and health data protection have been addressed. For this reason, our case study discusses these contexts in regard to Turkey, with the argument that, in order to create and maintain a responsible health landscape, governmental authorities need to be aware of the importance of data protection as well as the patient's right to confidentiality in the implementation of healthcare policy.

The Health App e-Nabız

The case study focuses on the widespread use of a Turkish multifunctional personal health record application, "e-Nabız" (e-Pulse). Promoted by the Turkish Ministry of Health since May 2015, the app e-Nabız stores health data and measures various vital parameters. It is possible via e-Nabız to set up hospital appointments or register for organ donation.

The app also facilitates blood donation and access to the ambulance system. Furthermore, every health service provider, hospital and physician in Turkey has been required to share health records of their patients with the e-Nabız system. This app is indicative of a trend towards the digitization of the medical treatment as well as personalized medicine. According to the Turkish Ministry of Health, more than five million users have been registered since October 2015 (Kahvecioğlu 2018). Yet, as the Turkish Medical Association has pointed out, e-Nabız presents ethical dilemmas regarding the rights to data protection and privacy. Not surprisingly perhaps, a lawsuit was filed for stopping the execution of e-Nabız.

By the beginning of 2015, the Turkish Ministry of Health made a public notification about the health app e-Nabız and the renewal of the health network system. A month later (5 February, 2015) it declared in the announcement 2015/5 that the aim of the new health system would be to give patients a mobile access to their health data. This system would also be integrated into the Sağlık.Net system until 1 March, 2015. The Turkish Ministry of Health defines Sağlık.Net as

> an information and communication platform that is integrated, safe, fast and expandable and the first aim of which is to collect the data produced in health institutions online, in compliance with the standards and directly from where produced. The second aim is to enhance efficiency and quality in the first, second and third level healthcare services by producing proper information from collected data for all stakeholders. ("Turkey Clinical Quality Program", 2013)

The integration of e-Nabız and the new health system includes patients' health data from public and private clinics as well as from university hospitals, including data transmission of all known personal health data. Especially, emergency data sets are of interest, while for all other data sets the consent of the patients is to be obtained. The Turkish Ministry of Health furthermore declared that all information regarding these issues would be available on the websites "enabiz.gov.tr" (website of e-Nabız) and "sys.sagliknet.saglik.gov.tr" (which is not available anymore: for further information, see http://saglik.gov.tr/). The lawsuit mentioned above was between the NGOs (Turkish Medical Association (Türk Tabipleri

Birliği, TTB) and Turkish Dental Association) and the Ministry of Health and concluded in the first quarter of 2016. NGOs sued e-Nabız on the violation of the privacy of personal information rights in February 2015, even though it is written on the website of e-Nabız that accessing, storing and sharing of information are only possible with the permission of the patients (e-Nabız 2015). In 25 February, 2015, the TTB announced on their webpage about the public notification that there was no information available on the e-Nabız pages indicating what emergency records were and how to obtain the consent of the patients. In their online message TBB has also referred to the scandal of 2013 when the Social Security Institute (Sosyal Güvenlik Kurumu, SGK[5]) sold personal health data to 5 companies (pharmaceutical industry, foreign companies) for 65,000 TL (about 30,000 USD in 2013). They further referred to previous decisions of the Turkish Council of State (similar to French Conseil d'Etat or German Federal Administrative Court and Ministry of Justice) that the Ministry of Health may not collect personal data. The TTB complained that the Ministry of Health places doctors in difficult positions regarding their medical confidentiality. They indicated that the TBB will file a claim in court (5 February, 2015). In fact, on 24 November, 2015, the Turkish Council of State declared it would stop collecting personal data and close down the e-Nabız project by the Ministry of Health. So, the case resulted in their favour (TTB 2016). However, irrespective of the Council's decision, the requests from the TTB remain unsuccessful and the e-Nabız project continued and even won the World Summit Award-Mobile (WSA[6]) 2016 in the category "health and well being" (WSA 2016). Moreover, the Turkish Ministry of Health declared in its public

[5] On the website of the SGK, the Social Security Institution is described as "Institution established with the objective of the realization of a social security system at the contemporary standards that will provide individuals with social insurance and universal health insurance, based on the principles of social insurance, effective, equitable, easily accessible, actuarial and sustainable in financial terms. The duties of SSI are as follows according to Article 3 of the Law No. 5502" ("Social Security Institution", 2016).

[6] The evaluation criteria of WSA are as follows: content (quality and comprehensiveness), functionality (ease to use, user experience, appropriate interactivity), design (navigation, orientation and visual appeal), technology (state of the art in technology and quality of technical realization) and innovation (originality and newness to targeted users, business model society and market). Besides the mentioned technical evaluation criteria, there are also strategic evaluation criteria such as impact (local impact/impact on society) and global/UN value (WSA 2016).

announcement in 2016 (2016/6), with reference to Article 56 of the constitutional law, that the State has to protect the physical and mental health of its citizens and that its task is to implement this efficiently in the form of centrally managed health services. Additionally, the Turkish Ministry of Health declared with reference to Article 20 of the constitutional law that the right to protection of personal data is maintained and that the right for rectification or deletion of personal data may be requested. It is interesting that there was no discourse in Turkey regarding health data protection and that the affected group was unconcerned and trusted in technology, as data protection remains theoretical in part only. In Germany, for instance, data protection officers were assigned to oversee the collection and maintenance of its citizens' sensitive information ensuring strict standards for the protection of privacy of the individual while, at the same time, collecting essential data for the improvement of their healthcare systems. In Turkey, on the other hand, the Ministry of Health opposes such measures. Although the TTB won the case, changes to legal and governmental bodies for the effective implementation of data protection are yet to be initiated. Instead, physicians continue to take on the sole role of privacy advocates and data protectionists without much backup from the state (Şahinol and Kirschsieper 2016).

Surprisingly, Turkish media do not report critical but rather informative and technically affirmative items about e-Nabız. For instance, Turkish media reported (Medimagazin 2016) about an award ceremony "e-Türkiye" for e-Nabız as innovative technology awarded by TÜSIAD, the Association of Turkish industrialists and business people, and TBV, the Turkish Foundation for Computer Science, that e-Nabız is the best health app on a worldwide level ("e-Nabız'a dünya çapında ödül", 2017). The public television channel Turkish Radio and Television (TRT) broadcasted an information programme on 25 April, 2016 "İyiFikir—E-Nabız Nedir?" (see https://www.youtube.com/watch?v=ldSHJittU38)—meaning "Good Idea: What Is e-Nabız?". And there are a number of informative YouTube videos from the Turkish Ministry of Health promoting e-Nabız as a fast and safe system to access personal health data, however, with no information about how one's health data is protected against misuse ("e-Nabız—Kişisel Sağlık Sistemi", see https://www.youtube.com/watch?v=qlYNnvNJZaE). Undoubtedly, the safety concept in the YouTube video refers to data access, to get the right personal health data in emergency cases—which seems plausible at first. The safety concept with regard to data protection must not be contradictory with data access. Lastly, the health system must be secure and ensure the protection of personal health data. To create transparency and effective online solutions for the dissemination of health- and medical-related information would mean to have legislation protecting privacy of individuals' health-related data (as specified by the WHO) as well as implementing them in practice. However, sharing health data, especially via social networks, is essential to increase the health awareness of the patient and so foster a self-regulated health management (in the long term, which is crucial for the national health system). However, if there is no awareness of protecting data—or, if there is a more or less naive faith in technology (Şahinol and Kirschsieper 2016)—even governance structures could fail. Here, NGOs like medical associations could have the power to reshape technological applications—or legal regulations—through their more critical perspective on eHealth.

To understand what we can learn from this case, it is worth looking at a more technocritical country like Germany. A recent study by the Federal Ministry of Health (Germany) comes to the conclusion that a "consistent implementation of the existing regulations and the creation of appropriate clarity and transparency in information and consent would promote the exercising of the individual right to informational self-determination" (Albrecht 2016, p. 26). Especially in connection to data protection most Germans are very critical. In Germany, eHealth-related developments are publicly discussed much more critically. Şahinol and Kirschsieper (2016) describe the differences of the usage of health apps in Turkey and Germany within different historical pasts and different visions and scenarios for the future. In Germany, scenarios of the "transparent person/patient" (Rosenbach et al. 2015; Züst 2014) and the "surveillance and control state" are dominant, but in Turkey visions of a healthy society within a technologically optimized world are central. "On the individual level, technophilia as a socio-cultural determinant lead to neglect data security issues, thus health data security awareness is not built up" (Şahinol and Başkavak 2020a, p. 41). In Germany, the value of health has to be subordinated to the value of the private (in the informational and decisional sense). In Turkey, on the other hand, there is an optimistic, technology-friendly culture that moderately fears the loss of privacy (Şahinol and Kirschsieper 2016).

Discussion: Cultural Impacts as Navigation Shift in Knowledge Landscapes?

In this chapter I have discussed eHealth applications in knowledge landscapes providing a brief historical overview and, in pointing out key factors and values, showed which systems are used for what purpose. Dependent on socio-technical, socio-cultural and socio-political aspects, person-centred applications to health-related knowledge[7] affect the way applications are used. The case study of Turkey gives a special insight into the interdependencies of the socio-technical, socio-cultural and socio-political shaping of knowledge landscapes and its relations to personal properties. I found that knowledge landscapes are not only shaped by the impact of these mentioned factors but are an immediate reflection of the unavoidable mingling of socio-cultural and socio-political norms and practices that dictate any form of socio-technical advancement and practice (see also Şahinol and Başkavak 2020b). These case-specific findings are associated with concerns and ethical and governance issues raised by eHealth in general, because in an ideal setting, these factors lead to improved social, cultural, political and technical systems designed to protect its citizens' interests. In presented case study of Turkey, however, one could see that cultural factors strongly influence governance practices that in return dictate the standards for all forms of knowledge gathering, storage, maintenance and distribution (sharing) and, thus, form the very basis of shaping knowledge landscapes as such.

eHealth applications in particular should be considered as socio-(bio-) technical systems, as health knowledge landscapes are directly shaped by social factors that, in combination with personal (biological) factors, are shaped by technical possibilities, which in return form knowledge

[7] The concept of health and all aspects related to preserving and restoring health as defined by the WHO in Official Records of WHO, no. 2, p. 100.

landscapes. These continuously ongoing interdependent and interconnected spirals are a complex system that needs strict standards to ensure safe and responsible handling of all data. Legal regulations and governmental certificates should help to create effective solutions for the dissemination of health- and medical-related information, but NGOs also play a significant role, as engaged in eHealth-related issues they can significantly shape eHealth knowledge landscapes. To foster a more responsible health landscape and its structures of communication, a cooperation in eHealth assessment with representatives of patients, consumers, clinicians, nurses, health insurers and healthcare companies would be beneficial to all parties—and for safe travelling in eHealth knowledge landscapes.

References

Abouelmehdi, K., Beni-Hessane, A., & Khaloufi, H. (2018). Big healthcare data: Preserving security and privacy. *Journal of Big Data, 5*(1), 1.

Al-Shorbaji, N. (2013). The World Health Assembly resolutions on eHealth: eHealth in support of universal health coverage. *Methods of Information in Medicine, 52*(06), 463–466.

Albrecht, U.-V. (2016). *Chancen und Risiken von Geshundheits-Apps / Chances and Risks of Mobile Health Apps (CHARISMHA).* In U.-V. Albrecht (Ed.). Retrieved from http://www.digibib.tu-bs.de/?docid=00060000

Ambinder, E. P. (2005). Electronic health records. *Journal of Oncology Practice, 1*(2), 57–63. Retrieved from http://www.ncbi.nlm.nih.gov/pmc/articles/PMC2793588/.

Anderson, J. G. (2007). Social, ethical and legal barriers to e-health. *International Journal of Medical Informatics, 76*(5–6), 480–483.

Andrews, E. L. (1998). European Law Aims to Protect Privacy of Data. *The New York Times*. Retrieved from http://www.nytimes.com/1998/10/26/business/european-law-aims-to-protect-privacy-of-data.html

Baker, L., Wagner, T. H., Singer, S., & Bundorf, M. K. (2003). Use of the Internet and e-mail for health care information: Results from a national survey. *JAMA, 289*(18), 2400–2406. https://doi.org/10.1001/jama.289.18.2400.

bitkom. (2017). Fast jeder Zweite nutzt Gesundheits-Apps. Retrieved from https://www.bitkom.org/Presse/Presseinformation/Fast-jeder-Zweite-nutzt-Gesundheits-Apps.html

Boulos, M. N. K., Brewer, A. C., Karimkhani, C., Buller, D. B., & Dellavalle, R. P. (2014). Mobile medical and health apps: State of the art, concerns, regulatory control and certification. *Online Journal of Public Health Informatics, 5*(3), 229–229.

Bravo, P., Edwards, A., Barr, P. J., Scholl, I., Elwyn, G., & McAllister, M. (2015). Conceptualising patient empowerment: A mixed methods study. *BMC Health Services Research, 15*(1), 252.

Carroll, J. K., Moorhead, A., Bond, R., LeBlanc, W. G., Petrella, R. J., & Fiscella, K. (2017). Who uses mobile phone health apps and does use matter? A secondary data analytics approach. *Journal of Medical Internet Research, 19*(4), e125.

CHP kişisel verilerin korunması kanunun iptali için AYM'ye başvurdu. (2016). *Sözcü*.

Confessore, N. (2018). Cambridge Analytica and Facebook: The Scandal and the Fallout So Far. *The New York Times*. Retrieved from https://www.nytimes.com/2018/04/04/us/politics/cambridge-analytica-scandal-fallout.html

Costa, Â., Castillo, J. C., Novais, P., Fernández-Caballero, A., & Simoes, R. (2012). Sensor-driven agenda for intelligent home care of the elderly. *Expert Systems with Applications, 39*(15), 12192–12204.

Della Mea, V. (2001). What is e-health (2): The death of telemedicine? *Journal of Medical Internet Research, 3*(2), 6–7. https://doi.org/10.2196/jmir.3.2.e22.

Diamond, C. C., Mostashari, F., & Shirky, C. (2009). Collecting and sharing data for population health: A new paradigm. *Health Affairs, 28*(2), 454–466.

Elbert, N. J., van Os-Medendorp, H., van Renselaar, W., Ekeland, A. G., Hakkaart-van Roijen, L., Raat, H., et al. (2014). Effectiveness and cost-effectiveness of ehealth interventions in somatic diseases: A systematic review of systematic reviews and meta-analyses. *Journal of Medical Internet Research, 16*(4), e110.

E-nabiz. (2015). Retrieved from https://enabiz.gov.tr/Yardim/Index

e-Nabız'a dünya çapında ödül. (2017). Retrieved from http://www.ensonhaber.com/e-nabiza-dunya-capinda-odul-2017-03-21.html

Ernsting, C., Dombrowski, S. U., Oedekoven, M., O'Sullivan, J. L., Kanzler, E., Kuhlmey, A., & Gellert, P. (2017). Using smartphones and health apps to change and manage health behaviors: A population-based survey. *Journal of*

Medical Internet Research, 19(4), e101–e101. https://doi.org/10.2196/jmir.6838.

EU GDPR Portal. (2017). *Key changes with the general data protection regulation*. General Data Protection Regulation (GDPR). Retrieved from https://www.eugdpr.org/the-regulation.html

European Commission. (2018). *EU Turkey 2018 report*. Retrieved from Strasbourg: https://ec.europa.eu/neighbourhood-enlargement/sites/near/files/20180417-turkey-report.pdf

European Commission. (2019, March 15). *eHealth: Digital health and care*. Retrieved from https://ec.europa.eu/health/ehealth/overview_en

Eysenbach, G. (2001). What is e-health? *Journal of Medical Internet Research, 3*(2), 1–5. https://doi.org/10.2196/jmir.3.2.e20.

Farr, C. (2018). *Facebook Building 8 explored data sharing agreement with hospitals*. Retrieved from https://www.cnbc.com/2018/04/05/facebook-building-8-explored-data-sharing-agreement-with-hospitals.html

FDA. (2018). *Mobile medical applications*. Retrieved from https://www.fda.gov/MedicalDevices/DigitalHealth/MobileMedicalApplications/default.htm

Freude, A. C. H., & Freude, T. (2017). *Echoes of history: Understanding German data protection*. Retrieved from http://www.bfna.org/wp-content/uploads/2017/04/Echoes_of_history_Understanding_German_Data_Protection_Freude.pdf

Fromholz, J. M. (2000). The European Union data privacy directive. *Berkeley Technology Law Journal, 15*, 461.

Garavand, A., Samadbeik, M., Kafashi, M., & Abhari, S. (2017). Acceptance of health information technologies, acceptance of Mobile health: A review article. *Journal of Biomedical Physics & Engineering, 7*(4), 403–408. Retrieved from http://www.ncbi.nlm.nih.gov/pmc/articles/PMC5809934/.

Geib, C. (2018). *Facebook sought medical data. Yes, this should raise red flags*. Retrieved from https://futurism.com/facebook-sought-medical-data-red-flags/

Gemalto. (2017). *The year of internal threats and accidental data breaches. Findings from the 2017 Breach Level Index*. Retrieved from https://breachlevelindex.com/assets/Breach-Level-Index-Report-2017-Gemalto.pdf

Greenleaf, G. (2017). *Countries with data privacy laws – By year 1973–2016 (Tables)*. Retrieved from https://ssrn.com/abstract=2996139

Healy, J. (2007). The WHO eHealth resolution-eHealth for all by 2015? *Methods of Information in Medicine, 46*(1), 2–4.

Heyl, C. (2004). A passion for privacy. Untersuchungen zur Genese der bürgerlichen Privatsphäre in London (1660–1800). *Revue de l'IFHA, Date de parution de l'œuvre.*

Houdek Von Holtz, L. A., Hypolite, K. A., Carr, B. G., Shofer, F. S., Winston, F. K., Hanson, C. W., & Merchant, R. M. (2015). Use of mobile apps: A patient-centered approach. *Academic Emergency Medicine: Official Journal of the Society for Academic Emergency Medicine, 22*(6), 765–768.

Istepanian, R., Laxminarayan, S., & Pattichis, C. S. (2006). *M-health.* Springer.

Kahvecioğlu, A. (2018). Sağlık Bakanlığı dijital atılımda. *Milliyet Gazetesi.* Retrieved from http://www.milliyet.com.tr/saglik-bakanligi-dijital-atilimda-gundem-2589440/

Kay, M., Santos, J., & Takane, M. (2011). mHealth: New horizons for health through mobile technologies. *WHO, 64*(7), 66–71.

Kim, J., Jung, H., & Bates, D. W. (2011). History and trends of "personal health record" research in PubMed. *Healthcare Informatics Research, 17*(1), 3–17.

Kişisel verilerin korunması kanunu. (2016).

Krebs, P., & Duncan, D. T. (2015). Health app use among US mobile phone owners: A national survey. *JMIR mHealth and uHealth, 3*(4), e101. https://doi.org/10.2196/mhealth.4924.

Küzeci, E. (2010). *Kişisel Verilerin Korunması.* Ankara: Turhan Kitabevi.

Lupton, D. (2018). *Digital health: Critical and cross-disciplinary perspectives.* London: Routledge.

Madden, M., & Rainie, L. (2015). *Americans' attitudes about privacy, security and surveillance.* Pew Research Center. Retrieved from Washington, DC: www.pewreserach.org

Massicotte, A. (2015). When to trust health information posted on the Internet. *Canadian Pharmacists Journal (Ott), 148*, 61–63.

McIntosh, J. R. D., Jay, S., Hadden, N., & Whittaker, P. J. (2017). Do E-health interventions improve physical activity in young people: A systematic review. *Public Health, 148*, 140–148.

Medimagazin. (2016). E-nabız projesine E-Türkiye ödülü. Retrieved from https://www.medimagazin.com.tr/hekim/saglik-bak/tr-e-nabiz-projesine-e-turkiye-odulu-2-13-69743.html

Merolli, M., Gray, K., & Martin-Sanchez, F. (2013). Health outcomes and related effects of using social media in chronic disease management: A literature review and analysis of affordances. *Journal of Biomedical Informatics, 46*(6), 957–969.

Newzoo. (2018). *Top countries by smartphone penetration users*. Retrieved from https://newzoo.com/insights/rankings/top-50-countries-by-smartphone-penetration-and-users/

Oh, H., Rizo, C., Enkin, M., & Jadad, A. (2005). What is eHealth (3): A systematic review of published definitions. *Journal of Medical Internet Research, 7*(1), e1.

Özkan, Ö. (2011). *Attitudes and opinions of people who use medical services about privacy and confidentiality of health information in electronic environment*. Middle East Technical University.

Peters, B. (2007). *Der Sinn von Öffentlichkeit*. Frankfurt am Main: Suhrkamp Verlag.

Pohl, M. (2017). *325,000 mobile health apps available in 2017 – Android now the leading mHealth platform*. Retrieved from https://research2guidance.com/325000-mobile-health-apps-available-in-2017/

Powell, J., Newhouse, N., Boylan, A.-M., & Williams, V. (2016). Digital health citizens and the future of the NHS. *Digital Health, 2*, 1–3.

Rainie, L., & Anderson, J. (2017). *The fate of online trust in the next decade*. Retrieved from http://www.pewinternet.org/2017/08/10/the-fate-of-online-trust-in-the-next-decade/

Rammert, W. (2007). Technik, Handeln und Sozialstruktur: Eine Einführung in die Soziologie der Technik. In W. Rammert (Ed.), *Technik – Handeln – Wissen* (pp. 11–36). Wiesbaden: VS Verlag fürSozialwissenschaften | GWV Fachverlage GmbH Wiesbaden.

Reichardt, C., & Gastmeier, P. (2013). "Patient Empowerment" Wie viel können Patienten zu einer verbesserten Compliance des Personals beitragen? *Krankenhaushygiene up2date*, 157–164.

research2guidance. (2017). *mHealth App Economics Report 2017/2018*. Retrieved from www.research2guidance.com

Rosenbach, M., Schmergal, C., & Schmundt, H. (2015). Der gläserne Patient. *Der Spiegel, 50*(2015), 10–18.

Rossi, M. C., Lucisano, G., Funnell, M., Pintaudi, B., Bulotta, A., Gentile, S., et al. (2015). Interplay among patient empowerment and clinical and person-centered outcomes in type 2 diabetes. The BENCH-D study. *Patient Education and Counseling, 98*(9), 1142–1149.

Rössler, B. (2001). *Der Wert des Privaten*. Frankfurt am Main: Suhrkamp Verlag.

Şahinol, M., & Başkavak, G. (2020a). *Between empowerment and disempowerment: A qualitative analysis of (voluntary) digital health (self-)tracking in*

Turkey. Unpublished Report: Orient-Insitut Istanbul for German Ministry of Health (#ZMV | 1 - 2517 FSB 016).

Şahinol, M., & Başkavak, G. (2020b). Türkiye'de Biyomedikalizasyon: Sağlığın Dijitalleşmesi ve Öz-Takip Pratikleri (engl. Biomedicalization in Turkey: Digitalization of Health and Self-Tracking Practices). In A. Turanlı, M. Şahinol, & A. U. Aydınoğlu (Eds.), Türkiye'de STS: Bilim ve Teknoloji Çalışmalarına Giriş.(engl. STS in Turkey. Introduction to Science and Technology Studies) (pp. 103–117). Istanbul: ITÜ Vakfı Yayınları.

Şahinol, M., & Kirschsieper, D. (2016). *Die Privatheitskultur in Deutschland und der Türkei – untersuchtan den Diskursenüber Gesundheits-Apps*. Paper presented at the Smart New World Conference, Wien.

Şahinol, M. (2016). Das techno-zerebrale Subjekt: Zur Symbiose von Mensch und Maschine in den Neurowissenschaften. Bielefeld: transcript.

Sankar, P., Mora, S., Merz, J. F., & Jones, N. L. (2003). Patient perspectives of medical confidentiality: A review of the literature. *Journal of General Internal Medicine, 18*(8), 659–669.

Schaar, P. (2014). *Überwachung total: Wie wir in Zukunft unsere Daten schützen*. Aufbau Digital.

Scholz, S., & Roth, N. (2017). Determinanten der E-Health-Akzeptanz bei Verbrauchern. In S. Müller-Mielitz & T. Lux (Eds.), *E-Health-Ökonomie* (pp. 333–357). Wiesbaden: Springer Fachmedien Wiesbaden.

Schriver, R. R. (2001). You cheated, you lied: The Safe Harbor Agreement and its enforcement by the Federal Trade Commission. *Fordham Law Review, 70*, 2777.

Sherman, C., Iannopollo, E., Shey, H., & Spiliotes, A. (2016). *Forrester's 2016 interactive data privacy heat map. Landscape: The data security and privacy playbook*. Retrieved from https://static.ftitechnology.com/docs/third-party/forrester-2015-data-privacy.pdf

Social Security Institution. (2016). Retrieved from http://www.sgk.gov.tr/wps/portal/sgk/en/detail/obj_duties

statista. (2017a). Global mHealth app downloads 2013–2017 | Statistic. Retrieved from https://www.statista.com/statistics/625034/mobile-health-app-downloads/.

statista. (2017b). [Usage of health apps and smart health devices in Turkey 2017].

statista. (2018a). *Biggest online data breaches worldwide 2018*. Retrieved May 24, 2018, from https://www.statista.com/statistics/290525/cyber-crime-biggest-online-data-breaches-worldwide/

statista. (2018b). *eHealth Turkey Statista Market Forecast*. Retrieved from https://www.statista.com/outlook/312/113/ehealth/turkey#market-arpu

Stevovic, J. (2017). [Pseudonymization vs. Encryption of Health Sensitive Data].

te Boveldt, N., Vernooij-Dassen, M., Leppink, I., Samwel, H., Vissers, K., & Engels, Y. (2015). Patient empowerment in cancer pain management: An integrative. *Patient Empowerment, 23*, 121.

Thompson, A. G. H. (2007). The meaning of patient involvement and participation in health care consultations: A taxonomy. *Social Science & Medicine, 64*(6), 1297–1310. https://doi.org/10.1016/j.socscimed.2006.11.002.

Tucker, C. (2011). Public health-related apps growing in number, popularity: Smartphones, tablets used for health. *The Nation's Health, 41*(8) Retrieved from http://thenationshealth.aphapublications.org/content/41/8/1.3.

Türk Tabipleri Birliği. (2016). *e-Nabız Projesinin yürütmesi durduruldu*. Retrieved from https://www.ttb.org.tr/haber_goster.php?Guid=67aba954-9232-11e7-b66d-1540034f819c#

Turkey Clinical Quality Program. (2013). Retrieved from http://www.klinikkalite.saglik.gov.tr/EN,2210/what-is-sagliknet.html

WHO. (2005). *WHA 58.28 – WHO eHealth Resolution*. Retrieved from http://www.who.int/healthacademy/media/WHA58-28-en.pdf

WHO. (2016a). *From innovation to implementation: eHealth in the WHO European Region 2016*. Copenhagen: WHO Regional Office for Europe. http://www.euro.who.int/__data/assets/pdf_file/0012/302331/From-Innovation-to-Implementation-eHealth-Report-EU.pdf

WHO. (2016b). *Global diffusion of eHealth: Making universal health coverage achievable: Report of the third global survey on eHealth*. Retrieved from http://apps.who.int/iris/bitstream/10665/252529/1/9789241511780-eng.pdf

WHO. (2018). *Health and sustainable development, Telehealth*. Retrieved from http://www.who.int/sustainable-development/health-sector/strategies/telehealth/en/

Wiederin, E. (2003). Der grundrechtliche Schutz der Privatsphäre: Eine Entwicklungsgeschichte. In W. Peissl (Ed.), *Privacy: Ein Grundrecht mit Ablaufdatum? Interdisziplinäre Beiträge zur Grundrechtsdebatte* (pp. 31–57). Wien: Verlag der Österreichischen Akademie der Wissenschaften.

Wildenbos, G. A., Peute, L. W., & Jaspers, M. W. M. (2016). Impact of patient-centered eHealth applications on patient outcomes: A review on the mediating influence of human factor issues. *Yearbook of Medical Informatics*, (1), 113–119.

Wilson Kwong, (2015) What is government's role in medical apps?. *Canadian Medical Association Journal, 187*(11), E339–E339.

WSA. (2016). *Turkish National Personal Health Record System: e-PULSE*. Retrieved from https://www.worldsummitawards.org/winner/turkish-national-personal-health-record-system-e-pulse/

Zapata, B. C., Fernández-Alemán, J. L., Idri, A., & Toval, A. (2015). Empirical studies on usability of mHealth apps: A systematic literature review. *Journal of Medical Systems, 39*(2), 1.

Züst, P. (2014). Gläserne Patienten, gläserne Ärzte. *Health & Science, 5*, 8.

11

Social Work, Children and the Digital Knowledge Landscape: New Possibilities and Challenges

Siv-Britt Björktomta and Heidi Aarum Hansen

Introduction

The nature of social work—how it is done, how it is understood and how it is conceptualized—changes over time. This chapter explores the ways in which social work with children is affected by both the digital transformations and possibilities created by social media. The chapter examines the concerns and experiences of social work professionals as they seek to engage with and navigate this digital landscape. Our interest here is how social workers understand, shape and make use of information and knowledge circulating within this landscape, an arena which has been

S.-B. Björktomta (✉)
Centre for Social Work, Department of Sociology, Uppsala University, Uppsala, Sweden
e-mail: siv-britt.bjorktomta@soc.uu.se

H. A. Hansen
Faculty of Health and Welfare Sciences, Østfold University College, Halden, Norway

A. L. Svalastog et al. (eds.), *Navigating Digital Health Landscapes*, Health, Technology and Society, https://doi.org/10.1007/978-981-15-8206-6_11

defined as a 'three dimensional knowledge distribution in both off- and on-line areas' (Svalastog et al. 2018): how might existing and new forms of knowledge be organized and operationalized in present and future social work through an engagement with social media? And how might the current understanding of professional social work expertise and practice, as well as wider socio-political considerations, shape this engagement? In doing so, the chapter contributes towards the analysis of the digital knowledge landscape found throughout this book. It does so through the disciplinary lens of social work, within which both authors are located.

More specifically, in frontline social work, present and future challenges include children's growing use of social media. Even so, children's Internet use is rarely examined in social work with children. The fact that children and adolescents have access to the Internet has a direct impact on their family life and everyday experiences. Children and adolescents (over 13 years of age) are often identified as the group that can benefit most from online social services while international research also shows that it is primarily this group that expresses a strong desire for online contact with professionals (Löfberg and Aspán 2011; Simpson 2017). How might social work respond to both the opportunities and challenges this poses? In the following sections of the chapter, we provide a detailed discussion of empirical work we have undertaken with social workers in Norway with a theoretical framing of the children/social media relation, an outline of the ways in which welfare state services in Nordic countries have become increasingly digitalized and how children's use of the Internet can be empowering but also creating new vulnerabilities. We then go on to present and discuss the implications of our empirical inquiry.

Theoretical Framework

Children's everyday communication practices online create expectations of how the adult world should communicate with them (Simpson 2017). If social workers are to communicate with children on social media, it will change the requirements for that communication, moving the boundaries of knowledge development in the field of social work (Hansen et al. 2017). Children's online communication and practices, together with the social worker's online practice, generate a highly complex situation. We need to map social workers' discrete knowledge landscape, in the online environment, and the use of it. We also need to understand the relation between social workers' discrete use of the online environment and the relation between online and offline communication and social work. Crucially, we need to understand how this can inform the context of each new generation's childhood.

It is in childhood and adolescence that the individual's identity and self-image are formed. In terms of the ecology of human development (Bronfenbrenner 2002), a dynamic, child-centred ecosystem operates on various levels and in both direct and indirect relations. Bronfenbrenner's theory describes the child's various environments: in the microsystem are family, preschool and relatives, representing relationships that are all directly related to the child or between adults in the child's proximity; in the 'exosystem' are indirect relationships between local authorities, schools, social services and parents' workplaces; and in the macrosystem are indirect relationships at the national level, furthest from the child as an individual—welfare systems, political decisions, legislation and norms.

An ecosystem of this type is predicated on specific conditions for how childhood evolves and, historically, the importance of parents and family (Ericson 1993). Home and school are the places where adults' norms, power and control have substantial bearing on children's lives. In addition, the Internet is an arena where the adult world's norms are present, but children, in navigating a wide-ranging knowledge landscape, have greater scope to design childhood and their sense of it on their own. We know that children use the Internet on a daily basis (Davidsson 2016). Children also often have a greater knowledge of and familiarity with social media than many of the adults who are part of the children's social networks; they have been born into the digital era and raised in a world of different knowledge landscapes, and a digital language is part of their native tongue. This new generation, Prensky's (2001) 'digital natives', is a challenge for child welfare professionals.

The Internet and the knowledge landscape therein add therefore another level to Bronfenbrenner's ecosystem: a global level where contact is *virtually* direct. When digital natives navigate the knowledge landscape, new opportunities present themselves. Direct and indirect relations are conducted in a digital language with like-minded people, who have shared interests, but come from other contexts. This gives young people opportunities of a kind not seen before to form alternative cultural identities, independent of their parents, family and school (Shifflet-Chila et al. 2016).

Viewed in terms of the sociology of childhood, digital natives, far more than former generations, are children and adolescents described as 'a being child', that is, subjects and social actors, rather than 'a becoming child', that is, passive objects and adults in the making (James and James 2004; Qvotrup 1994; Uprichard 2008). As a phenomenon, the Internet is two-edged. The Internet may be seen as being both good and bad, for the better or worse, and it could be both legal and illegal. The concepts of risk, vulnerability, protective factors and resilience (Rutter and Taylor 2002; Unger 2011; Werner 1995) from developmental psychopathology take on new dimensions—and demand new understanding.

The Digitalization of the Welfare State

All the governments in Nordic countries share a vision of their national health services and social services as digitalized. Technological progress has not been uniform, however. The private sector has taken the lead, followed by public health services, in such areas as online counselling and therapies. The digitalization of local authority social services has not advanced as far, being characterized by a certain inertia (Granholm 2016; Svensson and Larsson 2018).

Digitalization, however far it has progressed, affects social workers' jobs. Indeed, it appears to change social work as a whole. It is not merely a question of designing new digital tools, using algorithms and automated decision processes to perform routine tasks, thus freeing social workers to work with citizens, provide support and assistance and assess complex cases; it is also a question of professional development, which, in turn, will create new ways of working with citizens and clients. Thus Mishna et al. (2012) identify five core elements in social work that have been affected: boundaries (time and space), disclosures of information (practitioners' and clients'), therapeutic relationships, ethical and legal issues and dilemmas and policies and procedures. The digitalization of social work stands out as a turning point. Just as the Internet has shaped how people of all ages communicate, the digitalization of welfare services and social work has changed the premises for communication between practitioners and clients, even those engaged in traditional, face-to-face therapy (Ringstad 2016). So, there have been changes, but not all have been welcomed.

The physical meeting with clients is usually described by social workers as lying at the heart of social work itself (Svensson and Larsson 2018; Granholm 2016). Though there is a growing body of research on online therapy, studies of the impact of social media on traditional, face-to-face social work practices are limited (Mishna et al. 2012), and opinions vary among social workers about whether or not the Internet and social media are suitable tools for social work practice (Granholm 2016). In essence, digitalization sees power shift from social workers to clients. Although a participatory approach to clients is a legal right, the Internet has enabled clients to become active subjects in an entirely new way given greater opportunities to choose according to their own needs and wishes (Mishna et al. 2012; Svensson and Larsson 2018). The provision of online services can lower the threshold to clients initiating contact with social services, while some seem to find it easier to discuss sensitive matters online rather than face to face (Granholm 2016). Either way, citizens, clients and other stakeholders have new expectations of digital tools as the norm for modern social work practices (Simpson 2017).

Children and the Internet

Children today have grown up with social media; even very young children (from one year) use social media as a way to communicate (Småungar and Medier 2017). In the European Union, the recent General Data Protection Regulation (GDPR) sets the age threshold within a range of 13 to 16 years for children and adolescents to download apps and open online accounts, but it is for member countries to decide which age from within that range (European Commission 2013). Previously, this was regulated in user agreements between the companies and account holders by each new user submitting their name and age; however, findings show that a large proportion of children under 14 years give neither their name nor their correct age when they set up accounts on Twitter, Facebook, Instagram, WhatsApp and the like (Lareki et al. 2017). Among its numerous ramifications, GDPR places the responsibility on parents, since children must have parental permission to use social media—which can be difficult to check.

The Internet is one of several arenas for young people to socialize with friends and manage relationships in everyday life. However, there is a group of young people who report high levels of vulnerability (Björktomta and Hansen 2018). The Internet can also be an arena with forums fostering negative behaviour that may adversely affect young people's mental health (Hamm et al. 2015). The accessibility and mobility of social media generates new platforms for ill-treatment and has created new forms of abuse, bullying and violence. The Cybercrime Convention Committee (2018) uses the concept *cyberviolence* comprising the use of computer system to cause, facilitate or threaten violence against individuals using different forms of violence, for example, physical, sexual, psychological and economic violence as well cyberbullying. Cyberviolence is an increasing phenomenon and although its specific forms only recently have begun to be identified and understood, it is often a continuum of offline violence (ibid.). Øverlien (2018), for example, argues that teenage intimate partner violence in the digital arena is not new per se, but rather should be understood as a subcategory of psychological violence. BRIS (Children's Rights in Society), a Swedish NGO, reports that children contact them in writing about being exposed to online threats and violations (BRIS 2014). Children up to age 18 can approach BRIS anonymously by email or online chats when they need the support of an adult. BRIS's reports show that children have always asked about family conflict, anxiety, mental illness, bullying and sexual offences and now also have questions about personal integrity and how to handle security and online protection.

Boundaries for Exercising Public Authority Online

Based on three focus group interviews with social workers in three Norwegian local authorities, we look more closely at social workers' actions and their thoughts on the challenges of children's use of social media. Based on the social workers' responses, we examine the advantages and disadvantages of using digital aids in the exercise of their public authority. Our focus is the element of social work that concerns child welfare, from when social services receive notification that children are in some way being neglected, the investigation of the children's situation (both verbal communication with children and families and written documentation), to the implementation of measures under the provisions of Norway's Child Welfare Act.

Since the mid-1990s, the Internet has been a part of daily life. This means that public access to the Internet is in one sense a relatively new phenomenon; on the other hand, it is a tool that has been available to the majority of people for over 20 years. A whole generation has grown up not knowing what it is like to live in a society where one is not 'connected'.

In frontline social work, it has long been the view that access to the Internet is a relatively new phenomenon. The natural sciences and medicine were quick to see its possibilities, far ahead of the social sciences' interest in social media and its impact on human relations and communication patterns, whether private or professional (Daneback and Sorbring 2016). Today it is accepted that Internet use has implications for individuals, groups and professionals alike. The majority of those who live in welfare states today have access to information and expertise, and access to the Internet serves as both a means and an opportunity to access and build forms of knowledge and to exert influence.

Digital society thus challenges the present discourse of public sector services. The changes that the digital environment has generated in society have to be understood in terms of all public services, including child welfare services. Which digital tools, then, are available to Norwegian social workers in their work with children and families? The following two extracts from our focus groups address this issue:

1. 'We send texts if the parents want us to, but we don't send sensitive information; we can't do that. We can text children, yes, but only if they're teenagers, and only with times and short messages'.
2. 'There are times we get emails from people, and then we can answer briefly by email, but with a formal letter, because we aren't allowed to say anything else as we're bound by confidentiality. We don't answer by email, we just don't, because of the risk it might end up in the wrong place. That's how we handle contacts [e.g.] schools and other relatives. NAV [the Norwegian Labour and Welfare Administration] we often send emails as it's really difficult to catch them on the phone. But parents, it's mainly by letter, text, or phone'.

The quotes above show that social workers use texts and email differently in communication with parents, relatives and the public bodies they cooperate with. They were not uncritical of the various reasons for strengthening and legitimizing their use of texts and emails to communicate with clients. As the quotes show, they primarily problematized its legal aspects, singling out the requirements for confidentiality and the correct handling of personal information. They point out that whatever social workers do and do not do online, it has to be seen in the light of the guidelines for social work with children and young people in general; in this context, they are limited to non-personally identifiable information—the opposite of sensitive information—and are bound by the requirements for written documentation under the Norwegian Public Administration Act.

What defines the boundaries for the exercise of public authority online, then, can be issues that are fundamental to social work, such as secrecy, mentioned above, or building relationships, but equally can extend far beyond the issues that regulate social work with children and adolescents. For example, the legal aspects of Internet use by the various professions have required new guidelines and praxis in Europe. One change is the introduction of minimum ages for when children are allowed to set up online accounts, while at the same time recognizing that it is difficult to ensure the law is obeyed, a responsibility that falls to parents (Lareki et al. 2017). This was, however, not a theme in the focus group explaining that they had hands-on experience of using Facebook in their work. They described themselves as advanced in their use of digital tools. Child welfare service in their local authority had a project for children for whom a child protection referral had been made, but the child protection investigation was not yet complete. All children over the age of 13 (Norway's age of consent for digital services) are invited to join a Facebook group where one of the social workers has set up a personal profile with both name and email address visible. The aim of the project is to gauge children's and adolescents' opinions, while it also serves to evaluate how children feel about being the object of a child protection investigation. Questions were sent out as private messages (chats) to ensure confidentiality, and the children's feedback has become a regular theme at the social workers' team meetings.

> I set up a new profile, and it was really important that it was my photo, because there's something about being able to see for yourself exactly who you're talking to; I think it's young people, children and teenagers, who get the most out of it; families I'm not so sure, but children and teenagers really focus on it.

The social workers underlined how important it is that child welfare officers with an online presence for work are identified by name and photo. This Internet praxis is best understood as a way to create predictability for the child. Such openness offers children the chance to picture who will respond to their chat messages. Predictability and openness also help establish a basis for trust between children and social workers. An important aspect, although not mentioned in the focus groups, is that social workers can never be sure of who is responding to their profile. Using Facebook as a way to reach children also means a trust in technology, hardware and software. Another aspect is how cultural differences, that is, languages, religion and traditions, affect communications and trust building between social workers and clients.

Today's generation of children and adolescents has grown up with the Internet, and it is a natural part of their daily lives. For them, the Internet can be an opportunity to get in touch with professionals who are interested in their needs and opinions (BRIS 2014; Daneback and Sorbring 2016). Not all the child welfare officers in the focus groups had personal experience of using Facebook, but all had an opinion on how Facebook could be used to complement the relationships built in face-to-face meetings.

> I think a bit more preventatively; [if we] had an advisory service where you could get in touch and be given good advice about how you could move forward. If it could be a low-threshold offer; you know, information that made it a bit less scary to get in touch, made it easy to be accessible, to be contacted, because it's not us contacting them, but them us, according to where they are right now, and when they want to.

The social workers' comment illustrates their belief that an anonymous, low-threshold line of communication can fulfil at least two functions. First, it can be an opportunity for children and adolescents who otherwise hesitate to make direct contact with child welfare services: for many of those in need of support, meeting in person can be a worry that stops them from getting in touch or seeking the necessary help, and taking the first step online can reduce the significant stress factors. If children have the opportunity to decide themselves when to get in touch and how—by writing instead of speaking to someone—that gives them a greater say in when and how to act in contacts with social services. From the perspective of child welfare services, participation is about having control over their own circumstances. It also means that the child's understanding of the problem has, or should have, an impact on what happens to the child in future—what measures social services choose, in other words. However, research points to difficulties showing that children's and young people's stories of, for example, exposures to violence often are renegotiated and/or get lost during social services investigations (Heimer et al. 2017). Online contact can thus serve as one of several tools with which to develop child welfare services on the child's terms. Second, it can help promote child welfare services as a source of help. Child welfare services have a societal mandate that ultimately can see children removed from their families, so it is easy to think of child welfare services as being 'coercive'. Under such circumstances, many social workers do not dare attempt prevention and support work. This was why they turned to the Internet as an arena where child welfare services could be presented, but in a harmless or benign light. In sum, the social workers were on the horn of a dilemma between closeness and distance, that is, social workers need to be close to clients, building trust, and at the same time, they need to uphold a distance as a practitioner and embodiment of public authority.

Along with the focus on sort of knowledge seen as appropriate and an awareness of how the Internet can be used, digital tools were also seen by social workers to ensure that children's rights are better protected.

> It is we ourselves who are the tools of our job, and that worries me slightly. We shouldn't replace the digital tools, we should add to them. There shouldn't be any difference between children who are placed far away and those close to home. You should be able to talk to your contact regardless. And then you can use Skype and video [FaceTime] as alternative ways to get in touch. But when we choose to use digital tools, there should be an awareness of it, and we should know why we're doing it.

The social workers referred to factors that depend on having the correct qualifications in child welfare services. The fact that even small children use the Internet and have a greater knowledge and familiarity with social media than many adults who are part of their social networks (including social workers) is a source of fresh challenges for child welfare services. The social workers said they feared children and adolescents were developing modes of communication that are difficult for welfare professionals to interpret. In order to have a dialogue, social workers need to use the same channels as teenagers. Prensky (2001), as noted above, describes all those born after 1994 as 'digital natives'—that is, they have always lived in a digitally connected world. Parents and social workers, on the other hand, are in effect 'digital immigrants' (Prensky 2001)—adults who know about the new technology, but who have not internalized it. In practice, this means that children and adolescents take precedence as experts in a field where much of the adult population does not have sufficient knowledge to be able to guide or support the young. This is in line with the findings of Shifflet-Chila et al. (2016) that young people have little confidence in their parents' ability to protect them from online dangers, as adults are themselves dependent on young people's competence in order to navigate the Internet.

Another theme was how online accessibility can complicate the monitoring of children taken into care. Child welfare services have strict rules about children's contact with their parents by limiting telephone calls and supervised visits. At the same time, the child welfare officers described the Internet as a world they did not have a proper overview of and where children and parents can have close contact on social media. Children are drawn into the doings of their biological families and find it difficult to settle in foster care. As one of the child welfare officers put it, there can be 'a hundred reasons why a 14-year-old girl wants to talk to her mother or father on Facebook or chat'.

> Because even if they're living at different ends of the country and have four agreed visits a year, they can have a lot of contact between supervised visits. The more strictly it's enforced, the harder it is for the children to be open about it. Social media are not covered by it; what is still covered by it are meetings in person and telephone contact. We [social services] haven't included other developments. They [the children] can sit all day watching clips their parents have sent them, at the same time as telephone contact is controlled. We're years behind; hardly anyone makes phone calls these days.

The quote above summarizes the very essence of social work—social workers and clients meeting in person. It shows a contrast between the professional landscape and its control and the digital one and reveals a dilemma embodied in the welfare services' focus on meeting in person as against recent digital advances. The law on contact between children in care and their biological parents does not coincide with the boundaries for the exercise of public authority online. Thus, when child welfare services, after due investigation, judge that children must be separated from their parents and home environment and taken into care, a plan is agreed in which the children's contacts with their parents are limited in terms of physical meetings. Yet because the use of social media is not included in the plan, the reason for child welfare services taking children into care is negated.

Pleasures and Worries: Risks and Possibilities

Digital society has created new arenas, complete with opportunities and risks, for the young. Online activities offer them the chance to socialize with friends they meet in school and in their free time. Navigating a digital landscape also brings interaction with new acquaintances, both nationally and globally. In the main, the younger generation's daily life online is ordinary and filled with mundane routines, however, fairly often may also contain all the tragedy of adolescence. In this regard, young people report a high level of vulnerability, varying according to the modality used, with, for example, the public channels of social media versus more individually targeted modes such as email or text messages. For example, the accessibility and scope of the Internet can mean that children who are bullied at school no longer find any respite at home. Online, it is possible for the bullying to continue around the clock (Hamm et al. 2015).

From the social worker's perspective, that same accessibility and scope can make it easier to reach young people with information and guidance about the help social services can provide. In the focus group interviews, however, several social workers expressed their concern at what children and adolescents can be exposed to when they are active online.

> There are a lot of children who are bullied at home on social media; I think there are lots of children sitting at home in their rooms, feeling both shame and guilt because they've been picked on online, and it never stops, they take it with them everywhere; I think there are lots of children who share the same painful experiences. Snapchat is the worst of them, or at any rate has been the worst channel for bullying.

The quote shows social workers'concern about the young leaving themselves open to considerable danger, which can lead to loneliness and isolation, and in worst cases various forms of abuse or bullying. This exemplifies a key function of welfare services, which is to identify and protect children from potential risks, and sometimes this requires that they intervene in vulnerable children's lives. Moreover, protecting children also involves professionals having to understand the new communication patterns in a digital landscape that is constantly changing.

The social workers problematize how they can safeguard children's rights online. Several refer to adults' online activities that are risk factors for children and adolescents. It is not unknown for parents to text photos of their children's medical certificates or post video clips of them. The children probably never had the opportunity to consent to their parents sharing any of it online.

> You can't be sure a 12-year-old will think it's ok for mum to discuss something about child welfare services on Facebook, or to have opinions about child welfare services. It's really the same as for a great many of these groups on Facebook that discuss child welfare services—it can cut both ways. That's why I think there can be a lot of things about children being made public without it doing them any good. Many [parents] are cognitively weak and don't understand the consequences of what it means for their children to be posted online, for examples copies of decisions or things like "I'm going to fight for you, my child".

In the quote social workers discuss a group of parents who unwittingly expose their children to risk. This can be viewed as a continuum of parental neglect offline, a well-known phenomenon in social work. So, old risks such as bullying and parental neglect take on a new form on the Internet. The social workers are familiar with the phenomenon, but need to develop new skills to handle it if they are to fulfil their mandate of protecting children.

A similarly standard element in social work, which in the digital era calls for a different skill set than the social workers currently have, is online communication. To communicate online, they need to use formulations that are different to those used in traditional personal meetings.

> We must dare to use the words that are used online. We cannot package it in adult words; we have to use the words that the young people use online, we have to meet them where they are.

This comment indicates how important it is for social workers to express themselves in writing online and to dare to use the same language as young people. It is the encounter with the other that is central to social work, and for that both parties must have a common language. This idiom will be confirmation that one is being listened to, accepted and ultimately recognized.

As the social workers said, they want to be wherever children are in order to act on the child welfare services' social mission.

> If we want to have a dialogue with children and teenagers, we have to use the channels they use. Even small children use social media; they sit with their iPads from when they're small and learn how to use them young. They are better at it than we are, and if we don't keep up I think we're going to fail in how children and teenagers communicate.

The importance of meeting in person is a crucial theme for social workers. In the focus group interviews, there were concerns that social media will replace human contact in general, and the emphasis was on putting in place a well-thought-through strategy for the Norwegian child welfare services' use of social media in their work with children and adolescents.

> I think we should use the tools available, but I think a lot about this business of human contact and direct contact; children today grow up with the digital realities and spend a lot of time on their own. Now I'm not just talking about children in care—lots of children say they miss adult contact. So, if we are going to use it [social media] more, we need to think it through carefully so we don't kill off what the children really miss—adult contact.

Although our respondents were positive about starting to use digital tools at work, some concerns were raised. For example, there was the question of communication by text in ways that were unfamiliar to the child welfare officers and a degree of uncertainty about how they were to interpret and understand the children's texts.

> I feel that there is an opening there because we can communicate by text, but even though it's set out in black and white I feel there's still a big chance of misunderstanding. When they use emojis or smileys we can't be completely certain what they mean by it, and you can't see their facial expressions or body language when they communicate, not like when you meet.

The child welfare officers' concerns were about failing to grasp the nuances of textspeak. Interpreting body language and facial expressions in verbal communication was something they had mastered after years of courses and learning on the job. Gauging people's emotions from emojis and smileys was more difficult.

The social workers quoted have identified the problems of written, non-verbal communication. Social work turns on relationship-creating work, which is mainly concerned with interpersonal encounters, face to face. In such relationships, social workers can evaluate a child's part in proceedings from their body language. It is about opportunities: the child should have the opportunity to determine how the situation is read and what action should be taken; the social worker should have the opportunity to interpret and evaluate others' impact on the child from their body language. Written communication makes it harder for the social worker to interpret the child's body language, intonation or facial expression, which in a child protection investigation is necessary in forming a picture of the child's care and general situation. This is problematic, but equally it paves the way for the development of new practices. Working from written communication, the social worker can only see the information that the child chooses to write and which is visible on screen. It can be an advantage for the social worker not to be guided by first impressions, as can happen in face-to-face relations. Written contact is different and thus requires a different approach. Immediate follow-up questions are unhelpful, for example. Typing instead of talking can also recast the social worker as a coach of sorts, empowering the child, strengthening the child's self-belief through guidance, encouragement and support—'Well done!'

Organizational Challenges

The digitalization of social services in the Nordic countries has been notable for its inertia (Svensson and Larsson 2018). According to our informants, online social work poses organizational challenges. Social services keep the standard local authority opening hours of 8 a.m. to 4 p.m. All local authorities are required to have an out-of-hours service, with child welfare officers on call to deal with emergency cases, but they do not monitor ongoing cases or families who are already in the system.

The social workers reflected on their online availability and pointed out that the immediate need to talk to someone is often greatest in the evenings, at night and at weekends, yet given the way their work is currently organized, it is impossible to be available 24/7. They pointed to a considerable organizational challenge for the professionals: the demand for services will tend to be higher than supply, resulting in an imbalance between demands and resources. Theirs will necessarily be a dual role, as they will have to act as both problem solvers and gatekeepers in a situation characterized by a large amount of work but limited time and resources. As one social worker indicated, organizational factors can prevent or destroy the necessary trust, if social workers offer approaches that are difficult to implement on the ground:

> As soon as you're available, and make yourself available, you create an expectation of what you'll do, but you shouldn't create expectations without following through on them. You have to have some rules for how long it should take to get an answer, and a bit about how requests are handled, so that we don't make ourselves available and promise things, and then nothing happens. That would be wrong. So if we're going to use it to reach out to children and teenagers on their terms, we also have to be clear about how we can contribute.

This social worker was thus addressing trust and credibility. Trust is at the heart of social work and what trust does in interpersonal relationships—in the relationship between those who provide and those who receive social services' help. If child welfare services are to use social media in their professional work, guidelines will be needed for how social workers should relate online with children and adolescents.

However, the question is whether an organizational framework would merely add to the practices that obstruct professionalism, when it is the individuals and their encounters that are in fact the tool. One example of an organizational change on an individual level was social workers' access to an iPad or tablet. The idea was that if all social workers in a local authority had an iPad, it would make them more mobile and possibly more efficient. One of them said she found it had become a means of contact with children, especially at times when they had to discuss difficult subjects: the children were interested in the iPad, which facilitated contact with the social worker, and together they could explore the iPad's possibilities. Some showed the social worker what they used iPads for, while others were curious and wanted to know more. With the help of her iPad, the social worker could invite children to participate on their own terms.

The question here is how organizational changes can meet the needs of clients. Accessibility is central to social work, but, so far, it has been within regulated working hours, which makes it difficult for clients to contact social welfare services when they need to. In meetings with children, one key word is participation, and here digital tools, such as iPads, can be used to facilitate the interaction between the social worker and the child.

Discussion

This chapter illustrates the tension between professional practice, governance and accountability when mediated by social workers'engagement with digital systems. In the digital era the concepts from childhood studies are operationalized in new ways; children are 'being' in a real sense (James and James 2004; Uprichard 2008). The crucial question is how child welfare services will be able to cope with this?

The Internet creates new opportunities for children to form and develop identities on a global level and at a distance from the adult world's norms. Direct contacts in the home, in school and with friends have fanned out to comprise virtual contacts as well. This is a challenge for parents, social welfare services and society as a whole. However, when it comes to digitalization, in particular concerning children, welfare services have been characterized by a certain inertia (Granholm 2016; Svensson and Larsson 2018).

Focus groups interviews with Norwegian social workers demonstrate the existence of a three-dimensional space representing knowledge communication and exchange among children, parents and professionals (social workers).

Three key dilemmas are outlined in this chapter. First, there is a legal dilemma in striking a balance between information and secrecy. It touches the core of social work, namely to meet in person, as against recent digital advances. In other words, where are the boundaries for the exercise of public authority online? One of the Internet's foundations is openness and accessibility. However, social workers are bound by the requirements of the law and to follow the guidelines for social work with children and young people in general. New guidelines need to be developed that take into account the particularities of the Internet where it intersects with the social services' exercise of public authority.

Second, there is an ethical dilemma in the tension between children's need for protection, provisions and participation. The Internet offers both pleasures and worries, risks and possibilities. It is complex, a different arena for children to navigate and for social workers to follow in the digital landscape. One aspect to this is that even very young children have access. Another fact is that risk factors, such as bullying and parental neglect, as well as protecting factors, such as communicating with friends, take new forms that demand not only new skills but also a new understanding of how to fulfil the societal mandate of protecting children.

Third, there is an organizational dilemma about regulated working hours and digital technology's accessibility. One aspect that needs to be considered is regulated working hours and the Internet's availability 12/24. Another is that social workers have to have both resources and knowledge to meet new expectations from children and young people who use digital tools to communicate (Simpson 2017). They will need to develop skills in understanding digital languages and communicating in a way that children and young people do, using their idiom, emojis and all.

Finally, one general dilemma is about the gap between children's competence to navigate social media (the Internet) and the professional competence on one side and parents' lack of competence on the other. Social work is a profession in movement within the surrounding society and political and policy decisions. Digitalization is ongoing and grows apace. The findings reported here show a contrast between the professional landscape and its controls and the digital one and its short-circuiting of these controls. To fulfil its societal mandate, social work, as a profession, needs to map discrete knowledge landscapes to be able to follow, get in contact and communicate with children and young people, the 'digital natives' found in these landscapes. How these natives themselves navigate, understand and use these digital systems is of central importance to the future of social work.

References

Björktomta, S.-B., & Hansen, H. (2018). Child welfare services and social media: Childhood, being and becoming in a digital society. *Croatian Medical Journal, 59*(2), 90–92.

BRIS. (2014). *Children, Bris and IT: Young people's everyday lives online.* Available at https://statensmedierad.se/download/18.3f6a618014fefeab4b6a9527/1444207963439/Bris-2014-eng-webb.pdf. Accessed 1 May 2018.

Bronfenbrenner, U. (2002 [1979]). *The ecology of human development.* London: Harvard University Press.

Cybercrime Convention Committee. (2018). *Mapping study on cyberviolence with recommendations adopted by the T-CY on 9 July 2018.* Available at https://rm.coe.int/t-cy-2017-10-cbg-study-provisional/16808c4914. Accessed 15 Oct 2019.

Daneback, K. & Sorbring, E. (red.) (2016). *Socialt arbete och internet: att förstå och hantera sociala problem på nya arenor.* (1. uppl.) Stockholm: Liber.

Davidsson, P. (2016). *The Swedes and the Internet 2016: Summary.* Stockholm: Internetstiftelsen. Available at http://www.soi2016.se/theswedes-and-the-internet-2016-summary/. Accessed 1 May 2018.

Ericson, E. H. (1993). *Childhood and society.* New York: Norton.

European Commission. (2013). *European strategy for a better Internet for Children*. COM(2012) 196 final. Available at https://eur-lex.europa.eu/legal-content/EN/ALL/?uri=CELEX:52012DC0196. Accessed 6 June 2019.

Granholm, C. (2016). *Social work in digital transfer: Blending services for the next generation*. Dissertation, University of Helsinki, Faculty of Social Science Department of Social Research, Helsinki.

Hamm, M., Newton, A., Chisholm, A., Shulhan, J., Milne, A., Sundar, P., & Hartling, L. (2015). Prevalence and effect of cyberbullying on children and young people: A scoping review of social media studies. *Clinical Review & Education: JAMA Pediatrics, 169*(8), 770–777.

Hansen, A. H., Björktomta, S.–. B., & Svalastog, A. L. (2017). Digital society generates new challenges on child welfare services. *Croatian Medical Journal, 58*, 80–83.

Heimer, M., Palme, J., & Näsman, E. (2017). *Rättighetsbärare eller problembärare? Barns rättatt komma till tals och socialtjänstens insatser*. Stockholm: Stiftelsen Allmänna Barnhuset.

James, A., & James, A. L. (2004). *Constructing childhood: Theory, policy and social practice*. New York: Palgrave Macmillan.

Lareki, A., Altuna, J., Martinez de Morentin, J. I., & Amenabar, N. (2017). Young people and digital services: An analysis of the use, rules and age requirement. *Children & Youth Services Review, 79*.

Löfberg, C., & Aspán, M. (2011). *Digitala erbjudanden: Ungas erfarenheter av information, stöd och samspel med vuxna online*. Stockholm: Institutionen för pedagogik och didaktik, Stockholms universitet.

Mishna, F., Bogo, M., Root, J., et al. (2012). 'It just crept in': The digital age and implications for social work practice. *Clinical Social Work Journal, 40*, 277.

Øverlien, C. (2018). Våld mellan ungdomar i nära relationer: Digitala medier och utövande av kontroll. *Socialvetenskaplig tidskrift, 25*(1), 67–81.

Prensky, M. (2001). Digital Natives, Digital Immigrants. *On the Horizon, 9*(5), 1–6.

Qvotrup, J. (1994). *Childhood matters: Social theory, practice and policies*. Aldershot: Avebury.

Ringstad, Ø. (2016). Patient autonomy in a digitalizedworld: Supporting patients' autonomouschoice. *Croatian Medical Journal, 57*, 80–82.

Rutter, M., & Taylor, E. A. (2002). *Child and adolescent psychiatry* (4th ed.). Oxford: Blackwell Science.

Shifflet-Chila, E., Harold, R., Fitton, V. A., & Ahmedani, B. K. (2016). Adolescent and family development: Autonomy and identity in the digital age. *Children & Youth Services Review, 70*.

Simpson, J. E. (2017). Staying in touch in the digital era: New social work practice. *Journal of Technology in Human Services, 35*(1), 86–98.

Statens Medieråd. (2017). *Småungar & medier*. Available at https://www.statensmedierad.se/download/18.30c25b3115c152ee8f82fe95/1495204277588/Sm%C3%A5ungar%20och%20medier%202017%20tillg%C3%A4nglighetsanpassad.pdf. Accessed 19 Aug 2019.

Svalastog, A. L., Allgaier, J., & Gajovic, S. (2018). Navigating knowledge landscapes in the digital society: A look back and visions for the future. *Croatian Medical Journal, 59*, 274–278.

Svensson, L., & Larsson, S. (2018). *Digitalization of social welfare service*. Helsingborg: FoU Helsingborg.

Unger. (2011). The social ecology of resilience: Addressing contextual and cultural ambiguity of a nascent construct. *American Journal of Orthopsychiatry, 81*(1), 1–17.

Uprichard, E. (2008). Children as 'Being and Becomings': Children, childhood and temporality. *Children & Society, 22*(4), 303–313.

Werner, E. (1995). Resilience in Development. *Current Directions in Psychological Science, 4*(3), 81–85.

Part III

Travelling Safely

This third and final part of the book draws on a range of quite specific disciplinary expertise from those versed in socio-linguistics and natural language processing, electronic engineering and data visualisation. The section has been called 'travelling safely' to point to the contribution these areas of expertise can make in practical and policy terms to enable a more transparent, safe and socially robust knowledge landscape. Ulrich Beck's concept of the 'risk society' (Beck 1992) focused on how modernity and the technologies associated with it generate new forms of risk and insecurity in part through their role in trying to reduce risk. This paradox is evident in the chapters in this third part of the book where risks and opportunities are relative and linked to our understanding and handling of technological systems as well as our ability to cope with and organise the overload of online information. To reduce risk and gain knowledge, the authors propose that we need new types of understandings to ensure that the complexity of the technology at work (engineering and informatics) is understood and that software that can extract relevant knowledge from online information can be deployed by citizens. While the discussions are quite technical in places, the authors have sought to make their arguments as accessible as possible. The chapters point to ways in which it is possible to reduce some of the risks, mis/dis-information and complexities of health seeking, and add important insights to Part I on frames and characteristics of health and well-being in present digital society, and add content and context to the journeys presented in Part II.

There are, as noted in other introductions to each part, a number of shared meta-themes that can be found across the three chapters.

The first relates to the ways in which system architectures operate in generating the huge volume of information found on the web and in turn the ways in which both the users and the very systems themselves are subject to various forms of vulnerability. This is made more apparent when, as in the chapter by Simunic and Pale, these architectures combine to form a digital 'ecosystem' at a global scale, with interlinkages that surround and shape human action and understanding—'parahuman' systems, such as in the 'Internet of Things' (IoT). While these are in principle designed to improve and bring greater precision to our understanding (of health and other areas), the ecosystem is sufficiently unstable to generate new forms of risk, in particular regarding private everyday practice.

Connecting disparate, discontinuous sources of information using digital systems to interrogate, marshall and compare data sources, is another broad theme seen across the three chapters. Seeing where and how information can provide the basis for knowledge, a greater sense of where and how to judge competing claims on the web is a vital issue for those navigating it. Both the natural language processing technique reported in Vossen and Fokkens' chapter and the visualisation techniques discussed in Varga et al. show how it is possible to mine and organise diverse forms of information using data processing programmes and so enable more reliable understanding and informed decision-making.

In addition, greater reliability is dependent on how far system architectures are built upon shared standards and regulatory oversight—matters for state agencies and commercial actors. The safety and security of the IoT, and its form in the Internet of Medical Things, provides the broader socio-political context which needs to be considered if 'travelling safely' is to be made possible. To the extent that this is true, the techniques and recommendations offered in the three chapters are only part of the 'solution' to navigating knowledge on the web safely: wider aspects of the digital ecosystem need to be taken into account too, if we are to build more socially robust knowledge landscapes.

Reference

Beck, U. 1992. *Risk Society. Towards a new Modernity*. SAGE Publications Ltd. https://www.ark.no/boker/Ulrich-Beck-Risk-Society-9780803983465?as_templateId=4602761&gclid=EAIaIQobChMIiZ6npuG7QIVuSB7Ch2vwAfREAAYASAAEgKW9PD_BwE&gclsrc=aw.ds

12

Information Systems, Big Data and Knowledge Landscapes

Piek Vossen and Antske Fokkens

Introduction

In this chapter, we describe technical approaches that aim to address the challenges involved in finding accurate and up-to-date information. We focus on two challenges: the challenge of finding all relevant information and the challenge of determining the reliability of this information that might then form the basis of reliable knowledge.

The constant flow of information and the speed with which new things are discovered and shared bring many opportunities but also challenges. The Internet provides considerable information about topics such as health but also a lot of information that is less reliable or even false and

P. Vossen (✉)
Faculty of Humanities, Vrije Universiteit Amsterdam, Amsterdam, The Netherlands
e-mail: piek.vossen@vu.nl

A. Fokkens
Computational Lexicology and Terminology Lab (CLTL), Faculty of Humanities, Vrije Universiteit Amsterdam, Amsterdam, The Netherlands

A. L. Svalastog et al. (eds.), *Navigating Digital Health Landscapes*, Health, Technology and Society, https://doi.org/10.1007/978-981-15-8206-6_12

dangerous. The process through which people navigate knowledge landscapes is complex. Yet this book not only seeks to understand how this happens but also to provide methods to make this process more socially robust. As part of this, it is worthwhile to examine the potential contributions of current technical solutions for navigating available information. The first challenge, the challenge of finding relevant information, can be addressed by natural language processing (NLP) technologies that process text automatically and extract information from them at a highly detailed level. This includes the topic of the text, what is being claimed about this topic, by whom and based on what evidence. We describe the system architecture of tools providing this information and report on the accuracy of the technologies involved according to the latest state of the art.

The second challenge, the challenge of determining the transparency of the information found, can be addressed by representing the automatically extracted information using the Grounded Representation and Source Perspective (GRaSP) framework (Fokkens et al. 2017). The GRaSP framework is specifically designed to connect information from various sources. It maintains a clear registry of the sources of information and their perspective on the content. This does not only include the article the claim came from but also the sources that are mentioned in this article and their positions with respect to claims. Who was quoted in the article, what do they believe or claim and what does the author believe? What authorities were referred to? Which scientific studies were mentioned? GRaSP allows people to verify the original sources of claims, compare opposing views and positions and find out more about the sources behind a specific point of view. In other words, GRaSP provides people with more explicit information to judge the context and validity of individual claims and to obtain a more *transparent* overview of the different perspectives taken. The chapter offers, therefore, some important practical steps that can be taken in navigating the knowledge landscape more assuredly by deploying the NLP approach.

We illustrate how the technologies and representation format work and their current performance through the analysis of the online vaccination debate. People debate the pros and cons of vaccination since it was first conceived. Today, the debate is as vivid as it was back then, but the media have changed completely as discussions take place on the Internet and involve many more people and new ways of interacting and new modes for searching for and sharing information. There are a number of reasons to focus on the vaccination debate: (1) the topic is relatively focused as it mainly concerns the positive and negative effects of vaccination which makes it relatively easy to trace the content of the debate; (2) the debate is heated and involves a wide range of arguments and emotions and consequently different and complex ways of expressing these perspectives; (3) different truths, knowledge and information are spread within distinct filter bubbles; (4) the debate is relevant because it concerns the public health as well as the individual health and (5) the impact can partially be measured independently in terms of the vaccination coverage in different regions and periods in time.

This chapter is structured as follows. We first define the primary concepts in *information*, *knowledge*, *communication* and *natural language expression* in relation to specific knowledge exchange on online debates. We then introduce the GRaSP framework illustrating how this allows us to model differences in perspectives on a global and detailed level. Subsequently we provide an overview of NLP technologies that aim at extracting these perspectives automatically from text. We then go on to describe a data set on the vaccination debate that is currently under development and will allow us to assess how well these technologies perform when they are combined for one specific use case. We then conclude with a summary of the main points raised in this chapter.

Information, Knowledge Communication Through Natural Language on the Web

Information and knowledge are often used interchangeably, but as is argued in the Introduction to this book and in other chapters, it is important to make a distinction between the two. In this chapter, we do not use *knowledge* in its literal sense: *knowing about something* but in the sense of *generalised understanding of how things work*. We thus assume that knowledge is more generalised, rationalised and predictive than information.

Whereas people can be informed about specific cases of measles in specific places and moments in time, this information becomes knowledge when it is generalised to a categorial level and has predictive and explanatory value, for example, that certain people are more perceptual about the possibility of catching measles under certain conditions. As such information tends to address states of individuals that can change over time while knowledge tends to be associated with categories of things and possible states or relations. From a knowledge engineering point of view, knowledge focusses on the (formal) ontology of different things that *can* be out there and what is *possible* in the world (e.g. dinosaurs), whereas information focusses on what *is the case* and is *observed* in the current world (e.g. the current population of polar bears). Information can therefore be used to populate an ontology with instances and actual relations.

We expect reports to mainly contain information, because it is new and relevant. Opinions and emotions expressed by people can be considered as a form of information as well, as these inform us about their current inner state or state of mind. Knowledge accumulates slower and after some filtering or aggregation of evidence. In other words, we tend to base knowledge on logical *reasoning* and *authorised* evidence, and it is on the basis of this that personal or wider group action can be taken.

It should be noted though that, just like information can be false, knowledge can turn out to be incorrect. The difference between information and knowledge is, moreover, not always clear-cut. The intertwined relation between information and knowledge is what makes sharing and exchanging knowledge through the web and social media complex and often non-transparent: do people disagree about the number of deaths because of measles or about individual cases or do they disagree about the actual cause, the possible explanations or the evidence for these explanations? Furthermore, what does one believe and trust, how is evidence provided and is it cited correctly? What are the motivations of sources of information? The answers to these questions are often hidden and difficult to derive from the vast volume of dispersed information and knowledge that is posted on the web.

In case of debates on topics such as vaccination, we typically see that people mix information and knowledge. At the same time, they are very selective with respect to the information and knowledge they use in their communication. There are two possible explanations for this. First, people may (possibly unconsciously) only care about knowledge and information that fits their perspective. Second, they may not have an overview of all available knowledge and information, nor what different viewpoints exist and how they relate to available information. Both of these factors are likely to be shaped by the wider cultural resources and networks (on- and offline) within which people are embedded or entangled.

The following examples from the vaccination debate show two extreme positions in the debate and the way these are framed. In (1) Brian Shilhavy quotes an authority (Dr. and director of an official government body) stating that there have been no measles deaths in the US to argue that measles is not dangerous. In (2), the original Associated Press article from which the quote is taken argues the opposite that measles is dangerous and it is only a matter of time that the first people will be killed in the US despite there being no deaths in ten years.

(1) Source: http://vaccineimpact.com/2015/zero-u-s-measles-deaths-in-10-years-but-over-100-measles-vaccine-deaths-reported/. Website: Vaccination Impact. Author: Brian Shilhavy:

> According to a statement made by Dr. Anne Schuchat, the director of CDC's National Center for Immunization and Respiratory Diseases, in an Associated Press story picked up by Fox News on April 25, 2014: 'There has been no measles deaths reported in the U.S. since 2003'.[1]

(2) Source: Associated Press. Author: Mike Stobbe. Published Thursday, 24 April 2014:

> Wrapped into that estimate are 71 million measles cases, nearly 9 million measles hospitalizations and 57,000 measles deaths. There have been no measles deaths reported in the U.S. since 2003. 'But the way we're going, we feel it (another) is inevitable', Schuchat said.

[1] The citation taken from the *Vaccine Impact* website contains the spelling error "hs", whereas the original quote in the *Associated Press* has the correct spelling "has".

These two examples show many aspects of the debate: (1) evidence and arguments are used and even twisted to serve a purpose, (2) the authority of sources is used to substantiate claims and (3) a variety of linguistic constructions is used to express claims, sources and authorities. Messages such as the above can be found abundantly on the web, exploiting also other ways of argumentation, among which are included strong emotions (anger, disgust, frustration, sadness, sorrow), reporting individual cases (a specific child becoming autistic), allegations (scientists and government failing their duties) and conspiracies (Big Pharma causes regular outbreaks to sell vaccines).

Knowledge and information posted on the web has a source, which is either the writer/editor of the text or somebody cited by the writer/editor. In the default case, sources make simple affirmative statements. In that case, we can say that the source confirms or believes the information in the statement to be true. However, sources can also deny something, express a negative or positive opinion with respect to a claim or express that they are certain or uncertain about it. In example (3), we see a simple tweet that already contains a complex combination of claims, sentiments and sources, where we marked phrases with span boundaries "[" and "]" and labels to indicate sources, claims and sentiment:

(3) Source Twitter:

> [The new US president <SOURCE>] has <u>said</u> [he <SOURCE>] <u>believes</u> that [vaccines are harmful <CLAIM>] and has [repeatedly and erroneously <NEGATIVE>] <u>suggested</u> that [they cause autism <CLAIM>]
> [...] = span of text, <...> = label

In this tweet, *the new US president* is mentioned as a secondary source indicated by the predicate *said*. We read this source as confirming he *believes* a claim, where *he* co-refers with the president. The claim itself is a simple statement: *vaccines are harmful*. In this first part of the sentence, the opinion of the primary source (the twitterer) is not revealed. In the second part, the primary source expressed a negative sentiment towards another claim of the secondary source: *repeatedly and erroneously*. By doing this, the primary source takes positions against the president, directly with respect to the second claim, but indirectly also against the first. The interpretation that the tweeter does not believe the first claim made by the president, while denying the second, comes from the semantic relation between the claims. Readers automatically conclude that *causing autism* also implies *being harmful*. Finally, the predicates *believes* and *suggested* indicate a level of doubt and uncertainty with respect to the president's claims. Above all, this tweet mainly informs us about the positions of the twitterer and the US president in relation to the debate, but it is unlikely that it contains any new knowledge for people reading the tweet: vaccines can or cannot cause autism.

Many linguistic constructions to express positions and arguments are clearly marked. This provides handles to develop tooling for analysing the debates and how people exchange knowledge and information on a large scale. In the next sections, we show how we model information as to provide a comprehensive overview and transparency and outline how such information can be obtained automatically from text using NLP tools.

Modelling Claims, Attributions and Perspectives

The examples in the previous section illustrate some of the main challenges in finding reliable information and to enrich knowledge. The Internet is full of contradictory claims, factual statements that are not made based on evidence, misquotations, researchers that are careful in the statements they make and laypeople who are confident despite lack of scientific foundation. Formal modelling and automatic text analysis cannot determine whether a claim is true or not, but it can help people navigate through the wild growth of information in order to improve their knowledge for future decisions. We first outline the facilities we aim to provide and then describe how the GRaSP model introduced in this section supports these facilities.

Let us consider parents who want to inform themselves of the benefits and dangers of various vaccinations. Our goal is to provide them with all relevant information and avoid that they only find information supporting one specific vision, without the possibility of verifying the claims this vision is built upon. This means that they first and foremost need to receive an overview of relevant information on the topic (e.g. so that they do not only find information on the risks without gaining insights on the benefits nor information that is biased towards recommending any existing vaccination). Secondly, we want to give them as much evidence as possible for verifying the claims they find on a specific topic. This requires various kinds of information. When the information comes from a primary source (a direct claim), they need information on the source: what is the background of the individual or institute making the claim. In case of a claim based on external reference, they need a link to the information provided by the original publication, so they can verify whether the secondary claim correctly displays the information provided by the original primary source and check the background of this source. As part of the verification process, we also want to indicate sources that provide alternative views on the claim, either contradicting the claim or assigning it a different level of certainty. These claims should also be connected to the original sources and provide background information on them. When information is displayed in this manner, they have the means to compare different visions and examine the evidence they are based on.

It follows from the above that a central point in providing full insight in a topic lies in connecting pieces of information in a more transparent way. We therefore propose to represent information as Linked Data following Semantic Web standards. Linked Data represents information in RDF (Resource Description Framework),[2] an extensible knowledge representation model specifically designed to connect information and reason over it. The RDF schema presents information in triples consisting of a subject, predicate and object. Entities, classes and relations are represented by unique identifiers called internationalised resource identifiers (IRIs).[3] We provide a simple example to explain the principle. Consider

[2] https://www.w3.org/RDF/

[3] RDF versions prior to RDF 1.1 used *uniform resource identifiers*. The term URI is therefore also commonly used to indicate identifiers in RDF.

the following triples from DBpedia,[4] a database representing information from Wikipedia as Linked Data:

http://dbpedia.org/resource/Amsterdam http://dbpedia.org/ontology/isPartOf http://dbpedia.org/page/North_Holland
http://dbpedia.org/page/North_Holland http://dbpedia.org/ontology/isPartOf http://dbpedia.org/page/Netherlands

These triples state that Amsterdam is part of North Holland and that North Holland is part of the Netherlands. Because we can define being part of something as a transitive relation, we can infer that Amsterdam is part of the Netherlands. Imagine two other (made-up) resources (historic1 and historic2) that contain the following triples:

http://historic_resource_1/cities/Amsterdam http://historic_ontology.org/cityRightDate "1300"^^xs:date.
http://historic_resource_2/locations/Amsterdam http://historic_ontology.org/cityRightDate "1306"^^xs:date.

These resources were created independently and each introduced their own IRI to refer to Amsterdam. They do make use of the same (also made-up) generic ontology that includes the relation of the date on which a place obtained city rights, where one source places this in the year 1300 and the other in 1306. The value is a literal, specified as a date. If we find out that the IRIs ending with /Amsterdam in all three resources, DBpedia and both historic resources, refer to the same city, we can link them as follows:

http://dbpedia.org/resource/Amsterdam owl:sameAs http://historic_resource_1/cities/Amsterdam
http://dbpedia.org/resource/Amsterdam owl:sameAs http://historic_resource_2/locations/Amsterdam

[4] https://wiki.dbpedia.org

The relation *owl:sameAs* explicitly states that two IRIs denote the same thing and that, thus, what is true for the referent of one also is true for the other. By linking information from all three resources, we now have information about the location of Amsterdam (being part of North Holland and the Netherlands) as well as when it received city rights.

Amsterdam only received these rights once, but we have two conflicting values for this. The Semantic Web has no problem with conflicting information standing next to each other, though, naturally, researchers have tried to find solutions as to help users determine the reliability of information. An important contribution in this aspect came from PROV-O (Lebo et al. 2013), an ontology for modelling the provenance of information. With GRaSP, we build on top of this basic information on provenance and introduce a framework that is targeted towards citing information and pointing back to textual sources. In addition, GRaSP provides the means to indicate which level of uncertainty a source attributes to a statement and whether they express a specific sentiment or emotion. Figure 12.1 illustrates how the perspectives on vaccines cause autism expressed in the tweet above (Example 3, Section 3.2) can be represented through GRaSP.

The statement that vaccines cause autism is represented at the top of the image. We typically use the Simple Event Model (SEM, Van Hage et al. 2011) that is designed to model events and states as a generic framework for statements. We use DBpedia IRIs to denote "vaccine" and "autism" and they are related to each other through the causal relation defined in SEM. The statement is linked to a component of the aforementioned tweet using the GRaSP relation denotedBy.[5] Next, we model the perspective on the statement expressed by a specific source in this text. Recall from Example 3 that according to the tweet, Trump asserted that vaccines cause autism and that the twitterer qualified this statement as "erroneous". In this case, we have thus two separate attributions linked to the same statement, indicated by the leftmost and rightmost blue circles. The left circle represents Trump confirming it (without expressing

[5] The tweet itself as well as its components can also be represented by IRIs, which then point to the exact text that expresses a statement and can be resolved through the Twitter API. This is not done here for reasons of simplification.

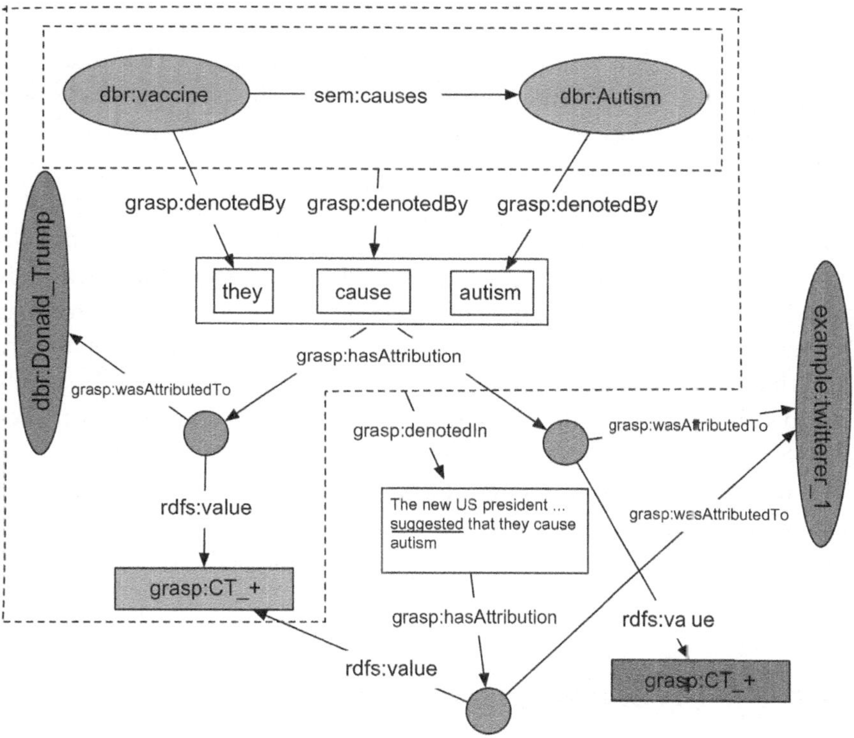

Fig. 12.1 Schematic representation of GRaSP of previous example from the vaccination corpus

doubt), indicated by value CT_+. The right circle represents the twitterer confidently denying it (value CT_-). Finally, Trump's view is expressed by a secondary source in this case. Figure 12.1 illustrates that we can link the entire representation of Trump asserting that vaccines cause autism (without expressing doubt) is represented in the tweet and that the twitterer is the source of Trump's view. If we find Trump's original tweets on the subject, we can directly compare their content to the reported content in Example 3 and thus automatically verify whether his view is reported correctly.

Figure 12.1 merely provides a simplified and partial illustration of what can be achieved by GRaSP: we can also make explicit that the twitterer's opposed view is expressed erroneously, that vaccines causing autism is a more specific statement supporting the view that they are harmful and so on. More importantly, though, because we also use IRIs to denote the source, we can provide information about this source: what other statements does this source make? What is known about their background? This is a vital component in determining how reliable information is and how it should be interpreted. Recall Examples 1 and 2 where a text correctly reported that there had been no measles deaths in the US since 2003. The reporting text suggested that this meant that measles is not dangerous. It is through the other statements by the same source that we learn that the statement is meant to indicate that vaccines keep us safe and that, without them, measles can become dangerous again. This ability to connect statements, background information and sources makes GRaSP an extremely powerful framework for modelling perspectives. This leaves us with the challenge of how to obtain these detailed representations from large amounts of text. The next section discusses natural language processing (NLP) technologies designed to extract this information.

NLP for Assessing Claims from Dispersed Sources

The information we intend to extract from individual texts consists of the following components: the statement itself, or content of the claims made, the source of the statement, any indication of (un)certainty or negation and emotion or sentiment. In addition, we need to link claims to other texts that provide perspectives on the same statements. This requires precise and detailed analysis by a system consisting of multiple natural language processing (NLP) components, which we refer to as a reading machine. In Fig. 12.2, we see a schematic overview of such a reading machine that was developed in the NewsReader (Vossen et al. 2016) and BiographyNet (Ockeloen et al. 2013) projects to extract perspectives.

Different aspects of the information are extracted by different specialised NLP components, called modules. We apply named entity

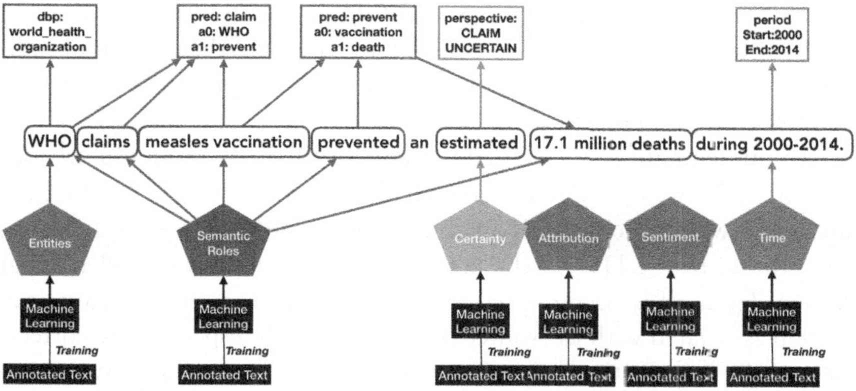

Fig. 12.2 Range of NLP modules for extracting claims and perspectives from a single text sentence

recognition to find entities such as WHO and entity linking to connect them to IRIs of resources such as DBpedia. We use event extraction to identify events such as claim, prevent and death. A semantic role labeling system identifies participants in these events such as measles vaccination and 17.1 million deaths and indicates which role they are playing in this event (e.g. vaccination receives an a0 role as the agent and deaths receives role a1 as the undergoer of prevent). Factuality detection aims to identify the level of certainty through expressions such as estimated. A special module for detecting attribution focuses on finding whether a statement comes directly from the author or the text mentions some other source. Modules that detect and normalise time expressions indicate the date or the period of time in which an event takes place or holds.

Finally, we use coreference modules for entity coreference and event coreference in order to identify which expressions in a text refer to the same entity or event. This module tells us that they refers to vaccines in Example 3 and Fig. 12.1 above.

Most modules make use of supervised machine learning (AI) models, which are trained on texts for which people have manually indicated the correct interpretation (annotations). They are typically trained on data sets specifically created for the task: only few data sets provide annotations for multiple tasks. For a complete representation of an article in

GRaSP, we need to apply all these modules to each sentence in the text and combine the outcome in a single representation. The content of individual texts then needs to be linked in order to provide perspectives expressed by various articles.

We implemented a specialised module for this task. From our attribution module, we derive that WHO is the secondary source cited by the author to which the claim is attributed. The word claim is used to connect the source WHO to the actual knowledge that is provided. That knowledge itself is decomposed into a specific proposition. Uncertainty is then associated with the source of the claim with respect to the correctness of the information because of the use of estimated. All these pieces of information are identified by our interpretation module, which generates the structure of the statement and identifies if the same statement has already been found elsewhere. If so, the module links the existing statement to the newly identified text and assigns the attribution values and source. Each individual article thus contributes attribution information of its own. If the statement is not found elsewhere, it is added to the model.

The above analysis can be applied automatically to a large volume of texts, potentially providing computers systematic access to any claim made anywhere at any moment in time. In Fig. 12.3 below, we give a

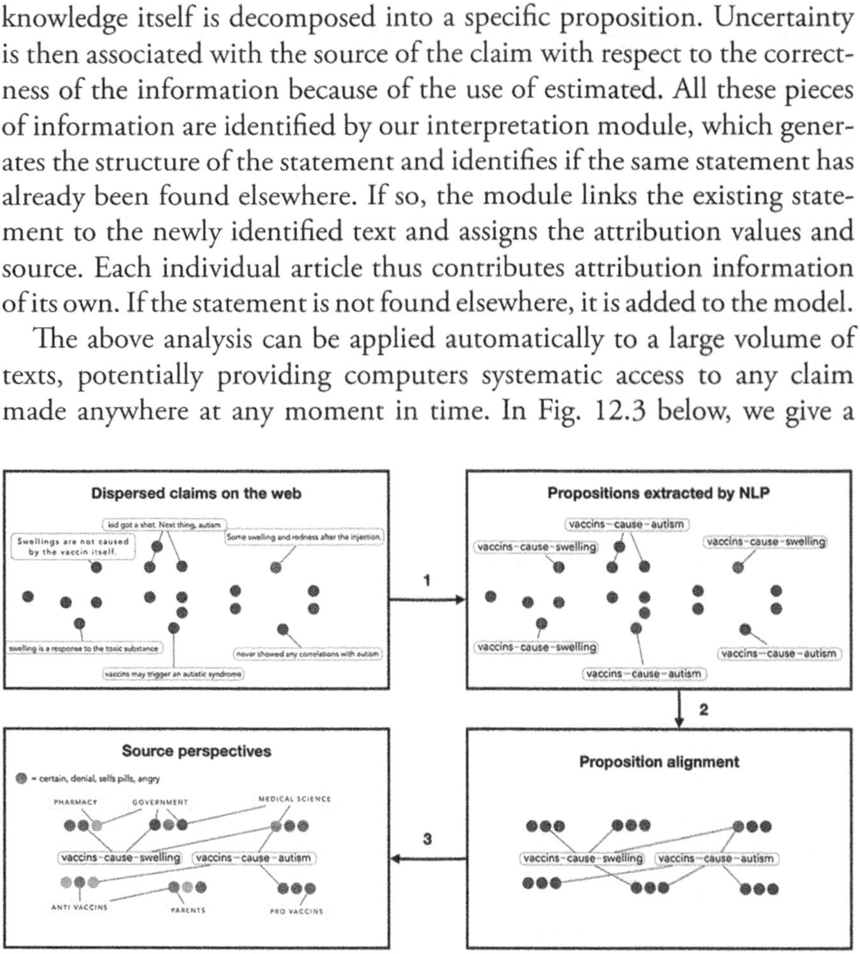

Fig. 12.3 Building a web of perspectives

schematic overview how a web with dispersed claims expressed on different websites (represented by the circles) or a network of referencing websites can be processed to provide an overview in source perspectives in three steps:

1. First, the NLP software interprets the claims made on each source in terms of the proportional content, normalising the content across the varied ways in which it is expressed.
2. In the second step, all different sources can now be aligned for their shared content, regardless of their perspective.
3. In the final third step, we determine for each source what the perspective is with respect to each claim, such as denying, confirming, certainty, emotions and so on.

On the basis of meta information, we can further group sources according to their authority or background but we can also group them by their shared perspectives.

We call the final result the Perspective web, as it organises knowledge and information in terms of perspectives on claimed propositions. The actual propositions are represented only once and sources are represented through their shared perspective or any other meta information that is provided, such as their professional role or background (van Son et al. 2014). To obtain all propositions, it is no longer necessary to read all sources, while a simple overview is given of all different views. Users can then easily trace these sources and judge the authority for their own position. In Fig. 12.4, we show how the same data can be organised by source,

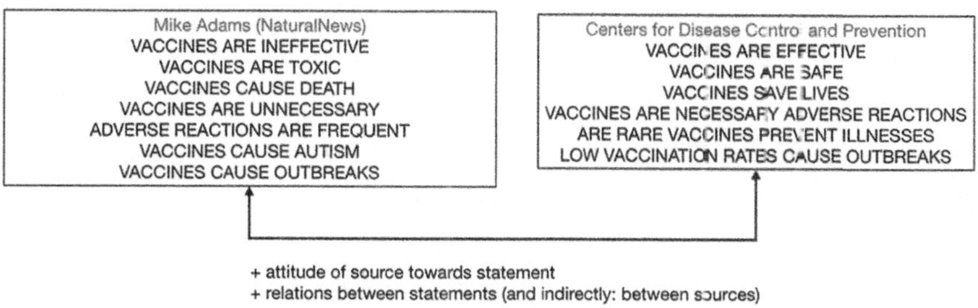

Fig. 12.4 Comparing claims and perspectives across different positions

showing all claims made by one source, or contrasted across pairs of sources by analysing how claims and perspectives relate to each other.

Finally in Fig. 12.5, we show how we can build a network of sources that make reference to each other to illustrate where they obtain their claims or point to further evidence. The graph shows three clusters of Dutch websites. The top cluster has a single website as a hub to which others point for evidence that vaccines cause side effects that can be cured using a homoeopathic treatment. The left-bottom graph also has one website as a hub to which others point for evidence and news on negative effects of vaccination. Both networks seem highly connected. The green cluster to the bottom-right side shows official government websites that advocate vaccination. Remarkably, these sites do not point to others and nobody points to them, which isolates them from the debate.

Analysing such networks can show silos of knowledge or bubbles within which information is filtered or shared, while no information is shared or connected across these clusters. Combining the propositional representation with these clusters sheds more light on what information, knowledge and argumentation resides where and can potentially be used to improve sharing of knowledge and the quality of the deliberation by providing more transparency.

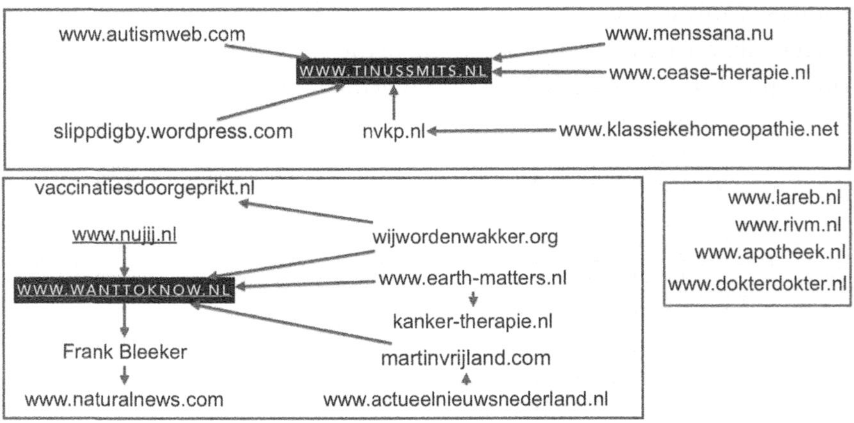

Fig. 12.5 Tracing knowledge in a web of sources

Perspectives on the Vaccination Debate

We mentioned in the previous section that data sets exist for each individual NLP module, but that these sets typically only cover one or few tasks, for example, named entity recognition or sentiment analysis. To develop and test the software that can generate the complete overviews shown in the previous section, we created a data set with 294 web documents around the vaccination debate (528,727 words and 23,467 sentences in total, Morante et al. 2020). The documents contain a large variety of sources: news, blogs, editorials, governmental reports and science articles. They represent supporting, opposing and neutral views with respect to vaccinations. The data can be downloaded from the following website: https://vaccinationcorpus.wordpress.com.

We applied our "reading machine" to the text to extract some basic propositional information. The next list gives a readable overview of what we automatically extracted:

- CAUSE things:

- death, harm, side effects, mild symptoms, autism, SIDS, seizures, abortion, neurological disorders, brain damage, diabetes mellitus, immune dysfunction, outbreaks of diseases, spread of chickenpox, severe allergic reactions
- PREVENT things:
- disease, rabies infection, measles, hepatitis A, potentially fatal diseases, the onset of AIDS, replication, 6 million deaths worldwide
- PROTECT/SAVE things:
- babies' immature immune system, people, children, our lives, you
- CONTAIN things:

- ingredients, antigens, germs, a live virus, thimerosal (mercury), unsafe toxins, a cancer-causing monkey virus, the dangerous pertussis toxin with unsafe additives

We see that many different claims are made with respect to positive and negative effects of vaccination. Given such lists, software can reason over all specific aspects and generalise these to classes, which adds predictive power to the data and allows for further generalisations.

We annotated the data manually to test and benchmark software. The next table shows an overview of the data layers that are annotated. We first annotated all mentions of events that relate to the debate. The annotators were instructed to exclude verbs such as says, claims, believes and states (so-called speech act verbs that indicate that some source is making a claim). In total 65,865 events have been annotated. Claim-related expressions are annotated as attribution relations, where students annotated the cited sources if present (the author is the default source), the expression that marks the attribution relation (e.g. the above speech acts), the paragraph that contains the claim and the specific content of each attributed claim. On top of this, we annotated any sentiment expressed with respect to persons, groups and organisations. There are 26,996 of these entities mentioned in the documents. We annotated 2222 opinions on these entities in 168 documents.

In future work, we will extend the annotations with propositional information. The events mentioned within a claim will form the basis for aligning propositions across different sources. For these propositions, we will annotate whether the source is certain, denies or confirms. For pairs of propositions across sources, we annotate whether these are related and if so if there is some entailment or a contradiction. The annotations will be used to evaluate the software that aims at generating the perspectives and propositional content. The vaccination data set is publicly available under a Creative Commons license and published on the Perspectives website (Table 12.1).[6]

[6] https://vuaperspectives.wordpress.com

Table 12.1 Overview of the annotations of the vaccination corpus

	Annotation type	Total
Events		65.865
Attribution	**Content**	4.894
	Sources	4.009
	Cues	4.579
	Claims	4.693
Sentiment	**Entities**	2222

Conclusion and Discussion

In this chapter, we provided a high-level description of how current Semantic Web and NLP technologies can be used to obtain an overview and provide transparency to online debates. We discussed that information and knowledge in online debates are dispersed and difficult to grasp as many different sources post information discontinuously and do not address each other's claims. We showed how the GRaSP framework can be used to connect claims that express the same or different perspectives on a statement and that it provides the means to find the original source of a claim, verify the claim itself or find background information on the person or organisation that made the claim. We described the NLP software needed to derive propositional relations from articles and identify the sources of a claim and their perspectives. The propositional relations can be used to find different sources making related claims to contrast perspectives across individual sources and groups. The software is capable of processing a massive amount of information at any moment in time and likewise can provide a more transparent landscape of knowledge and information over large amounts of online data but also monitor the dynamics and relate the claims to networks of websites and communities that form silos and filter bubbles. So far we are testing the software on a specific data set on the vaccination debate, but in the future we hope to extend this to other debates and apply it on a larger scale.

Our technical framework can be used to capture the textual and linguistic debate but still requires some interface for non-experts to navigate the resulting knowledge landscape as complex graph. The design of such an interface is out of the scope of this paper but can be inspired on the various graph exploration solutions, for example, Gephi,[7] GraphViz[8] and SocioViz,[9] that have been used for other data sets.

References

Hage, v., Robert, W., Malaisé, V., Segers, R., Hollink, L., & Schreiber, G. (2011). Design and use of the simple event model (SEM). *Journal of Web Semantics, 9*(2), 128–136.

Lebo, T., Sahoo, S., McGuinness, D., Belhajjame, K., Cheney, J., Corsar, D., Garijo, D., Soiland-Reyes, S., Zednik, S., & Zhao, J. (2013). Prov-o: The prov ontology. *W3C Recommendation, 30.*

Morante, Roser, Chantal van Son, Isa Maks, & Piek Vossen, 2020. Annotating perspectives on vaccination. *In Proceedings of international conference on language resources and evaluation* (LREC 2020).

Ockeloen, N., Fokkens, A., Ter Braake, S., Vossen, P., De Boer, V., Schreiber, G., & Legêne, S. (2013). BiographyNet: Managing provenance at multiple levels and from different perspectives. In *LISC@ ISWC* (pp. 59–71) Australia, Springer, ISBN 978-3-642-41338-4.

okkens, A., Vossen, P., Rospocher, M., Hoekstra, R., & van Hage, W. R. (2017). Grasp: Grounded representation and source perspective. In *Proceedings of the workshop knowledge resources for the socio-economic sciences and humanities associated with RANLP 2017* (pp. 19–25).

van Son, C., van Erp, M., Fokkens, A., & Vossen, P. (2014). Hope and fear: Interpreting perspectives by integrating sentiment and event factuality. In *Proceedings of the 9th international conference on language resources and evaluation (LREC 2014)* (pp. 26–31).

Vossen, P., Agerri, R., Aldabe, I., Cybulska, A., van Erp, M., Fokkens, A., Laparra, E., et al. (2016). NewsReader: Using knowledge resources in a cross-lingual reading machine to generate more knowledge from massive streams of news. *Knowledge-Based Systems, 110*, 60–85.

[7] https://gephi.org

[8] https://www.graphviz.org

[9] https://socioviz.net

13

Safety and Security in Knowledge Landscapes

Dina Simunic and Predrag Pale

Introduction: Safety and Security

This chapter explores the meaning of, and ways of managing and responding to, issues surrounding safety and security in digital systems and how these need to be considered from a technical perspective when trying to understand knowledge landscapes. Digital health information has a range of risks and challenges as seen in earlier chapters in this book: here we discuss risks associated with the development and use of the Internet of Things (IoT) and in particular the Internet of Medical Things (IoMT), devices and systems increasingly seen in healthcare. The chapter draws on

D. Simunic (✉)
Wireless communications, Faculty of Electrical Engineering and Computing, University of Zagreb, Zagreb, Croatia
e-mail: dina.simunic@fer.hr

P. Pale
Faculty of Electrical Engineering and Computing, University of Zagreb, Zagreb, Croatia

A. L. Svalastog et al. (eds.), *Navigating Digital Health Landscapes*, Health, Technology and Society, https://doi.org/10.1007/978-981-15-8206-6_13

the authors' disciplinary expertise in electrical engineering and computing. As with the other two chapters in this section, it offers some practical ways forward in regard to managing risks.

In spite of the fact that many languages do not in practice differentiate between 'safety' and 'security', it is crucial that we clarify their difference. This is especially important in the context of information and communications technologies (ICT) and their role in health systems. In broad terms, 'safety' covers events caused by the environment, technology or unintentional accidents caused by people, while security relates to incidents intentionally caused by people (M-W Dict, safety 2020a). For example, a user may accidentally erase a digital file and in most cases it will be possible to recover the content. This can also happen through disc malfunction, computer malfunction, water spillage, and so on. These unintentional events are covered by the term 'safety' and procedures that help avoid them. In contrast, a malicious attack by a hacker can erase a file on purpose and in such a way that it cannot be recovered by any means (except if backed-up): such attacks can be prevented by appropriate 'security' measures (M-W Dict, security 2020b).

The IoT gathers pace across many societies and, related to IoT wireless security, surveys show that a high percentage (39%) of respondents think that it 'remains a huge concern' (Weissman 2015) as is amply demonstrated by the recent fallout over the use of Facebook data. The European Union seeks to develop a legal solution to this problem, at least in regard to key concerns which are to be addressed through new provisions in the General Data Protection Regulation (e.g. developing privacy by design) (GDPR 2016). However, policing and enforcing these policies calls for considerable financial and human resources that have to be effectively planned and harmonized at all the levels, involving both strategic and tactical domains. While 'pure' IoT sensors will in general be oriented mostly to the broad human environment, the IoMT system (Marr 2018) is built on improved precision to facilitate effective interaction between medical expertise and the human body. An example would be remote health monitoring for illness, diagnostics and prevention. Another example is remote surgery that enables precision medical care outside a shared geographical location for the medical expert and patient. Unfortunately, all these devices and their communication systems and structures, enabling their 'connectivity', can be extremely vulnerable.

As a result, the possibility of individuals or organizations hacking the IoMT could have a significant impact on the health of an individual or even of a wider population, raising crucial ethical, legal and technological issues. In this context, a multi-stakeholder discussion between the four most important parties—citizens, medical professionals, government and private industry—on the governance of the 'smart human society' and its related connectivity has to be pursued, aiming to create a consensus over the meaning of connectivity security. The most powerful defence against and prevention of abuse is to educate users, especially younger people, about the possible risks and threats they may have to deal with. As noted above, this chapter explores the dangers, risks and threats in the existing and near-future healthcare environments, related to digital systems.

Some Basic Principles

Measures to achieve safety are based on three pillars: (i) backing-up data at two or several remote locations and in different types of media; (ii) building redundancy into solutions, systems and infrastructures; and (iii) closely monitoring systems, components and activities and promptly alerting users/others about risk-related events or discrepancies. However, measures to achieve desired security level are much more complex.

Security depends on three different stakeholders: (a) designers, developers and producers, (b) solution and maintenance providers and (c) end users.

(a) Designers of devices and systems are focused on functionality, flexibility, ease of use and cost-effectiveness. These are in direct opposition to security, because security and comfort are reversely proportional—the more a system is secure, the more cumbersome and slower it is to use it.

Developers should be given time, resources and knowledge to implement a 'security by design' concept. Industry should be forced by regulation and standards to deliver safe and secure devices from the beginning. For example, every device delivered should have a globally unique identifier and authentication token(s).

(b) Those who design, install and maintain custom solutions should have an in-depth knowledge of both ICT and a client's local domain needs and processes. They are struggling in particular with equilibrium of usability and security. They need to monitor their devices and networks for any sign of vulnerability or accident and quickly respond to them. Especially they need to patch, update and replace software or their components in order to reduce their vulnerability.

(c) Users also have the responsibility to purchase secure products, to wisely choose competent consultants and trainers, to update software and licenses, to promptly respond to requests and instructions from technical personnel and above all not to share their credentials with anyone. They are also responsible for their own awareness and competence in computer security.

While social media reports the growth of hacking and cybercrime, many users neglect more common issues involving damage to data and/or financial risk which are in fact due to safety incidents. Quite a significant proportion of information-related safety incidents are caused unintentionally by people, due to their lack of awareness or competence or mere mistakes.

Security incidents in contrast are believed to be predominantly caused by hackers and other malicious sources outside of any organization. IBM defines an attack as 'malicious activity that is attempting to collect, disrupt, deny, degrade or destroy information system resources or the information itself'. However, in reality the majority of attacks (c.60%) are executed by insiders: current or recent ex-employees (IBM X-Force Cyber Security Index 2016). IBM X-Force studies, monitors and reports on the latest threat trends. The first goal of the X-Force's activity is to understand the threats in order to provide a higher security content to its customers but also to warn customers and the general public about emerging and critical threats. It is also important to keep in mind the observation that the 'typical hackers sit inside a network for 254 days before they make themselves known' (Joy 2019).

Compared to 2015, when the healthcare sector was globally most likely to be hit by data breaches, by 2019 the sector was the tenth most targeted industry, accounting for 3% of all attacks within the top ten sectors (IBM X-Force Threat Intelligence Index 2020). The most usual motivation of cybercriminals is financial with the aim to steal and sell medical records, or to disrupt activity of hospitals and nursing home networks for ransom. In the summer of 2018, what was known as 'Ryuk' attacks started to appear in a public malware repository with the aim of targeting enterprise environments. In 2019 Ryuk attacks in the USA demanded more than $7.5 billion from at least 966 government agencies (113 state and municipal governments and agencies, 764 healthcare providers and 89 universities, colleges and school districts, with operations at up to 1233 individual schools potentially affected) (Taylor 2019). Thus, the healthcare sector has a clear interest in improving security within current and emerging medical systems. The Herjavec Group in its 2019 Official Annual Cybercrime Report (Herjavec 2020) estimates that healthcare companies will experience approximately $6 trillion in damages (e.g. data loss) in 2021.

Safety and Security Navigating Knowledge Landscapes

There is a whole range of information safety and security risks, threats and vulnerabilities, while navigating knowledge landscape [Svalastog et al. 2020]. Most commonly these relate to outdated, incomplete, damaged, poorly transformed, inadequately stored, poorly described or inappropriately structured data. Then there is user's inability to find the source of information, root data, evaluate trustworthiness, validate, verify, attribute or simply identify who said something, to whom, why and in which context. Finally, there are cases of intentional misinformation, lies, spin, fake news, deep fake videos, plagiarisms and logic violations.

Each of these problems deserves at least a whole chapter.

The above-mentioned problems have one common denominator: the individual user as the one most likely to encounter the problem. Thus, intuitively it is often hoped that if effective and trustworthy machines were the source of data, we would have no or much less information security problems.

The Internet of Things (IoT)

In 2018 more than 8.4 billion 'things' joined the 'Internet of Things' (IoT), making the total worldwide number of active IoT devices in 2019 to 26.66 billion [Statista 2019]. Projections say that by 2025 there will be 75 billion of IoT devices worldwide.

Every second, 127 new devices are connected to the Internet. The majority of healthcare providers have increasingly become engaged with IoT in the medical world, hence referred as the 'Internet of Medical Things' or sometimes the 'Internet of Health Things' (IoHT). By 2020, 40% of all IoT devices will be used in the healthcare industry. Estimates from Deloitte (Deloitte 2019) are that the global IoT market will reach $7.1 trillion and within it the global IoMT market a '$158 billion valuation in 2022, up from $41 billion in 2017'. Thus, all the theories of 'big data' hold (Mayer-Schönberger and Cukier 2013).

Internet of Medical Things (IoMT)

The IoT changes almost any object into a source of information ('thing') that can be used for further processing. Since IoMT comprises only devices that are used in medical assistance, IoMT is clearly a subgroup of IoT that covers almost all activities of human society.

This means that the IoMT consists of medical devices, software applications, health systems and services connected by a communication infrastructure. The IoMT ecosystem is very special due to its enabling role of remote patient monitoring with sensor-based tools and the possibility of coupling gathered patient data with patient information. The rise of IoMT is driven by 'an increase in the number of connected medical devices that are able to generate, collect, analyze or transmit health data or images and connect to healthcare provider networks, transmitting data to either a cloud repository or internal servers', as noted by Deloitte (2019).

Ultimately, this connectivity between medical devices and sensors is streamlining clinical workflow management and leading to an overall improvement in patient care, both inside care facility walls and in remote locations.

The following IoMT examples show the full spectrum of existing applications that is growing every day. One of the most important features of the current IoMT world is the possibility of tracking in the operational area of healthcare, where, for example, tags are used to prevent baby theft or their misplacement (Centrak 2019). The IoMT is also used in regard to smart beds with the purpose of monitoring vital functions and preventing common patient problems such as bedsores (Wellsensevu 2019). Some applications (e.g. AutoBed by GE Healthcare) have helped to reduce emergency waiting times in New York hospitals by 50%. Some other applications take care of patient medications and blood samples (e.g. SensorMetrix 2019) to ensure that they are exposed to a required accurate temperature. No less important is a system of remote patient monitoring by sending an alert if the patient does not move or if he/she falls (e.g. Zanthion 2019). Even in an intensive care unit in a hospital, IoMT enables the responsible senior doctor on duty to have an immediate notification of any change in the vital parameters of his/her patient with all the required details without being close by. This is also the case while a doctor is 'on-call-duty', that is, not in the hospital (Binkowski 2016).

The IoMT contributes to a network of connected medical devices, which enables patients and healthcare providers access to data, and thus also to important information. In the information and communication society, there is a difference, as noted in other chapters, between data as information and how this can be processed to form tractable forms of knowledge. Data are unprocessed facts or figures, whereas knowledge represents the processed data. Furthermore, data doesn't depend on information, whereas the knowledge depends on data. Actually, data represent a single unit, whereas knowledge is based on data that carries news and meaning. For example, in IoMT, the 'Medical Thing' (MT) can be a medication, a wheelchair, a heart monitor or any sensor on or in the human body (Mole 2018; Meola 2020; Tung et al. 2015). Sometimes, when it is really of urgent importance to get a complete 'picture' of the patient and thus have a full and continuous flow of patient data, as for example in the smart city scenario, all the sensors and devices (so-called patient 'body area network(s)', BAN(s)) are connected to an internal hub. In this case, the hub of the patient can be considered as MT (Hammi et al. 2017). The main aim of IoMT is to increase the quality of life for all the citizens, but especially for the elderly and disabled, who often require specially designed healthcare (Chen et al. 2017). At the same time, the IoMT makes possible preventive care and improvement thereby in patient outcomes. In addition, it opens entirely new space for medicine and medical personnel given it is possible to identify higher health risk individuals in patient populations. This latter is the objective in the near future, where it is expected that IoMT systems will utilize not only sophisticated sensor technology and classical wireless communications systems but also artificial intelligence and novel wireless communications systems, as planned in the quickly growing smart cities (United Nations Department of Economic and Social Affairs 2018; European Smart Cities 2015; EC 2020). Finally, the IoMT makes the costs of healthcare lower due to the efficient management of medical assets.

The World Health Organization (WHO) acknowledges the arrival and application of new technologies by organizing regularly WHO Global Fora on Medical Devices (WHO 2019). While many are working towards ease of workflows and transformation of healthcare in practice, the IoMT is vulnerable to various cybersecurity threats as all the other ICTs. Unfortunately, the ICT in the medical sector (mostly IoMT, connected to the networks) is in general less protected, because of the wish and the need for simple and easy-to-use systems for non-ICT personnel and/or patients (Lynch and Farrington 2018).

It seems that IoMT already plays an important role, but it will play an even more important role in the near future, since the majority of relevant data can be collected via IoMT external to clinics. Recent studies (e.g. Pandor et al. 2015) show that some European clinics are piloting a system to remotely monitor patients to reduce re-admission rates. This could be very important in monitoring chronic conditions, shortening hospital stays and improving medication adherence.

Mobile health (mHealth), as a sub-area of eHealth, covers medical and public health practice supported by mobile devices (see also Chap. 10). mHealth uses applications and sensors connected to mobile communication devices for monitoring health and well-being of the individuals, that is, mHealth uses IoMT for remote monitoring of health status. This combination enables patients to actively monitor and manage their own health and, thus, a higher quality of life due to fewer required visits to a medical doctor or to a hospital. On the other hand, mHealth also enables healthcare professionals more efficient treatment of patients. As a consequence, patients are getting healthcare of a higher quality enabling them longer life, with less burden on the healthcare system. Consequently, the more precise determination of a patient's current health status opens the door to the possibility of providing tailored health recommendations and prediction of potential future issues (EC 2004). Examples of devices used in remote monitoring include glucometers, electrocardiography devices, wearable healthcare devices, smart pill boxes, insole sensors, smartwatch applications, activity trackers of patients' ambulatory abilities after surgery and fall detection devices. All these devices generate patient data that enable precious and precise clinical care external to clinics, often the best place for such a chronic patient, that is, in the home (such as a medically 'smart' home). Thus, the aim of the IoMT concept is to enable longer lives of a higher quality for all, allowing significantly shorter patient stays in hospital, enabling at the same time more efficient use of the existing health system for all users.

In spite of the increasing enthusiasm with the dawn of the ongoing IoMT revolution, society should not fall into the trap of believing that IoMT is a completely secure and safe system. On the contrary, as noted above, IoT and particularly IoMT actually create a completely new realm of information security problems.

IoT Threats, Vulnerabilities, Risks and Mitigations

Today a global awareness exists of the many possible threats to systems, especially to medical systems that are connected to the information and communication infrastructure, as is the case of the IoMT. Therefore, it is necessary to understand these threats. The definition of **threat** in Merriam-Webster dictionary is that it is an event with the potential to have a negative impact (M-W Dict, threat 2020c). In the context of IoMT, three main types of threats can have a negative impact on its operation:

(a) Natural threats (e.g. floods, hurricanes, earthquake, COVID-19)
(b) Unintentional threats (by a mistake of an employee who accidentally disrupts an IoMT)
(c) Intentional threats (by a virus arriving through exposure to automated attacks)

In this sense, our discussion on safety and security from the beginning of the chapter is related to unintentional threats and intentional threats, respectively.

The Merriam-Webster dictionary defines **vulnerability** as a quality of the environment that allows a realization of the threat [M-W Dict, vulnerability 2020d]. In our case, it means that it is a known weakness of the IoMT that can be exploited by hackers and succeed in their attack(s).

According to the Merriam-Webster dictionary, **risk** is the potential for loss or damage when a threat exploits a vulnerability. In the IoMT case, risks include loss of privacy in terms of a personal medical record or any other data and loss of connection that enables transfer from the patient to the medical doctor.

Therefore, the threat is outside of anyone's control. However, the weak points of the system can be assessed and the action plan for minimization of the impact on the system can be developed. If such a plan is not developed, this creates vulnerability. The risk is then, for example, the loss of a personal medical record. However, the risk can be prevented (or mitigated, if the prevention is not possible) by identifying potential threats and addressing vulnerabilities, that is, by developing a risk mitigation plan.

The IoMT consists of hardware and software systems, which means that the systems are vulnerable to a diversity of threats. As explained above, system functionality is based on understanding both: threats and vulnerabilities. In this game of balancing threats and ensuring safe and secure systems, three options are possible:

1. The system is not protected enough (so-called under protection).
2. The system is just-enough protected (optimum protection).
3. The system is over-protected (over protection).

Of all the options, the third option takes too many resources (often system memory and users' time), so the users may well be minded to disregard it. Therefore, the system has to be designed more towards the direction of providing optimum protection.

The fact that the IoMT encompasses many devices (as part of the hardware) and programs (as part of the software) opens the door to a high number of possible threats, The decision that has to be taken is whether every potential threat and corresponding vulnerability will be treated separately, or as a 'threat bulk'. One of the further procedures is based on understanding the potential vulnerabilities without a specific corresponding threat (e.g. media failure). The complete risk assessment process comprises a detailed approach to both the views; it is an intermix of threat and vulnerability of the digital asset.

In general, risk assessment is oriented towards the identification of hazards. The risk assessment tries to understand who/what is a possible cause, who/what is a possible 'victim' and how can the 'victim' be harmed.

In the case of IoMT, the risk assessment is oriented to the environmental, site-support, physical and technical issues that are given below with examples.

Environmental issues of the IoMT security are reflected in any undesirable environmental activity, being a hazard (Halkos and Zisiadou 2018), such as lightning, or sprinkler activation. The other environmental concerns include, inter alia, fire, tsunami, earthquake, flood, lightning, smoke, insects, dust, volcanic eruption, severe weather, chemical fumes, rodents, sprinkler activation, water leakage, vibration, electromagnetic interference, electrostatic discharge, explosion and nuclear disaster.

Site-support issues are related to the site aspects, such as electrical power or air conditioning. The other physical nature encompasses personnel action, such as vandalism or theft. A more detailed list comprises the following: site-support concerns include power outage, extreme or unstable humidity, extreme or unstable temperatures, facility inaccessibility, unsafe environment, electrical noise, improper maintenance, personnel unavailability, inappropriate fire suppression, inability to cut power during fire or flood, inappropriate trash disposal or telephone failure.

Physical issues (GlobalSecurity 2001) of the IoMT security encompass personnel action, such as vandalism or theft. They also include unauthorized facility access, sabotage, extortion, war, spillage or droppage, magnets or magnetic tools, collision, trip hazards, improper transportation, labour unrest, fire hazard, terrorism or improper mounting or storage of the equipment.

Technical concerns include specific events as a part of the technical system, and they include both the design and the use of the system. The fact that most of the technical devices and systems are typically thoroughly tested before arriving on the market is the basis for very few real threats. Interestingly, the most important threats are untrained users. The definition of 'untrained user' includes all the employees in an organization, who can, for example, typically click on a phishing email (Morin 2016). Therefore, it can be stated that the technical security concerns include improper operation, improper hardware and/or software configuration, improper or inadequate procedure, unauthorized software or hardware or their modification (Meidan et al. 2020), unauthorized logical access, unauthorized software duplication, unsanctioned use or exceeding licensing, malfeasance, malicious software, hardware and/or software error or failure related to functionality and/or security, communications error, data entry error, media failure, accidental software and/or data modification and/or deletion, over- or under-classification, repudiation, message flooding, electronic emanations, accidental data disclosure, message playback, data remanence, geo-location, masquerading, object reuse, line tapping and communications failure or overload. These are generic concerns, but they are often used in the system design. System-specific vulnerabilities can be treated only by automated tools that identify operating system-, application- and middle-ware-specific vulnerabilities.

All the risk assessments must be evaluated for the specific system, with extensive calculation of the probability of their occurrence, projected event impact and mitigation costs.

The US FDA recently issued (1 October 2019) 'URGENT/11 Cybersecurity Vulnerabilities in a Widely-Used Third-Party Software Component May Introduce Risks During Use of Certain Medical Devices: FDA Safety Communication', with the conclusion that there are no any currently confirmed adverse events related to the given vulnerabilities, but the software to exploit these vulnerabilities is already publicly available. Therefore, 'these vulnerabilities may allow anyone to remotely take control of the medical device and change its function, cause denial of service, or cause information leaks or logical flaws, which may prevent device function' [FDA 2019].

IoT Risks and Mitigation Techniques for the Special Case of IoMT

Even though the IoT has to provide a constant seamless connection, meaning that the security should always satisfy the highest standards, the special case of IoMT in the world of IoT has even higher security demands. This is the case, because the IoMT is directly related to human health and any kind of security compromise, especially in the case of connection of, for example, a breathing machine, can possibly lead instantly to a fatality for the individual under treatment. Thus, here are identified five IoT risks, together with the mitigation techniques for the risks removal. The identified risks with their description and mitigation are device discovery; processes of identification, authentication and authorization; IoT botnets, DDoS attacks and IoT and IoMT passwords; encryption and network security.

Let us start with the first risk and its mitigation.

1. Device Discovery

In a nutshell, there should be no IoMT powered and attached to the network that is not known and not included in tracking, updating and checking. Devices no longer used should be powered down and disconnected from the communication network. Their decommission needs to be promptly communicated with all systems they were exchanging data with.

The very first task related to the IoMT risk and mitigation is device discovery. For example, port scanning, protocol analysis and other detection techniques support determination of the connected devices to a specific network. Examples are free tools, like Nmap (Nmap 2019), Shodan (Shodan 2019) and Masscan (Masscan 2019). After understanding which devices are connected, it is necessary to know the purpose of all the connected devices in order to distinguish between connected devices with approval and devices without approval with a possible malicious intention. If some of the devices from the approved list are stolen or lost, action has to be taken in the form of remote wiping or disabling their connectivity. This is very important, because sometimes an old login to a connected seemingly unimportant device like a refrigerator or a printer that should have been wiped long ago can be misused by a hacker and it can cause a data breach of the whole system.

Device Tracking and Updating

The core of security practices embedded in sound security policy is updating and patching devices. 'Updating' is the process of replacing a device's software with a newer version. 'Patching' is the process where only a part of software is replaced with a newer component. The IoMT patching is very specific, because of the dispersed nature of the IoMT system. The other good reason for the IoMT patching is the critical nature of the IoMT systems. The IoMT is very sensitive to the use of insecure or outdated software and firmware. Also, it is very sensitive to a system failure that can appear due to a possible corrupted update. Therefore, as suggested previously, all the devices should be listed in the asset registers, together with the versions of software and hardware. The updates should be tracked in relation to their publishing date, with the decision of the personnel dealing with the system operation whether the update will be automatic or on a periodic schedule. The IoMT devices should be tracked when retired to overcome and deny any kind of malicious activity.

2. Processes of identification, authentication and authorization

In order to prevent an unauthorized device to replace a legal device or a completely new device to penetrate the landscape, measures need to be taken. They should uniquely identify an IoMT device and assign it a predefined, strict set of authorizations.

Identification is a process of understanding the context of future interoperation by sending a mutually known identifier for a person or device, typically a username or device ID. According to Turner (2016), **authentication** is an electronic process for confirming or verifying the identity of an individual or device. **Authorization** is the process of giving the access to the individuals or devices with the confirmed identity.

In practice this means that any device included in the IoMT should have a unique identifier (e.g. in the form of a device ID). According to AIOTI (2018), an identifier is a pattern to uniquely identify a single entity (an instance identifier) or a class of entities (i.e. type identifier) within a specific context. The authentication is based on the user's use of one or several credentials based on any one or combination of three possible factors: what they have (a device-token), what they are (biometrics: fingerprint, retina scan, etc.) or what they know (a password, an answer, an algorithm or a combination). While humans can use any of these three authentications, the devices can use only the knowledge-based technology. However, these passwords or algorithms can be much more complex than those for humans.

After the successful identification and authentication, the next step is the authorization. The authorization enables the exact operational management of the devices, that is, which devices are to be let in to work in the IoMT environment, what they can access and to whom they can communicate.

The first priority is to allow the IoMT devices to access only what is necessary for their full operation. The second priority is to change passwords in all devices that come with the factory-installed default passwords. The IoMT risks can be combatted by the strong passwords and by the two- or three-layered authentication, if we apply, for example, the device-token, fingerprint and a password. In principle, using cryptographic hardware together with digital certificates or biometrics issued from a trusted public key infrastructure (PKI) is the best solution. For the purpose of adjusting operations of the digital system for a specific need, the user or foreign device usually has initially to be identified, authenticated and authorized.

The Mirai attack in 2016 started with the connected cameras that had factory-default or hardcoded passwords, usually 1 from the 60 username-password combinations. Thus, it is of the utmost importance to understand that it is obligatory to update passwords by using strong passphrases or passwords. Manufacturers should also require changing default credentials before putting device into the function. Actually, manufacturers should be required to avoid using default passwords by any means.

3. IoT botnets, DDoS attacks and passwords

Botnet is a group of Internet-connected devices controlled by a central system. They usually all perform the same task controlled and synchronized by the botnet controller, the central system. The term is most often used in conjunction with malicious attacks, especially of the kind of Distributed Denial of Service (DDoS) attacks (Vishwakarma and Kumar Jain 2019). In DDoS, the Internet-connected devices in a large group flood a website or a network by sending many fake requests. The result is that the legitimate users cannot access it, since their requests are lost in the sea of the fake requests. Since hundreds or thousands of devices are involved trying to access the same number of unique IP addresses during the attack, it is impossible or almost impossible to stop it. The IoT and, especially, the IoMT can easily become a part of the botnet and co-execute attacks, since the market is full of inexpensive devices (webcams, thermostats and many others), having small or zero built-in security. Therefore, they can be easily broken into and programmed to do harm or merely become a 'home' for the attacker. However, the users' behaviour presents the most important vulnerability, because usually the users themselves are not paying any attention to the security. As an example, most of the users do not put any kind of password on their devices, which means that the devices are an easy target for any kind of attackers, especially for botnet specialists.

The impact of irresponsible user's behaviour is huge. For example, an integral Internet infrastructure provider, Dyn, was partially offline in October 2016, because attackers used a botnet of approximately 100,000 unsecured IoT devices to take it down (Hammons and Kovac 2019). The direct consequence was that many high-traffic websites (i.e. Netflix, Amazon and Twitter) disappeared from the Internet for a while. Moreover, there was not one specific hacker who wrote a new code; instead the malware was assembled from existing code on the net and entitled Mirai. Mirai automated the process of coopting all the unsecured devices in the attack and used them until the owners removed these hacked devices from their network. Of course, when the attacker has so many devices at their disposal, they can be used for various kinds of purposes: speeding up password guessing, mining Bitcoins or any other kind of illegal service that can be rented by criminal organizations to perform whatever task they like. The only possible mitigation of these attacks is that all the IoT and, especially, IoMT devices run on a secure software, which is quite a difficult task. One of the options is to use Intrusion Prevention Systems (IPS) and Intrusion Detection Systems (IDS) with DDoS features. The other is to take a partner with an Internet service provider that will detect and filter DDoS packets before reaching the considered network. Basic security hygiene encompasses changing default passwords. Nevertheless, it is quite important that all the users are aware of possible misuses, especially in the health sector, where any kind of misuse can cause hazardous consequences.

4. Privacy and Encryption

In relation to IoMT, **privacy** implies the need for legitimate data to be visible and readable only to those they are intended for. Privacy risks are usually mitigated by the encryption. The related cryptography protects the integrity of IoT and IoMT data. This is the crucial property required for the IoMT, having incorporated all the sensitive information of users. However, simple small sensors collecting data like environmental parameters are not equipped with processing and/or memory resources required for traditional **encryption** algorithms (e.g. Advanced Encryption Standard, AES). The IoT and IoMT with the aforementioned simple unsecured devices (such as cameras) must incorporate additional algorithms for high security and low computation (e.g. elliptic curve cryptography). The Public Key Infrastructure (PKI) can be embedded into devices at the manufacturing level, or later at the enterprise level. PKI can help in distributing and identifying keys that allow users and 'things' a secure exchange of IoMT data. PKI issues unique identity and digital certificate to 'things'. In this case, it is also very important to have a 'hygienic' approach towards the encryption of a key lifecycle.

The encryption is the key step towards privacy. However, the essential issue with cryptography is that it assumes a lack of resources, that is, there is often not enough processing power. The decryption is not possible without the proper key in a reasonable time-frame. However, detection of faults in encryption algorithms or their implementations as well as advances in the computer technology and principles (e.g. quantum computing) might create a possibility to break codes soon by exposing all the hidden content and rendering integrity of archived digital documents questionable. The hope is now seen in the quantum cryptography and the other advanced methods, but they are uncharted areas of science and there can be no realistic forecasts. Therefore, one of the important measures is to anonymize data referring to individuals as early as possible (GDPR 2016).

5. Network Security

Networks can be secured by traditional methods like the above-mentioned IPS and IDS programmes, anti-malware and firewalls. But, best practice suggests the separation of IoT devices in the network by segmenting them. In this way, the IoT devices are in one network and all the other systems are in another network segment. This is not always an easy task, because some of the non-replaceable legacy systems require different kinds of update and patching. The network segmentation offers a higher level of security, because different parts of networks are organized as subnetworks, with their own customized security policies. However, the nature of this kind of segmented network introduces additional latency and exposes the full system to more errors related to the connectivity, in comparison with the non-segmented network. The mitigation of the problem, especially related to the latency that is a critical parameter in every IoMT, but especially in the segmented IoMT, is use of a gateway. Thus, by using a gateway with more processing computing and memory power than the IoT devices in the network, the IoMT will be much more secure and without introduced much higher latency. Thus, a gateway can apply stronger security measures (like firewalls and antimalware), much closer to 'things'. Except for the mitigations noted above, it is of crucial importance never to open IoT ports when not needed and to disable them for port forwarding, thus, ensuring port security. Blocking unauthorized IP address is always a must. One of the known issues and risks in the IoT and IoMT networks is a lack of the bandwidth, which causes a slowdown of productivity and efficiency in the network. Therefore, an important task is to perform regular capacity assessments in network planning, in order to avoid any kind of issues related to throughput.

The Digital Devices as Non-human Communicating Agents in the Knowledge Landscapes

The account above in regard to those technologies involved in the communication of the Internet-connected devices illustrates just how complex an interaction this is. These interactions are performed mainly by machines, some of them were initiated at the request of a user, and some are completely independent of human influence. When discussing the knowledge landscapes, they are considered to be formed by the interactions of content, users and technology, where the users are people searching for knowledge (Svalastog et al. 2014, 2020). However, digital technology is far from offering a passive obedience in performing any given task. The levels of autonomy and independent interactions necessary to maintain the functionality of the system are in particular visible when discussing the issues of safety and security.

The human user is, in regard to safety and security, more a liability contributing to risks than an element allowing for the safe and secure functionality of the system. Consequently, the issues of safety and security depend mostly and substantially on the activity of the interconnected devices themselves. Ideally, especially in the near future within the environment of smart cities, digital systems should be able to confront threats automatically.

The functionality of all devices connected in the IoT depends on their ability to communicate. Subsequently they are part of the total communication within the digital environment involving all combinations of device-to-device, device-to-human, human-to-device and human-to-human interactions. When considering the digital society, the extent of digital communications and digital spaces where this communication occurs should recognize as well these non-human participants in the interactions. If we consider the whole of humanity to be connected in the very near future, the 8 billion humans will be in the communicating space with 26.66 billion communicating devices. Assuming the current growth of number of devices connected and the expected increase in their communicating and processing abilities, it becomes obvious that these digital entities are already members of digital society. With the onset of artificial intelligence, they would be further humanized with cognitive abilities (Hutter 2005). In Everitt and Hutter (2018) the 'autonomous agents' are presented in a way that they may have an ability to modify themselves but also that the 'present AI [artificial intelligence] systems are not yet close to exhibiting the required intelligence or "self-awareness"' (see also Luger and Stubblefield 2004).

Conclusions

It is currently predicted that urbanization, contributing to shifting the residence of the human population from rural to urban areas, will result with ca. 70% of the global population living in cities by 2050. Thus, it is necessary to plan the new paradigm of 'smart city'. The definition of the smart city is 'a place where traditional networks and services are made more efficient with the use of digital and telecommunication technologies for the benefit of its inhabitants and business' (EC, Smart City). Therefore, ICT becomes a backbone of the smart city: it extends horizontally across all the building blocks or key fields of a smart city; it develops itself only to support development of the key fields of the smart city; it interconnects them. The six key fields of urban development are smart economy, smart mobility, smart environment, smart people, smart living and smart governance.

All the components of the triad IoT-AI-5G belong to the ICT area. They enable development of smart cities. Our common vision is that all the smart cities on Earth, managed by AI, will be one day interconnected. AI is generated by human endeavour, and one scenario is that this global interconnection creates some sort of trans-human 'brain': as Nikola Tesla, approximately 100 years ago argued, 'When wireless is perfectly applied the whole Earth will be converted into a huge brain' (Tesla 1926).

Digital devices are partners in the communications and interactions of digital society. Although they can be very simple, their number and distribution create a complex world of para-human interactions, which directly involve humans in the case of IoMT. Consequently, the issues of safety and security illustrate the interdependencies and challenges within digital ecosystems populated by humans and digital devices.

IoMT represents a challenge within the health sector and its digital infrastructure, since it is expected that IoMT devices will be attached directly to a human body or they will be placed even within the body, in order to monitor or directly influence bodily functions. Any cyber-attack on them is an attack on human health. Here, we would like to stress that it is not only the IoMTs that control something that are at risk like pacemakers, brain stimulators, medicine-dispensing devices, breathing machines and so on. Even those that only measure parameters of the human body are important. For example, if a hacker manages to forge measurement data about any bodily parameter, the user or his/her doctors could prescribe or apply a deadly lethal dosage or dangerous combination of medicines.

Therefore, some of the regulatory measures that have been and can be established should regard any attack on the IoMT as an attack against the human body, yielding the heaviest penalties and punishments as well as requiring the highest precautions and responsibilities by producers and distributors alike—very secure default settings, clear and understandable instructions about achieving security for users, mandatory training and certification of IoMT designers for security by design. Technical measures could lead towards the concept of a 'personal health hub' (PHH), a device 'attached' to a human body which would be the sole device communicating with all IoMTs of that person. PHH would then need to be highly secure and restrictive in communicating with the outside world. Finally, the PHH should never be integrated with general-purpose devices like smartphones.

We have shown in this chapter that the highest form of awareness needs to be achieved in IoMT developers, medical personnel and end users. Here elaborated interconnectedness between humans and digital devices, specifically sensitive in case of health-related devices, shows how the digital society and knowledge landscapes are a symbiosis of human and non-human participants.

References

[ehealth-hub]. Internet page: www.ehealth-hub.eu. Retrieved February 8, 2020.

AIOTI. (2018, February). *Identifiers in internet of things (IoT), AIOTI version 1.0, AIOTI WG03 – IoT standardisation*. Internet page: https://euagenda.eu/upload/publications/identifiers-in-internet-of-things-iot.pdf, Retrieved February 18, 2020.

Binkowski, S. (2016). *Medical IoT use case: I care about you 'ICU' – App, EMEA, 2016 SAP SE or an SAP affiliate company*. Published: October 26th, 2016.

Internet page: https://open.sap.com/files/4bda64d8-1a14-4e00-b8b0-14b66046225a. Retrieved April 20, 2020.

Centrak. (2019). Internet page: www.centrak.com/solutions/newbaby-infant-protection/. Retrieved July 8, 2019.

Chen, T. L., Bhattacharjee, T., Beer, J. M., Ting, L. H., Hackney, M. E., & Rogers, W. A., (2017). Older adults' acceptance of a robot for partner dance-based exercise. *PloS ONE, 12*(10): e0182736. https://doi.org/10.1371/journal.pone.0182736. Retrieved February 8, 2020.

Deloitte. (2019). *Deloitte report.* Internet page: https://www2.deloitte.com/global/en/pages/life-sciences-and-healthcare/articles/medtech-internet-of-medical-things.html. Retrieved February 18, 2020.

European Commission. (2004). Green paper on mobile health ("mHealth") (SWD(2014) 135 final), COM(2014) 219 final. *Brussels, 10*(4), 2014.

European Commission. (2020). White paper on artificial intelligence – A European approach to excellence and trust. *COM*. 65 final. Brussels, 19.2.

European Smart Cities.4.0 (2015). Internet page: http://smart-cities.eu/?cid=2&ver=4. Retrieved April 20, 2020.

Everitt, T., & Hutter, M. (2018, January). Chapter 2: Universal artificial intelligence, practical agents and fundamental challenges. In Abbass, H. A., Scholz, J., & Reid, D. J. (Ed.), *"Foundations of trusted autonomy", studies in systems, decision and control 117*. Springer. Internet page: http://www.hutter1.net/publ/uaitas.pdf. Retrieved April 20, 2020.

FDA. (2019). URGENT/11 cybersecurity vulnerabilities in a widely-used third-party software component may introduce risks during use of certain medical devices: FDA safety communication. safety communications. Date Issued: October 1, 2019. Internet page: https://www.fda.gov/medical-devices/safety-communications/urgent11-cybersecurity-vulnerabilities-widely-used-third-party-software-component-may-introduce. Retrieved April 26, 2020.

Gehealthcare. (2019). Internet page: www.gehealthcare.com/about/healthcare-systems. Retrieved July 8, 2019.

Globalsecurity. (2001). Chapter 1: Physical security challenges. Field manual 3-19.30: *Physical security. Headquarters*, United States Department of Army. Archived from the original on March 13, 2013. Internet page: https://www.globalsecurity.org/military/library/policy/army/fm/3-19-30/ch1.htm. Retrieved February 18, 2020.

Halkos, G., & Zisiadou, A. (2018, July 7). Reporting the natural environmental hazards occurrences and fatalities over the last century. Munich personal

RePEc archive (MPRA). Internet page: https://mpra.ub.uni-muenchen.de/87936/1/MPRA_paper_87936.pdf. Retrieved February 18, 2020.

Hammi, B., Khatoun, R., Zeadally, S., Fayad, A., & Khoukhi, L. (2017). Internet of Things (IoT) Technologies for Smart Cities. *IET Networks*. 7. 10.1049/iet-net.2017.0163.

Hammons, R., & Kovac, J. (2019). *Fundamentals of internet of things for non-engineers* (1st Ed.). Auerbach Publications, 430 Pages, ISBN 9780429274992, Published June 7.

Herjavec Group, Steve Morgan, Editor-in-Chief, Cybersecurity Ventures. (2020). 2019 official annual cybercrime report. Internet page: https://www.herjavecgroup.com/2019-official-annual-cybercrime-report/. Retrieved April 21, 2020.

Hutter, M. (2005). *Universal artificial intelligence*. Berlin: Springer.

IBM X-Force Cyber Security Index. (2016). Internet page: https://www.slideshare.net/KanishkaRamyar/the-ibm-x-force-2016-cyber-security-intelligence-index. Retrieved April 19, 2020.

IBM X-Force Threat Intelligence Index, IBM X-Force Incident Response and Intelligence Services (IRIS). (2020). Internet page: https://www.ibm.com/security/data-breach/threat-intelligence. Retrieved April 19, 2020.

Joy, A. (2019). CHIME fall forum 2019: Securing IoMT devices requires collaboration and a culture shift. *HealthTech Magazine*, CDW LLC 200 N. Milwaukee avenue, Vernon Hills, IL 60061. Internet page: https://healthtechmagazine.net/article/2019/11/chime-fall-forum-2019-securing-iomt-devices-requires-collaboration-and-culture-shift. Retrieved April 22, 2020.

Luger, G., & Stubblefield, W. (2004). *Artificial intelligence: Structures and strategies for complex problem solving* (5th ed.). San Francisco: Benjamin/Cummings.

Lynch, R., & Farrington, C. (2018). *Quantified lives and vital data: Exploring health and technology through personal medical devices*. Basingstoke: Palgrave.

Marr, B. (2018). Why the internet of medical things (IoMT) will start to transform healthcare in 2018. Internet page: https://www.forbes.com/sites/bernardmarr/2018/01/25/why-the-internet-of-medical-things-iomt-will-start-to-transform-healthcare-in-2018/#4e7405c24a3c, Forbes.com. Published: January 25, 2018. Retrieved February 18, 2020.

Masscan. (2019). Internet page: manpages.org/masscan/8. Retrieved July 8, 2019.

Mayer-Schönberger, V., & Cukier, K. (2013). *Big data: A revolution that will transform how we live, work, and think*. Boston: Houghton Mifflin Harcourt.

Meidan, Y., Bohadana, M., Shabtai, A., Ochoa, M., Tippenhauer, N. O., Guarnizo, J. D., & Elovici, Y. (2020). *Detection of unauthorized IoT devices using machine learning technique*, Researchgate. Internet page: https://www.researchgate.net/publication/319736005_Detection_of_Unauthorized_IoT_Devices_Using_Machine_Learning_Techniques. Retrieved February 18, 2020.

Meola, A. (2020). *IoT healthcare in 2020: Companies, devices, use cases and market stats, business insider*. Published: February 13, 2020. Internet page: https://www.businessinsider.com/iot-healthcare?op=1. Retrieved April 20, 2020.

Merriam-Webster Dictionary. Internet page: https://www.merriam-webster.com/dictionary/safety. Retrieved February 18, 2020a.

Merriam-Webster Dictionary. Internet page: https://www.merriam-webster.com/dictionary/security, Retrieved February 18, 2020b.

Merriam-Webster Dictionary, Internet page: https://www.merriam-webster.com/dictionary/threat. Retrieved February 18, 2020c.

Merriam-Webster Dictionary, Internet page: https://www.merriam-webster.com/dictionary/vulnerability. Retrieved February 18, 2020d.

Mole, B. (2018). *With ingestible pill, you can track fart development in real time on your phone*. Internet page: https://arstechnica.com/science/2018/01/with-ingestible-pill-you-can-track-fart-development-in-real-time-on-your-phone/. Published: September 1, 2018. Retrieved February 18, 2020.

Morin, D. (2016, February 19). *Untrained IT users: Who they are might surprise you*. Global-ICT 2015, Article: 7. Internet page: https://connect-world.com/untrained-it-users-who-they-are-might-surprise-you/. Retrieved April 20, 2020.

Nmap. (2019). Internet page: https://nmap.org. Retrieved July 8, 2019.

Pandor, A. T., Gomersall, J. W., Stevens, J., Wang, A., Al-Mohammad, A., Bakhai, A., Cleland, J. G. F., Cowie, M. R., & Wong, R. (2015, April 28). *Remote monitoring after recent hospital discharge in patients with heart failure: A systematic review and network meta-analysis*. Internet page: heart.bmj.com (published on Researchgate). Retrieved February 8, 2020.

GDPR. (2016). Regulation (EU) 2016/679 of the European Parliament and of the Council of 27 April 2016 on the protection of natural persons with regard to the processing of personal data and on the free movement of such data, and repealing Directive 95/46/EC (General Data Protection Regulation) OJ L 119, 4.5.2016, p. 1–88.

SensorMetrix. (2019). Internet page: www.sensormetrix.com. Retrieved July 8, 2019.

Shodan. (2019). Internet page: https://www.shodan.io. Retrieved July 8, 2019.

Statista. (2019). Internet page: www.statista.com. Retrieved July 8, 2019.

Svalastog, A. L., Allgaier, J., Martinelli, L., & Gajović, S. (2014). Distortion, confusion, and impasses: Could a public dialogue within Knowledge Landscapes contribute to better communication and understanding of innovative knowledge? *Croatian Medical Journal, 55*, 54–60.

Svalastog, A. L., Gajovic, S., & Webster, A. (2020). *Navigating knowledge landscapes*. Basingstoke: Palgrave.

Taylor, H. (2019, December 13). The state of ransomware in the US: Report and statistics 2019, Emsisoft, security blog. *Journal of Cyberpolicy*. Internet page: https://journalofcyberpolicy.com/2019/12/13/state-ransomware-us-report-statistics-2019-emsisoft-security-blog/. Retrieved March 21, 2020.

Tesla, N. (1926). *When woman is boss, (1926) an interview with Nikola Tesla by John B. Kennedy, colliers*. January 30, 1926. Internet page: http://www.tfc-books.com/tesla/1926-01-30.htm. Retrieved July 8, 2019.

Tung, C. E., Su, D., Turakhia, M. P., & Lansberg, M. G. (2015). Diagnostic yield of extended cardiac patch monitoring in patients with stroke or TIA. *Frontiers in Neurology, 5*, 266.

Turner, D. (2016). *Digital authentication: The basics*. Cryptomathic. Archived from the original on 14 August 2016. Retrieved February 18, 2020.

United Nations Department of Economic and Social Affairs. (2018). *68% of the world population projected to live in urban areas by 2050*. 16 May 2018, New York. Internet page: https://www.un.org/development/desa/en/news/population/2018-revision-of-world-urbanization-prospects.html. Retrieved April 28, 2020.

Vishwakarma, R., & Kumar Jain, A. (2019, April). *A honeypot with machine learning based detection framework for defending IoT based Botnet DDoS Attacks*. The 3rd International Conference on Trends in Electronics and Informatics (ICOEI), 23–25. IEEE 2019.

Weissman, C. G. (2015). *Survey: We asked executives about the internet of things and their answers reveal that security remains a huge concern*. http://www.businessinsider.in/We-Asked-Executives-About-The-Internet-Of-Things-And-Their-Answers-Reveal-That-Security-Remains-A-Huge-Concern/articleshow/45959921.cms. Published January 21, 2015. Retrieved February 18, 2020.

Wellsensevu. (2019). Internet page: www.wellsensevu.com. Retrieved July 8, 2019.
WHO. (2019). Internet page: www.who.int. Retrieved July 8, 2019.
Zanthion. (2019). Internet page: www.zanthion.com. Retrieved July 8, 2019.

14

Visualization and Visual Analytics in Knowledge Landscapes

Margaret Varga, Helena Webb, Tomas Krilavičius, and Martin Maiden

Introduction

The data-information-knowledge-wisdom (DKIW) hierarchy represents the transformation of "data to information to knowledge to wisdom" (Ackoff 1987). Within DKIW, raw data only become useful when they

M. Varga (✉)
Department of Zoology, University of Oxford, Oxford, UK
e-mail: margaret.varga@zoo.ox.ac.uk

H. Webb
Computer Science, University of Oxford, Oxford, UK
e-mail: helena.webb@cs.ox.ac.uk

T. Krilavičius
Applied Informatics Faculty, Vytauto Didžiojo University, Kaunas, Lithuania
e-mail: tomas.krilavicius@vdu.lt

M. Maiden
Department of Zoology, University of Oxford, Oxford, UK
e-mail: martin.maiden@zoo.ox.ac.uk

A. L. Svalastog et al. (eds.), *Navigating Digital Health Landscapes*, Health, Technology and Society, https://doi.org/10.1007/978-981-15-8206-6_14

provide meaning, that is, information. Information in turn becomes knowledge when it is cognitively processed and assimilated into human knowledge construction. Knowledge becomes "wisdom" when it is capable of being used to make a decision. Elsewhere in this book, this is described as those affordances through which action might be taken. Decisions vary by individual and circumstances, as they are likely to be dependent on an understanding of the context including personal experience, geographical location, local healthcare policy and financial considerations. There are different versions of the DIKW model, which differ in their emphases; while some emphasize data, information and knowledge, others emphasize information, knowledge and wisdom (Rowley 2007). Zeleny mapped the elements in the DIKW hierarchy as (i) know-nothing, (ii) know-what, (iii) know-how and (iv) know-why (Zeleny 1987). Data, information and knowledge are in the past or present, while wisdom is for the future. This chapter, deploying expertise in data visualization, shows how it is possible to mine and organize data sources using visual analytics to see whether it is possible to identify or build more robust forms of knowledge in the digital knowledge landscape.

Visualization and Visual Analytics

A picture is worth a thousand words. The use of visual aids is a well-established practice to help humans define, understand, analyse, explore and navigate their way through tasks and problems, so as to understand "the situation" and make informed decisions (Heer and Shneiderman 2012; van Wijk 2005).

Visual analytics (VA) is the science of analytical reasoning facilitated by interactive visual interfaces (Thomas and Cook 2005). It enables the analysis of massive and complex data to support users in understanding the inter-relationships that exist within it. VA is an iterative process: it is an integration of automated analysis techniques such as data mining, statistical analysis and knowledge discovery with interactive visualization to provide users with an effective means to dynamically and visually interact with, explore and analyse big, complex and, at times, contradictory and uncertain data (Keim and Liew 2007). VA systems achieve this by exploiting human perception, thereby reducing cognitive load. They facilitate the understanding of data and situation, thus supporting informed decision-making. When applied to person-centred healthcare, VA provides an intuitive means that supports the users in their construction and navigation through digital health landscapes and so enable informed decisions that are relevant to their needs and circumstances.

Knowledge Construction Process

The knowledge construction process (Fig. 14.1, adapted from Varga and Webb (2017) starts with a search for the data of interest, for instance from the Internet, followed by the choice of potentially relevant information by zooming and filtering. This is followed by reading the retrieved data to understand and assess their relevance, that is, extract relevant information. Knowledge is constructed through analysis of the

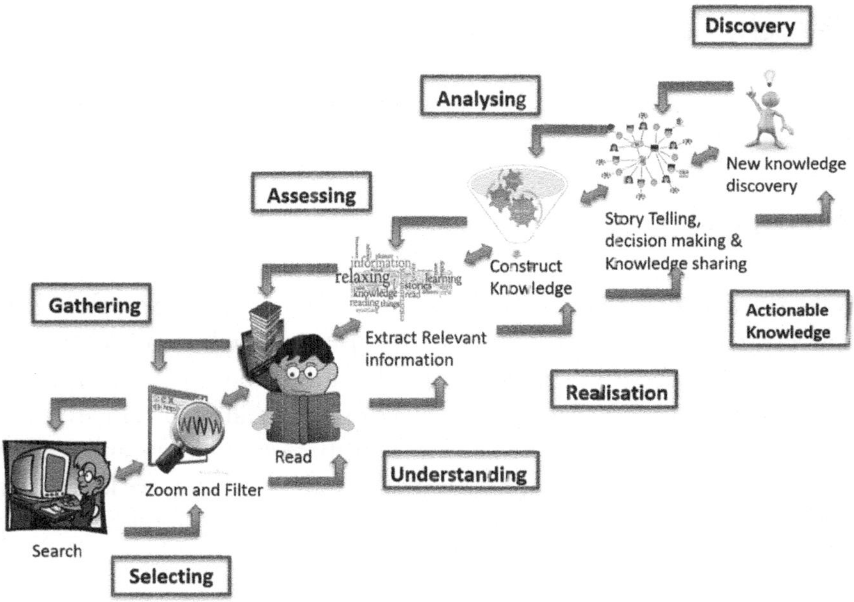

Fig. 14.1 Knowledge construction process

information and realization of its significance. Knowledge sharing ("storytelling") can then be achieved, which, in turn, enables informed decision-making and the discovery of new knowledge. This is an iterative process—the output from each stage can be improved through feedback between stages (Pirolli and Card 2005).

The following sections show example approaches of the various elements/stages of the knowledge construction process to demonstrate how digital content can be captured, recorded, exploited, represented and shared. Together, these result in a dynamic representation of a digital landscape that enables the user to interact and understand the data within it and to extract information and derive knowledge to support timely and informed decision-making. The representation evolves over time as more information becomes available, as or when the focus changes and so on. There are many variables that can influence the development and maintenance of the knowledge landscape, such as the individuals, their objectives, mental models, constraints, experience and environmental factors.

Search, Zoom and Filter

Here we discuss the search, zoom and filter stages of the knowledge construction process.

Search Engines

Whenever there is a need to find out about something, more often than not a search of the Internet is conducted using a search engine of preference such as Google or Bing. For example, at the time of writing, a search of Google for *Campylobacter* returned almost five million hits in less than half a second (Fig. 14.2). We benefit from these voluminous and readily available sources of data on *Campylobacter*, and, at a glance, we know that in the UK *Campylobacter* is the most common cause of food poisoning. The challenges we face, however, include:

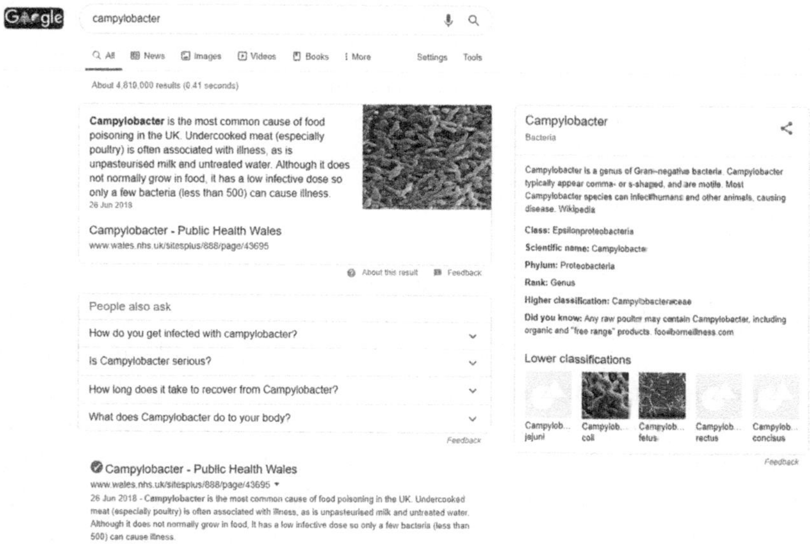

Fig. 14.2 Google search results on *Campylobacter* (19 July 2019)

1. It is infeasible to read all the retrieved results.
2. There are no means to identify their relevance without reading them—which is time and labour intensive.
3. There are no means to correlate the retrieved results.
4. Knowledge discovery, in any substantive or comprehensive sense, would require intense manual work that is likely not feasible.
5. We cannot save the search results, that is, they are ephemeral.

There is a need to address these challenges to provide a more robust and effective means of exploiting these amazing data sources—though caution is necessary as misleading data may also be present. Irrelevant or misleading data need to be filtered out and useful data need to be zoomed-in upon: information needs to be extracted and knowledge derived to support informed decision-making. We term this as *navigating the knowledge landscape.*

Searching for information online, for example about a health concern or a clinical intervention, thus typically produces an avalanche of data in a list form (Fig. 14.2). The problem is thus navigating the vast and complex knowledge landscape, which is contained within this online content (data). Visual analytic and visualization techniques provide a possible solution as they provide tractable and effective means for users to filter and analyse content in a way that is meaningful to them and coherent with their task objectives.

Carrot²

Carrot² is an open-source clustering engine for search results (Carrot² 2019). It provides document clustering algorithms such as Suffix Tree Clustering (STC), Lingo and k-means. Carrot² also provides mechanisms for retrieving data from search engines, indexing engines (Apache Solr (n.d.) or ElasticSearch (n.d.)), generic XML feeds and files. It can search in 19 different languages. It automatically clusters the retrieved documents into thematic categories on the principle that, through the overview of what is available, users can quickly find that in which they are interested. For example, using eTools,[1] a metasearch engine within Carrot², to search for "*Campylobacter*" (Fig. 14.3), there are 125 retrieved documents and 34 automatically identified themes, which are automatically displayed in a folder format. The number of retrieved documents for each theme is displayed. Other external search tools can also be used with

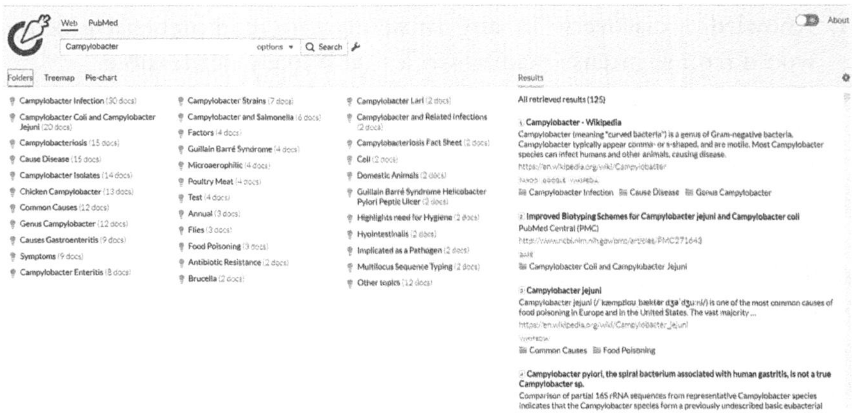

Fig. 14.3 Carrot² clustering of *Campylobacter* documents in folders

[1] search.carrot2.org

Carrot², for example, PubMed, which is a free search engine accessing mainly the MEDLINE database.

The retrieved documents can be visualized in different formats, in addition to the folder form, for example, a pie chart or a treemap (Fig. 14.4). The theme that is most covered, that is, "*Campylobacter* infection", has 30 documents and this is placed in the middle of the display, with the largest area. All other themes are displayed around it with their associated number of documents. Each theme is colour coded with a white boundary so that they are easy to differentiate. The right-hand side of the display shows the list of web-links with summaries; clicking on any of the listed items will automatically open the link in a new tab.

Within a treemap, an individual theme, for example, "Common Causes", can be chosen (Fig. 14.5) and identified with a black border: the documents (12 in this case) associated with the theme are automatically displayed on the right-hand side.

A stacked pie chart can also be used to display the same data (Fig. 14.6) with an inner circle showing the themes while the outer layers show the associated documents. Clicking the grey clockwise arrow displays more detailed information (drilling down) and clicking the anti-clockwise arrow reduces the information displayed (drilling-up). The display can be modified to focus on the top-most themes (Fig. 14.7) or on more details (Fig. 14.8).

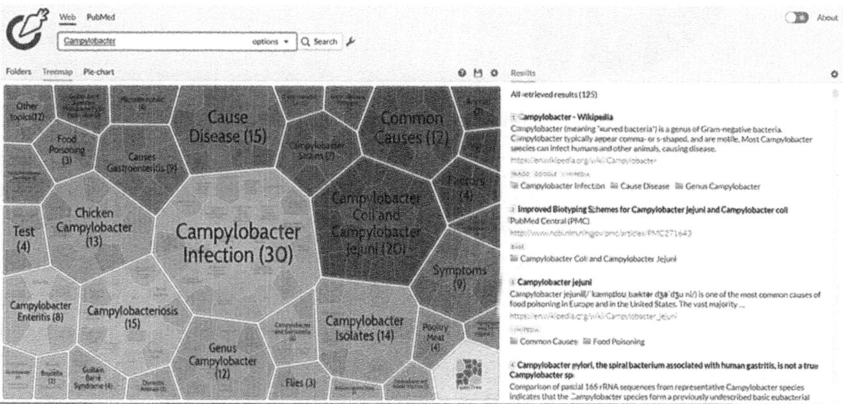

Fig. 14.4 Treemap of search results for "*Campylobacter*"

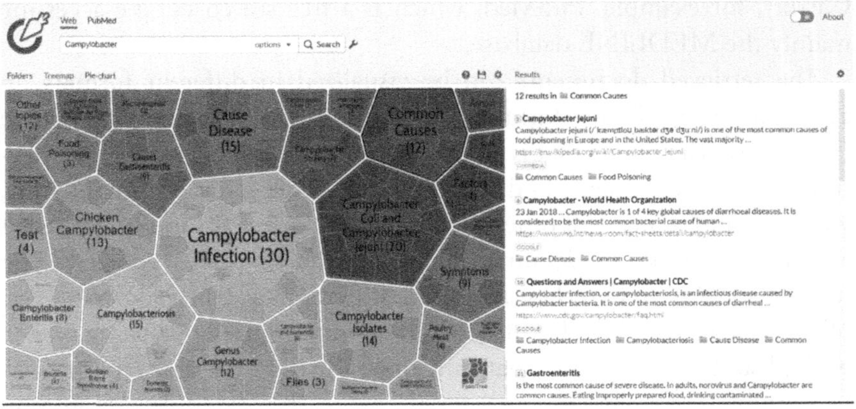

Fig. 14.5 Treemap with highlighted theme

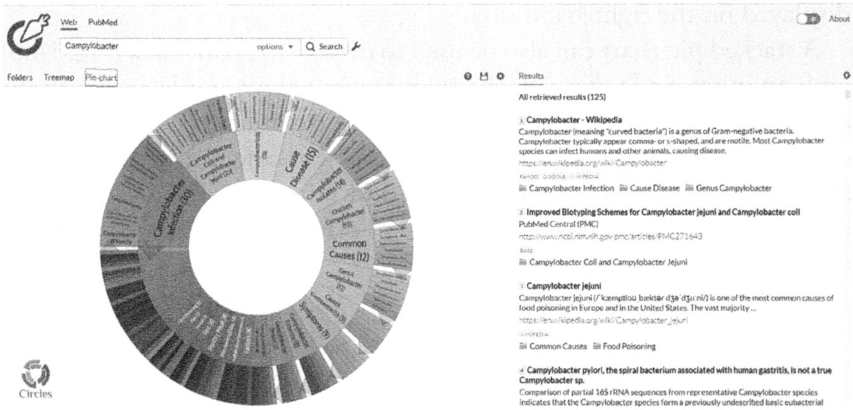

Fig. 14.6 Stacked pie chart display of retrieved documents

Users can discover "new" topics that are more relevant to them, for example, information on *Campylobacter* bacteria.

Users can navigate/explore the data effectively by revising their searches, for example, "*Campylobacter* bacteria" (Fig. 14.9). By these means users can retrieve documents with topics of which they might not have been previously aware and thus discover more relevant topics.

Carrot[2] can be used to organize data outputs from searches of large databases such as PubMed, which consists of more than 29 million

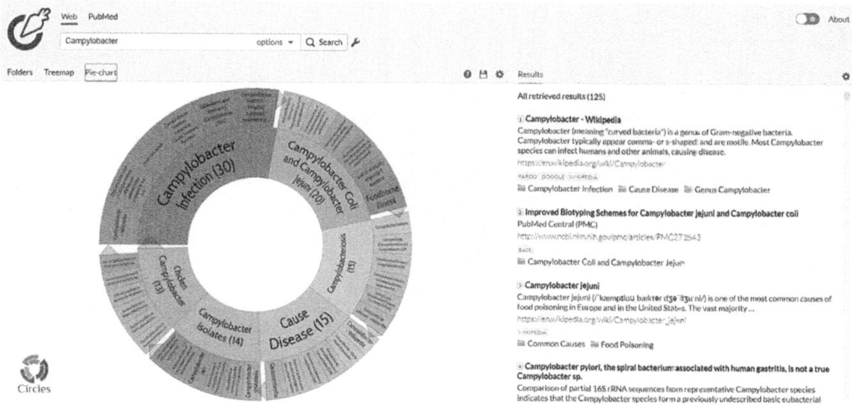

Fig. 14.7 Showing top six themes only, drilling-up by clicking on the anti-clockwise grey arrows

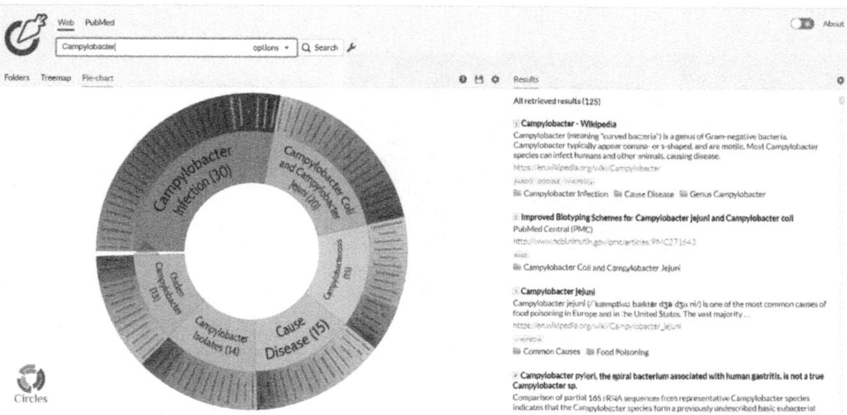

Fig. 14.8 Drilling down to show more detailed information on the outer-most ring by clicking on the clockwise grey arrows

citations for biomedical literature such as MEDLINE, life science journals and online books. For example, Carrot[2] can effectively and automatically cluster retrieved documents resulting from the search term "*Campylobacter*" within the PubMed database by themes/topics. This provides, at a glance, useful indication of document content and thus enables users to select documents of interest and of relevance to them and/or to discover new topics (Fig. 14.10).

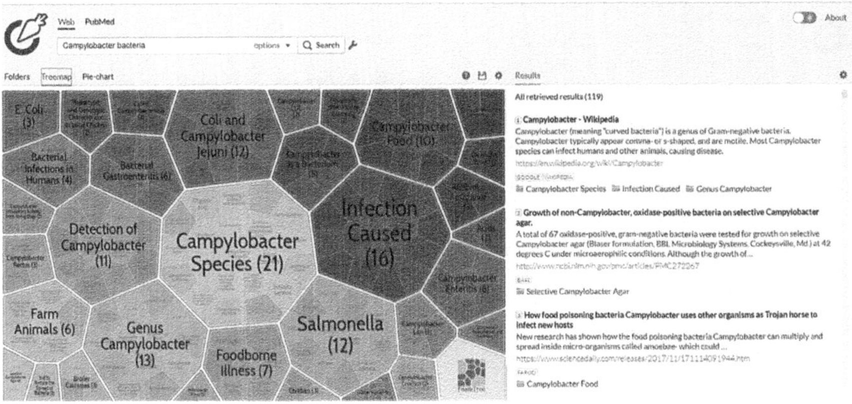

Fig. 14.9 Identification of topic of interests—*Campylobacter* bacteria

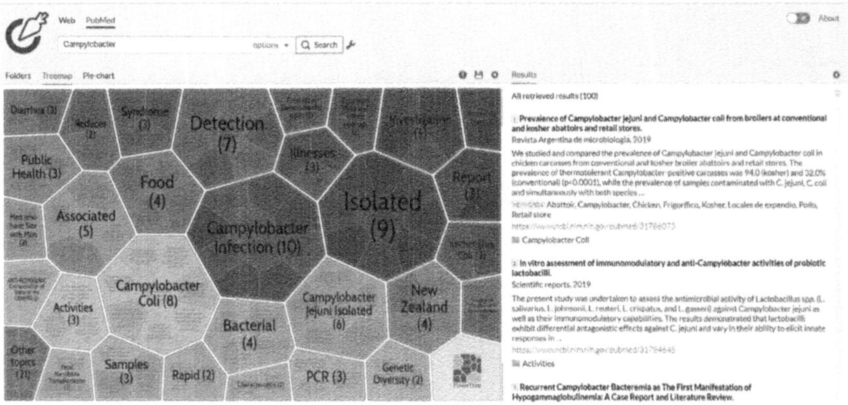

Fig. 14.10 PubMed search results for *Campylobacter* using Carrot[2]

Friskr

Friskr[2] is an open-source 3D conceptual search engine that extracts concepts and supports discovery by detecting the relationship between keywords, search results and concepts, in an interactive 3D display (Friskr n.d.). For example, the results for a single keyword *Campylobacter* can be

---

[2] https://friskr.com

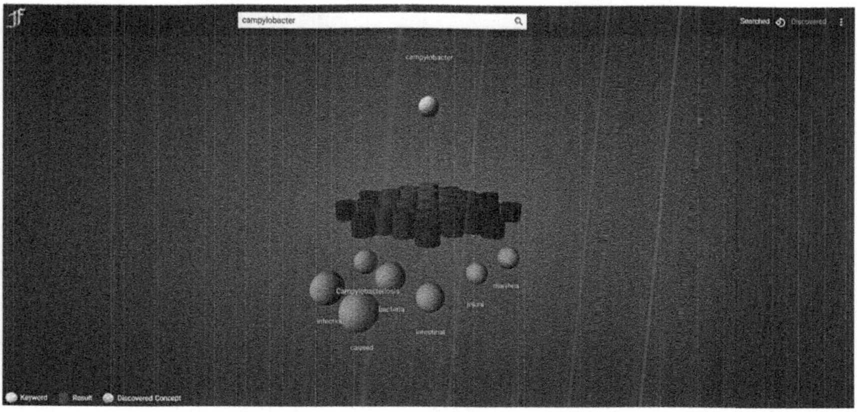

Fig. 14.11 Friskr—display of search results and discovered concepts/terms for *Campylobacter*

shown graphically (yellow ball, Fig. 14.11), with the documents containing the keyword *Campylobacter* shown as blue cylinders. Concepts discovered in the documents ("bacteria", "intestinal", etc.) are represented as orange balls whose sizes correspond to the number of documents that discuss the concept. Users can decide how many documents to retrieve, for example, 10, 20, 50 or 100.

It is possible to alter the display layout in Friskr to aid the user in assimilating/seeing the information, (Fig. 14.12). Friskr links the documents by their concepts in a different manner from Carrot[2].

Information Analysis and Extraction Stages

Once the data have been searched, zoomed and filtered by reading and analysing, relevant information can be extracted, and thence knowledge can be constructed. There are numerous conventional approaches to extracting and managing of relevant information, including highlighting the relevant parts in documents, creating a new document by extracting the relevant parts of different documents and using post-it notes. Notes can also be made with words, diagrams, drawings, URLs and so on based on the understanding developed about the information.

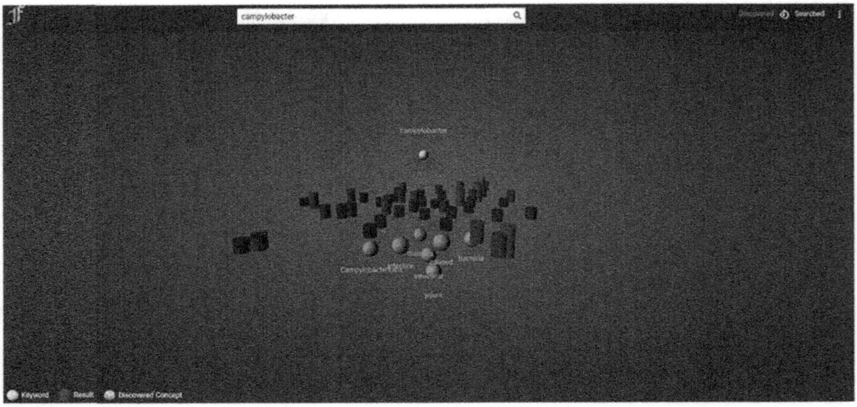

Fig. 14.12 Friskr—alternative display of retrieved documents from Fig. 14.11 in which the documents are clustered by their shared discovered concepts

It is, however, difficult to keep track of the information using the above conventional ad hoc approaches (Fig. 14.13). An alternative approach is to use a mind map to support the collection and integration of all the information in one place. Mind maps can be easily updated/revised as more information becomes available or interests change or re-focus.

Mind Maps

Mind maps are primarily used for brainstorming ideas and organizing thoughts (Buzan and Buzan 2006). The approach provides an effective and intuitive means to quickly organize taxonomies of inter-related information and thus show how things are related. Mind mapping enables users to conduct a brain dump quickly on a problem, question, idea and so on. They are very useful support tools for planning and decision-making.

Multiple nodes on a map can be used to record topics or ideas that are of interest; these can be grouped, connected, ordered, re-grouped, re-ordered, re-organized, removed and so on as more thoughts are given to them and relationships are developed. Furthermore, as users investigate or explore information, they can record the sources of information, for

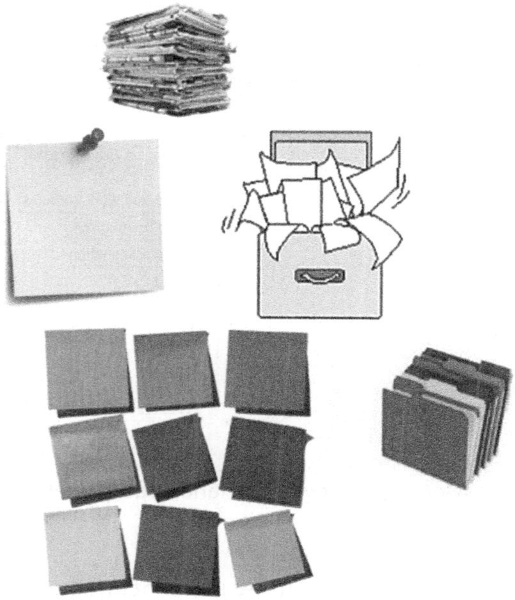

Fig. 14.13 Ad hoc note taking

example, URLs, as well as add notes inside copied content and link together local files, screenshots, thoughts, decisions and so on. Users can visually organize information to show hierarchical structure and interrelationships and thus capture knowledge and create a knowledge landscape. This is also an information management process through which users can put together what they know and what they do not know so as to create the knowledge landscape. This can be a collaborative process as users can create, view, edit and share mind maps with others (Zeleny 1987).

Information, data and notes extracted using, for example, Carrot[2] can all be captured using the mind map approach.

Freeplane

Freeplane (n.d.) is an open-source tool for mind mapping, knowledge management and project management that enables the development, organization and communication of ideas and knowledge.

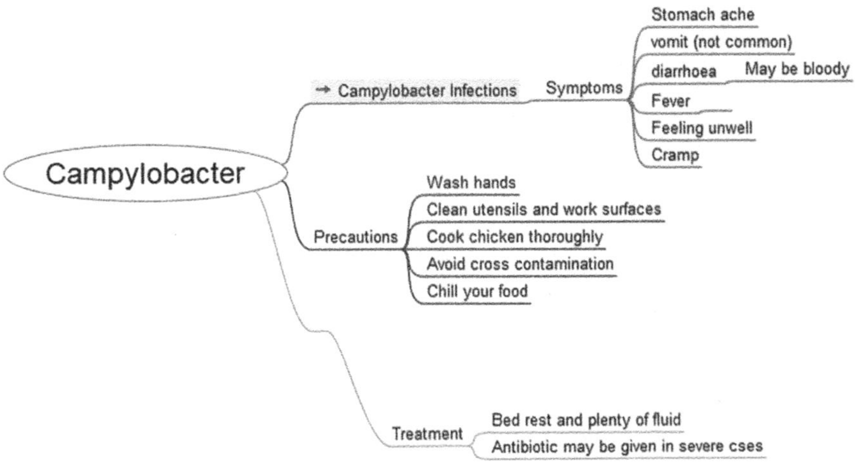

Fig. 14.14 A *Campylobacter* knowledge landscape presented as a mind map using Freeplane (n.d.)

A *Campylobacter* knowledge landscape generated using the Freeplane mind mapping tool (Fig. 14.14) shows three main topics, namely, *Campylobacter* infections, precautions and treatment. Each main topic has associated sub-topics. In the figure, the red arrow in the *Campylobacter* infections connection description indicates that there is an external URL link for more information. Users can share the output of their *Campylobacter* knowledge landscape with other people in their network or community.

Information Sharing: Storytelling

The preceding sections illustrate a process of knowledge construction and representation and how a knowledge landscape can be shared among users. Humans use storytelling to tell narratives about experiences and to report the effect of these experiences. Storytelling provides an effective means of communicating information so as to enable other users to gain insight and understanding, that is, situation awareness. Situation awareness plays an important role in the decision-making process. In the simplest terms, situation awareness means being aware of one's surroundings. Endsley's work on situation awareness (SA) is an established definition of SA, in particular for dynamic environments:

> Situation awareness is the perception of the elements in the environment within a volume of time and space, the comprehension of their meaning and the projection of their status in the near future. (Endsley 1995)

Endsley considered that there are three stages of situation awareness, namely, (1) perception, (2) comprehension and (3) projection (Endsley 1995). This links cognitive psychology with human factors in the explanation of making sense in complex situations such as person-centred healthcare. Endsley's definition of situation awareness encompasses the three stages. Storytelling provides a high-level contextual narrative view of what is happening.

The challenges for public-facing storytelling are to establish, for users of differing types and knowledge levels, how to (i) choose relevant information, (ii) organize and present information and (iii) transform any non-visual datasets into natural, intuitive and easily accessible visual forms. There are also, potentially, social context, cultural, operational, ethical and, indeed, philosophical considerations; however, these are beyond the scope of this chapter.

Campylobacter Storyboard

Visual analytic techniques can be used to present the *Campylobacter* story in the data, that is, a *Campylobacter* storyboard (Varga et al. 2017; Varga et al. 2019a, b). Such a storyboard enables users to interactively analyse recorded infection events and use deductive reasoning to gain situation awareness from the dataset. It consists of webpages with images, graphical displays and text presented in a sequence to tell a *Campylobacter* story wherein users can interactively explore topics of interest, the knowledge landscape, such as trends or patterns in gender, age group, *Campylobacter* species and so on.

The front page of this *Campylobacter* storyboard (Fig. 14.15), gives an overview on "what is *Campylobacter*" and other panels in the page provide further information on *Campylobacter*. There are two main types of panels: interactive exploratory panels and information panels. In the interactive exploratory panel, users can explore data on reported *Campylobacter* infections in relation to age, gender and *Campylobacter* species. These interactive exploratory panels are on the left-hand side of the page. While the information panels in the middle and the right-hand side of the webpage provide information on treatment, preventative precautions, access to data and links to relevant publications—drill-down to further detail can be achieved by clicking on the relevant panel.

Clicking, for example, on either the Gender tab at the top of the webpage or on the left-hand panel will cause the gender exploration page to be displayed (Fig. 14.16). This shows that in the UK the incidence of *Campylobacter* infection varies with age, being highest among those under five years of age. Males are more frequently affected, with a male-to-female ratio of 1.2–1. There are many different species of *Campylobacter*, including *Campylobacter jejuni* and *Campylobacter coli*, which cause most human diseases. Under each species there are different "sequence types" and "clonal complexes", some occurring more frequently than others. At the top of the page, some explanation of the gender and clonal complex is provided. In the visualization display, a Sankey visualization is used to show the relationship between the clonal complex (left-hand side of the display) and the gender where pink represents females and blue represents males (right-hand side). The size of the Clonal Complex bar corresponds with the number of infection cases. The user can use the time slider to explore the temporal patterns of the infections that affect males and females in relation to clonal complexes. Furthermore, information on the most recent five patient cases are displayed on the right-hand side and the associated data can be accessed by clicking to drill-down.

This web-based *Campylobacter* "storyboard" provides an effective means of enabling users of all levels to explore and gain understanding of the information contained within a very large, sophisticated and complex *Campylobacter* database, in an easy and yet detailed manner and without training or user manual. The users can thus be the general public, as well as policy/decision-makers, epidemiologists, researchers, genomics specialists and so on.

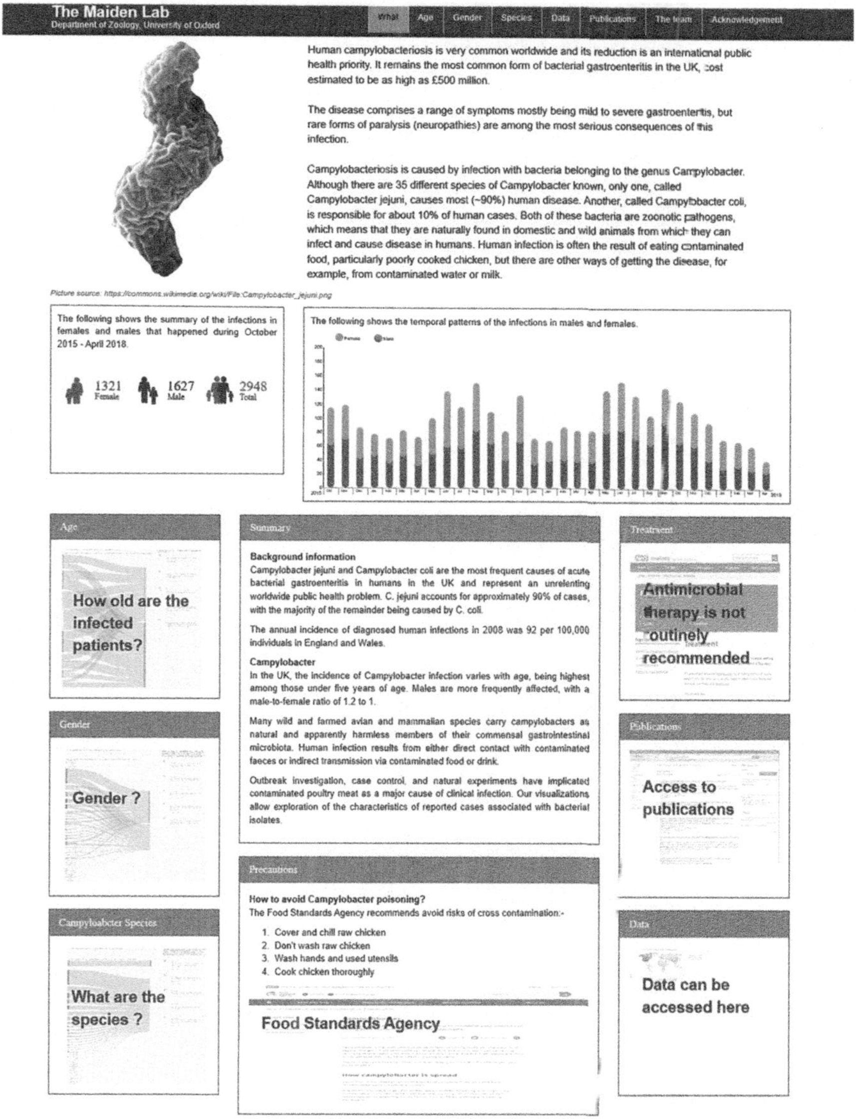

Fig. 14.15 *Campylobacter* storyboard front page

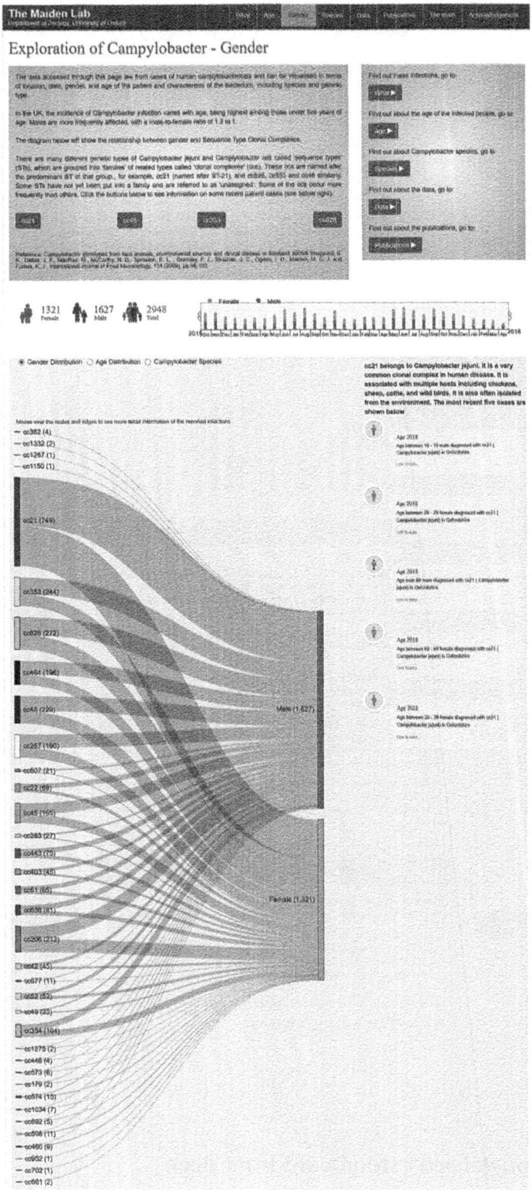

Fig. 14.16 Gender and clonal complex exploration

Conclusions

This chapter has discussed the exploration of visualization and visual analytics in the knowledge construction and navigation processes. A number of examples have been presented to demonstrate how digital content can be captured, recorded and shared as interactive visualization. We have illustrated a number of open-source tools, Carrot², Frisk and Freeplane, which are available for users to (i) retrieve data and extract information relevant their perspectives and needs and (ii) to construct relevant knowledge landscapes. This supports users in gaining understanding of the situation and thence in informed decision-making. In addition, storytelling provides an effective means of sharing knowledge with a wider community, for example, the general public.

Such methods allow users to handle ever-increasing amounts of data from heterogeneous sources, to perform deeper and wider analysis and to take data-driven decisions faster. When applied to health and person-centred care, they can bring many benefits. They can help users to work through the avalanche of content that typically follows an online search about a health condition in highly effective ways. Visual analytic techniques reduce the complexity of this online content and increase its meaningfulness. They allow users to filter content in a way that is personally meaningful to them—for instance in terms of relevance or trustworthiness—and to repurpose content to share amongst their own networks. This enhances user awareness and can be applied to support health- and wellbeing-related choices both online and offline.

There are many further issues and challenges to address over the application of visual analytic processes and the various ways in which meanings are attributed to visualizations. There is a growing body of work emerging from the field of science and technology studies that raises important questions in these areas (Baecker 1998; Bell 2005; Burri and Dumit 2007; Latour 1986). There are also, potentially, social context, cultural, operational, ethical and, indeed, philosophical considerations; however, these are beyond the scope of this chapter. The focus in this chapter has been to make a practical contribution by highlighting how visual analytics and visualization can enable users to show visually what they mean by their knowledge landscape. This approach allows users to utilize fully their cognitive and perceptual capabilities with the support of advanced computational capabilities in order to enhance the discovery process. We suggest that this contribution is not only beneficial to lay users and communities but it can also form a vital component of inter-disciplinary and multi-disciplinary research on health in the digital society. Visual analytic techniques can, for example, enable researchers—including those from non-technological backgrounds—to scope online content and analyse it in order to gauge the volume of information available to users about particular health conditions, its provenance and the kinds of recommendation being offered. This kind of analysis can be combined with other approaches in order to make connections between online and offline health behaviours and create exciting opportunities to explore the dynamics of knowledge landscapes. In this way we have shown how applications in visual analytics and visualization offer immense benefits to the lived experience and academic analysis of health-related knowledge in the digital society.

Acknowledgements NIHR: Health Protection Research Unit in Gastrointestinal Infections

FSA: Enhanced molecular-based (MLST/whole-genome) surveillance and source attribution of *Campylobacter* infections in the UK—FS101013

References

Ackoff, R. L. (1987). From data to wisdom. *Journal of Applied Systems Analysis, 16*, 3–9.

Baecker, R. (1998). Sorting out sorting: A case study of software visualization for teaching computer science. *Software Visualization: Programming as a Multimedia Experience*, 369–381. MIT Press.

Bell, K. (2005). Thirteen ways of looking at images: The logic of visualization in literature and society (review). *University of Toronto Quarterly, 74*(1), 336–338.

Burri, R. V., & Dumit, J. (2007). Social studies of scientific imaging and visualization. In E. J. Hackett, O. Amsterdamska, M. Lynch, & J. Wajcman (Eds.), *The handbook of science and technology studies, third edition* (pp. 297–318). Cambridge: MIT Press.

Buzan, T., & Buzan, B. (2006). *The mind map book*. Harlow: Pearson Education.

Carrot[2]. (2019) https://project.carrot2.org/index.html, website accessesd 2019.

ElasticSearch. (2019) https://lucene.apache.org/solr/, website accessed in 2019.

Endsley, M. R. (March, 1995). Toward a theory of situation awareness in dynamic systems. *Human Factors, 37*(1), 32–64.

Freeplane. https://www.freeplane.org/wiki/index.php/Home

Friskr. http://exocortex.com/blog/introducing_friskr

Heer, J., & Shneiderman, B. (2012, February). Interactive dynamics for visual analysis. *ACM Queue, 10*(2), 1–30.

Liew, A. (2007, June). Understanding data, information, knowledge and their inter-relationships. *Journal of Knowledge Management Practice, 8*(2), 1–16. ISSN 1705–9232.

Latour, B. (1986). Visualization and cognition: Thinking with eyes and hands. *Knowledge and Society: Studies in the Sociology of Culture Past and Present, 6*, 1–40.

Pirolli, P., & Card, S. (2005). *The sensemaking process and leverage points for analyst technology as identified through cognitive task analysis*. Proceedings 2005 International Conference *on* Intelligence Analysis (p. 6). McLean.

Rowley, J. (2007). The wisdom hierarchy: Representations of the DIKW hierarchy. *Journal of Information and Communication Science, 33*(2), 163–180. https://doi.org/10.1177/0165551506070706.

Solr. https://lucene.apache.org/solr/

Thomas, J. J., & Cook, K. (2005). *Illuminating the path: The research and development agenda for visual analytics*, 0769523234. ISBN13: 9780769523231. National Visualization and Analytics Ctr (January 1, 2005).

van Wijk, J. J. (2005). The value of visualization. In: 16th IEEE Visualization Conference VIS 2005 23-28 October, 2005, Minneapolis, MN, USA. pp. 11. https://doi.ieeecomputersociety.org/10.1109/VIS.2005.102. Editors C. Silva, E. Gröller, H. Rushmeier, published by Institute of Electrical and Electronics Engineers, ISBN 0-7803-9462-3.

Varga, M. J., & Webb. H. (2017, April 27). *The exploration of visual analytics in navigating knowledge landscapes, international conference on health and person-centered care in the digital society*. Halden, Norway.

Varga, M., Jansen van Rensburg, M. J., Colles, F., Jolley, K., McCarthy, N. D., & Maiden, M. C. J. (2017, September 10–14). *Exploring Campylobacter surveillance data with visual analytics.* 19th International workshop on *Campylobacter*, helicobacter and related organisms. Nantes, France (Poster).

Varga, M., Cody, A., Jolley, K.., McCarthy, N., Colles, F., Janssen van Rensburg, M., Douglas, A., & Maiden, M. (2019a, September). An Interactive *Campylobacter* Storyboard, CHRO, Belfast.

Varga, M., Cody, A., Jolley, K., McCarthy, N., Colles, F., Janssen van Rensburg, M., Douglas, A., & Maiden, M. (2019b, June 5–7). *Interactive Campylobacter storytelling, applied bioinformatics and public health microbiology. Wellcome Genome Campus Conference Centre*. Hinxton, Cambridge.

Zeleny, M. (1987). Management support systems: Towards integrated knowledge management. *Human Systems Management, 7*(1), 59–70.

Index

A. L. Svalastog et al. (eds.), *Navigating Digital Health Landscapes*, Health, Technology and Society, https://doi.org/10.1007/978-981-15-8206-6

The manufacturer's authorised representative in the EU is Springer Nature Customer Service Centre GmbH, Europaplatz 3, 69115 Heidelberg, Germany. If you have any concerns regarding our products, please contact ProductSafety@springernature.com

Printed and bound by CPI Group (UK) Ltd, Croydon, CR0 4YY
30/09/2026
02225243-0010